Seizures and Epilepsy in the Elderly

Seizures and Epilepsy in the Elderly

A. James Rowan, M.D.
Professor and Vice Chairman, Department of Neurology,
Mount Sinai School of Medicine, New York, New York;
Chief, Neurology Service, Department of Veterans Affairs
Medical Center, Bronx, New York

R. Eugene Ramsay, M.D.
Professor of Neurology and Psychiatry and Director,
International Center for Epilepsy, University of Miami School
of Medicine; Department of Veterans Affairs Medical Center,
Miami, Florida

Butterworth–Heinemann

Boston   Oxford   Johannesburg   Melbourne   New Delhi   Singapore

Every effort has been made to ensure that the drug dosage schedules within this text are accurate and conform to standards accepted at time of publication. However, as treatment recommendations vary in the light of continuing research and clinical experience, the reader is advised to verify drug dosage schedules herein with information found on product information sheets. This is especially true in cases of new or infrequently used drugs.

Recognizing the importance of preserving what has been written, Butterworth-Heinemann prints its books on acid-free paper whenever possible.

Library of Congress Cataloging-in-Publication Data
Seizures and epilepsy in the elderly / [edited by] A. James Rowan.
       p.   cm.
  Includes bibliographical references and index.
  ISBN 0-7506-9622-2 (alk. paper)
  1. Epilepsy in old age.   2. Convulsions in old age.   I. Rowan, A.
J.
  [DNLM: 1. Epilepsy—in old age. 2. Epilepsy—therapy. 3. Aging-
-physiology.   WL 385 S463 1996]
  RC372.S45   1996
  618.97'853—dc20
  DNLM/DLC
  for Library of Congress   96-28927
                                         CIP

British Library Cataloguing-in-Publication Data
A catalogue record for this book is available from the British Library.

The publisher offers special discounts on bulk orders of this book.

For information, please contact:
Manager of Special Sales
Butterworth-Heinemann
313 Washington Street
Newton, MA 02158-1626
Tel: 617-928-2500
Fax: 617-928-2620

For information on all medical publications available, contact our World Wide Web home page at:
http://www.bh.com/med

10 9 8 7 6 5 4 3 2 1

Printed in the United States of America

Contents

Contributing Authors

Judith C. Ahronheim, M.D.
Associate Professor of Geriatrics and Adult Development and Medicine, Mount Sinai School of Medicine; Attending Physician, Department of Geriatrics and Adult Development, Mount Sinai Medical Center, New York, New York

Frederick Andermann, M.D., F.R.C.P.(C)
Professor of Neurology and Pediatrics, McGill University Faculty of Medicine; Director, Epilepsy Service, Montréal Neurological Institute and Hospital, Montréal, Québec

Robert N. Butler, M.D.
Director of International Longevity Center and Professor of Geriatrics, Mount Sinai Medical Center, New York, New York

James Cloyd, Pharm.D., F.C.C.P.
Professor and Head, Pharmacy Practice, College of Pharmacy, University of Minnesota Medical School, and Senior Pharmacy Consultant, Minnesota Comprehensive Epilepsy Program, Minneapolis

Antonio V. Delgado-Escueta, M.D.
Professor of Neurology, University of California, Los Angeles, School of Medicine; Director, VA Southwest Regional Epilepsy Center, Neurology Services, West Los Angeles DVA Medical Center, Los Angeles

Robert J. DeLorenzo, M.D., Ph.D., M.P.H.
Professor and Chairman of Neurology, Virginia Commonwealth University, Medical College of Virginia School of Medicine; Neurologist-in-Chief, Department of Neurology, Medical College of Virginia Hospitals, Richmond

Marc A. Dichter, M.D., Ph.D.
Professor of Neurology and Pharmacology, University of Pennsylvania School of Medicine; Director, Penn Epilepsy Center, University of Pennsylvania Medical Center, Philadelphia

Carl B. Dodrill, Ph.D.
Professor of Neurological Surgery, University of Washington School of Medicine; Associate Director, Regional Epilepsy Center, Harborview Medical Center, Seattle

Howard Fillit, M.D.
Clinical Professor of Geriatrics and Medicine, Mount Sinai Medical Center; Corporate Medical Director for Medicare, New York City Care Health Plans, New York, New York

W. Allen Hauser, M.D.
Professor of Neurology and Public Health and Associate Director, Sergievsky Center, Columbia University College of Physicians and Surgeons; Attending Neurologist, Presbyterian Hospital, New York, New York

Kyusang S. Lee, M.D.
Assistant Professor of Neurology, Albert Einstein College of Medicine; Attending Physician, Department of Neurology, Beth Israel Medical Center, New York, New York

Ilo E. Leppik, M.D.
Clinical Professor of Neurology and Pharmacy, University of Minnesota Medical School and Director of Research, Minnesota Comprehensive Epilepsy Program, Minneapolis

Pierre Loiseau, M.D.
Emeritus Professor of Neurology, l'Université de Bordeaux, Bordeaux, France

Michael J. McLean, M.D., Ph.D.
Associate Professor of Neurology and Pharmacology, Vanderbilt Medical Center and Department of Veterans Affairs Medical Center; Associate Professor of Neurology, Vanderbilt University Hospital, Nashville, Tennessee

Patti D. Meyers
Department of Veterans Affairs Medical Center, West Los Angeles, California

Myron Miller, M.D.
Professor and Director of Medical Education, Department of Geriatrics and Adult Development, Mount Sinai Medical Center, New York, New York

Kenneth L. Minaker, M.D., F.R.C.P. (C), C.S.C.
Associate Professor of Medicine, Division on Aging, Harvard Medical
School; Chief, Geriatric Medicine Unit, Division of Primary Care,
Massachusetts General Hospital, Boston

Linda Ann Morrow, M.D.
Assistant Professor of Medicine, Harvard Medical School, Boston,
Massachusetts; Medical Director, Senior Health Center, Alexian Brothers
Hospital, San Jose, California

Timothy A. Pedley, M.D.
Professor and Vice Chairman of Neurology, Columbia University College
of Physicians and Surgeons; Director, Comprehensive Epilepsy Center and
Associate Chief, Neurology Service, Department of Neurology, The
Neurological Institute, Columbia-Presbyterian Medical Center, New York,
New York

John M. Pellock, M.D.
Professor of Neurology, Pediatrics, and Pharmacy and
Pharmaceutics; Chairman, Division of Child Neurology, Virginia
Commonwealth University, Medical College of Virginia School of
Medicine, Richmond

J. Kiffin Penry, M.D.
Professor of Neurology, Bowman Gray School of Medicine,
Winston-Salem, North Carolina

Charles E. Pippenger, Ph.D.
Clinical Professor of Health Sciences, Grand Valley State University,
Allendale, Michigan; Director, Peter C. and Pat Cook Health Sciences
Research and Education Institute, Grand Rapids, Michigan

Roger J. Porter, M.D.
Adjunct Professor of Neurology, University of Pennsylvania School of
Medicine, Philadelphia; Adjunct Professor of Pharmacology,
Uniformed Services University of the Health Sciences, Bethesda,
Maryland; Vice President of Clinical Pharmacology, Clinical Research
and Development, Wyeth-Ayerst Research, Radnor, Pennsylvania

A. James Rowan, M.D.
Professor and Vice Chairman, Department of Neurology, Mount Sinai
School of Medicine, New York, New York; Chief, Neurology Service,
Department of Veterans Affairs Medical Center, Bronx, New York

Tess L. Sierzant, R.N., M.S., CNRN
Clinical Nurse Specialist of Neuroscience, Minneapolis Neuroscience Institute, Abbott Northwestern Hospital, Minneapolis, Minnesota

Raymond Tallis, M.B., Ch.B., F.R.C.P.
Professor of Geriatric Medicine, University of Manchester, United Kingdom; Consultant Physician in Care of the Elderly, Department of Medicine, Hope Hospital (Salford Royal Hospitals Trust), Salford, United Kingdom

Rein Tideiksaar
Director, Department of Geriatric Care Coordination, Sierra Health Services, Inc., Las Vegas, Nevada

Paolo Tinuper, M.D.
Research Fellow, Institute of Clinical Neurology; University of Bologna, Italy

David M. Treiman, M.D.
Professor of Neurology, University of California, Los Angeles, School of Medicine; Co-Director, Epilepsy Center, DVA Medical Center, West Los Angeles

Nancy Y. Walton, Ph.D.
Assistant Research Neurologist, University of California, Los Angeles, School of Medicine; Research Physiologist, DVA Medical Center, West Los Angeles

Leonard M. Weinberger, M.D.
Assistant Clinical Professor of Neurology, Case Western Reserve University School of Medicine, Cleveland, Ohio

L. James Willmore, M.D.
Professor of Neurology, University of Texas Medical School, Houston

Denise Wolff, Pharm.D.
Clinical Assistant Professor of Pharmacy Practice, University of Minnesota College of Pharmacy; Pharmaceutical Care Coordinator, MINCEP Epilepsy Care, Minneapolis

Robert D. Zimmerman, M.D.
Professor of Radiology and Director of Outpatient Services, Mount Sinai Medical Center, New York, New York

Preface

The elderly represent the fastest-growing segment of the general population. Now 13%, the proportion of individuals in the United States older than age 65 is expected to reach 20% by the early part of the twenty-first century. The aging of the population is, in fact, a global phenomenon and carries with it profound implications for health care delivery. Combined with recent evidence that the incidence of epilepsy in the older population is two to three times that in children, it is clear that the management of seizures in the elderly poses a major challenge. In the past, epilepsy in the elderly generated little specific interest. This is unfortunate, for the elderly present unique challenges not found in younger populations. Aging is associated with important physiologic changes, increased incidence of systemic and neurologic disease, and multiple medications, all of which increase the complexity of diagnosis and treatment of seizures in this age group.

This volume brings together experts in the fields of epidemiology, epileptology, electrodiagnosis, radiology, pharmacology, pharmacotherapeutics, medicine, and geriatrics who present a broad and detailed picture of the elderly patient with seizures. Included are discussions of physiologic and pathologic changes in the aged, antiepileptic drug metabolism and its age-related changes, and drug-drug interactions. These concepts are applied to issues of seizure management, both with previously available and newly developed antiepileptic compounds. This synthesis of current knowledge is intended both to improve clinical management of the elderly patient with seizures and to provide a framework for future research.

AJR
RER

xiii

Acknowledgments

The editors are indebted to Dr. Myron Miller for his invaluable contributions to the international symposium, Seizures and Epilepsy in the Elderly, held in Coral Gables, Florida, on which this volume is based. We also are deeply grateful to Ms. Linda Tuchman and Ms. Esther Lopez, whose dedication and remarkable efficiency made possible both the symposium and this work. The assistance of Ms. Yolanda Gonzalez in preparing the manuscript is much appreciated. Thanks are also due to the American Epilepsy Society, the Epilepsy Foundation of America, and the American Geriatrics Society for their encouragement and support.

AJR
RER

I

The Scope of the Problem

1

Aging: The Challenge of Twenty-First Century Medicine

Robert N. Butler

The twentieth century has seen the beginnings of a revolution in longevity that has resulted in an unprecedented increase in the absolute number and relative proportion of older people. There has not only been a dramatic increase in the 65 and older age group but also an extraordinary increase in the 85 and older population, which includes the most rapidly increasing age group of all, the centenarians. How well prepared is medicine to deal with this extraordinary demographic event? Medicine itself has enjoyed a revolution in the twentieth century. For perhaps the first time, there is at least a 50% chance that physicians can be helpful to most patients. Modern biology, particularly since the advent of molecular biology and genetics, developed after the unraveling of the structure of DNA. More recently, we have seen the expansion of neurobiology. The Human Genome Project itself will help us elucidate the estimated 5,000 genetically based medical conditions. Thus, we can anticipate great contributions to understanding both health and disease. Has the revolution in longevity been adequately matched with the revolution of modern medical science? A successful joining of the two would be revealed in the structure and quality of the health care delivery system; however, there are serious problems.

Aging, along with genes (genes that cause defects) and the environment, broadly defined (including how we eat and how we behave), is one of the three great antecedents of health and disease. These three are interrelated. Yet we devote relatively little attention to aging per se. Benjamin Gompertz in 1812 described the equation that bears his name and spells out the fact that after about age 30 years an individual's mortality rises logarhithmically every 7 years of life. The force of mortality is a rough measure of the age-related increase in vulnerability to disease and therefore death. It tells us of the susceptibility that is created by the degradation of biological systems with age. Yet only approximately $44 million is devoted by the National Institute on Aging to understanding the basic biology of aging!

Although every medical school in Great Britain has a department of geriatrics, as do many medical schools in Scandinavia and an increasing number in Japan, there are perhaps only 20 significant programs in geriatrics in the United States in departments of internal medicine, family medicine, and psychiatry. There is only one full-scale department of geriatrics that endeavors to integrate the teaching of geriatrics throughout all of primary care and specialty medicine, conduct model inpatient and outpatient programs of patient care, and organize and conduct research on the various maladies associated with aging.

Although Medicare legislation was passed in 1965 to provide medical care for older people and the disabled, it was set up as though older people were 40-year-olds (and largely male). It was not established with the advice of geriatricians, and it does not meet the basic requirements of geriatrics: providing geriatric assessment, the team approach, long-term care (including institutional and community-based care), outpatient medications, and prevention. Medicare does not speak to the organization of care, only to its financing, and then in only a limited way. Medicare today pays for hardly more than 40% of the bills of older patients and only about 2% of nursing home costs.

The topic of seizures and epilepsy in the elderly is another example of various age-related medical problems that we have only begun to recognize and about which we know very little and cannot fully treat. The neurologic diseases of old age that have understandably received the most attention have been stroke, Alzheimer's disease, multi-infarct dementia, amyotrophic lateral sclerosis, and Parkinson's disease, but I believe we have much to learn about the many obscure and probably still unrecognized neurologic conditions of old age. Indeed, the three great reasons for institutionalization in old age are problems of mobility, dementia, and incontinence; all obviously have neurologic roots. The neurology of old age, or geriatric neurology, should become a more prominent field and body of knowledge as we move into the twenty-first century.

There is much pressure now for expansion of primary care physicians and the making of generalists. I hope that this does not come at the expense of attention to specialization, which has brought so much progress to worldwide medicine. Indeed, effective primary care physicians or generalists must also be specialists. They must be specialists in disease prevention and health promotion, in the early detection of disease, and in the ability to carry out a wide range of therapeutic activities. Part of the specialization of the generalist must include the knowledge and the wisdom to know when to refer the patient to the care of an organ specialist or system specialist. This must not be compromised by financial considerations, which can be the case in some health maintenance organizations and other forms of managed care.

The aging baby boomers will challenge twenty-first century medicine. This group is the largest generation in U.S. history. The baby boomers make up one-third of the population at present, and in the years 2011–2030 will constitute approximately 20% of the American population. Caring for one out of every five Americans who have special geriatric needs will surely provide a challenge! Young physicians and medical students today will find population aging to be the great challenge when they reach the prime of their careers. They should have the advantage of sophisticated integration of geriatrics knowledge related to various diseases and disabilities throughout all primary care and specialty medicine. This is especially true of neurology, since so many of the problems of aging are related to the central nervous system (and the peripheral nervous system as well). Certainly the topic of seizures and epilepsy counts among the special challenges.

SELECTED READINGS

Abrams WB, Berkow R (eds). The Merck Manual of Geriatrics. West Point, PA: Merck Sharp & Dohme Research Laboratories, 1990.

Brocklehurst JC, Tallis RC, Fillit HM (eds). Textbook of Geriatric Medicine and Gerontology (4th ed). London: Churchill Livingstone, 1992.

Butler RN. The Challenge of Geriatric Medicine. In JD Wilson, E Braunwald, KJ Isselbacher et al. (eds), Harrison's Principles of Internal Medicine (12th ed). New York: McGraw-Hill, 1991;16.

2

Epidemiology of Seizures and Epilepsy in the Elderly*

W. Allen Hauser

There is a general perception that convulsive disorders for the most part start in childhood and that onset in adults is rare. This perception is called into question by several recent population-based studies of epilepsy, all unprovoked seizures, or any seizure that all report an increasing incidence—at times dramatic—with advancing age. Population-based studies limited to elderly populations also report an incidence comparable to the high incidence reported in total population studies.[1-9] The incidence of epilepsy in those older than age 60 years exceeds that of children, and seizure disorders in general and epilepsy in particular are among the more commonly occurring neurologic disorders in the elderly.[2, 7]

This high frequency of seizures and epilepsy relates in part to the substantial risk for seizures in association with or as a consequence of conditions that occur with an increased incidence in the elderly. This includes conditions, such as stroke, brain tumor, or head injury, in which (acute symptomatic) seizures occur with a high frequency as part of the acute process. It also includes conditions, such as stroke or brain trauma, in which unprovoked seizures occur as long-term sequelae in a substantial proportion of cases, and progressive conditions, such as Alzheimer's disease, in which unprovoked seizures are a specific clinical manifestation. The importance of the seizures in the elderly is stressed in a British study in which almost 25% of newly identified seizures (not epilepsy) were accounted for by those age 60 and older.[10]

The epidemiologic data supporting an increased incidence of epilepsy in the elderly are reviewed in this chapter. The prevalence of epilepsy in the elderly and the potential causes of seizures and epilepsy are briefly discussed.

INCIDENCE OF ACUTE SYMPTOMATIC SEIZURES

Acute symptomatic seizures include seizures occurring in the context of an acute metabolic disturbance and those occurring at the time of an acute insult to the central nervous system (CNS).[11, 12] Seizures are frequently associated with acute neurologic disease and therefore complicate its management. They also may be associated with a number of systemic disturbances. Stroke,[13, 14] head injury,[15, 16]

*Supported in part by RO1-NS 32663 and NS 16308.

and infection of the CNS[17] all have relative or absolute peaks in incidence in the oldest age groups, and seizures occur at the time of insult in a substantial proportion of those affected. Metabolic conditions such as uremia, hyponatremia, and hypoglycemia also associated with an increased risk for seizures, are frequent in the elderly.

In many reports of studies of seizures or epilepsy in the elderly, it is difficult to separate patients with acute symptomatic seizures from those with unprovoked seizures. This distinction is important clinically. The underlying condition, which determines prognosis, must be the target of the primary treatment. Seizures are epiphenomena, however, and may complicate medical management, particularly if they manifest as status epilepticus. Seizures may also be an indicator of severity of the underlying disease[18] and are a predictor of subsequent epilepsy. Nonetheless, for these conditions, the occurrence of seizures per se will have little long-term impact on outcome.

Acute Symptomatic Seizures in the General Elderly Population

The incidence of "acute symptomatic" seizures in those older than age 60 years is approximately 100 per 100,000 population and increases with advancing age (Figure 2.1).[6, 19] Thus, approximately 50,000 Americans in this age group will have a first acute symptomatic seizure each year. Acute symptomatic seizures occur more frequently in males—probably because of the increased incidence of diseases associated with acute symptomatic seizures in this group.

The occurrence of acute symptomatic seizures is related to the frequency of the underlying condition in the target population. The highest proportion of these individuals (40–50%) will have acute symptomatic seizures attributable to a cerebrovascular insult. Next in frequency will be seizures with systemic metabolic disturbances (approximately 10–15%). Acute brain trauma, drug (alcohol) withdrawal, CNS infection, and toxic insults account for 5–10% each (Figure 2.2).[6, 19] Approximately 30% of those with acute symptomatic seizures will experience a seizure of sufficient duration to meet criteria for status epilepticus.[20] This is discussed in greater detail in Chapters 15 and 16.

Acute Symptomatic Seizures in Specific Conditions

Between 5% and 10% of individuals with an acute cerebrovascular insult will experience a seizure at the time of the stroke.[21, 22] The frequency with which these early or acute symptomatic seizures occur varies with the nature of the cerebrovascular insult. The proportion is highest in those with intracerebral hemorrhage, but seizures also occur at the time of thrombotic, embolic, and lacunar strokes. Approximately 6% of individuals with brain injury related to head trauma will experience one or more seizures at the time of the injury.[23–25] Regardless of how measured, this proportion increases with increasing severity

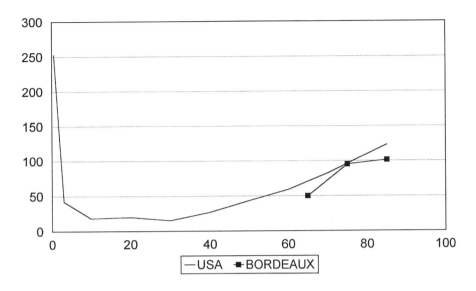

Figure 2.1 Incidence of acute symptomatic seizures.

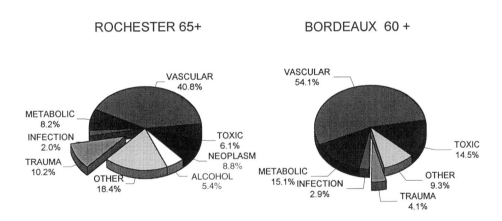

Figure 2.2 Causes of acute symptomatic seizures.

of insult. When compared with other adult populations, the elderly do not seem to be disproportionately affected with acute symptomatic seizures if one controls for severity. Approximately 5% of individuals with an infection of the CNS will experience acute symptomatic seizures.[26] This proportion seems consistent across populations.

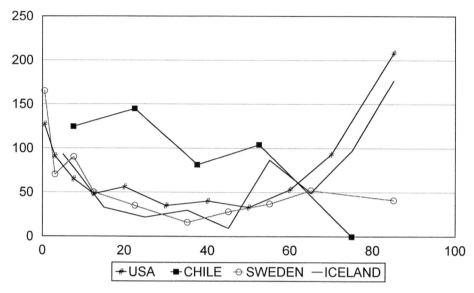

Figure 2.3 Incidence of unprovoked seizures.

For each of these conditions, those with early or acute symptomatic seizures have a substantial increased risk for subsequent epilepsy when compared with those without early seizures. For example, the absolute risk for epilepsy after stroke or head injury may exceed 30% in survivors with early seizures, compared with 10–15% for those without.

INCIDENCE OF UNPROVOKED SEIZURES AND EPILEPSY

Unprovoked seizures, or epilepsy, are frequent long-term complications of static encephalopathies resulting from stroke or head injury, and also occur in association with progressive degenerative conditions such as Alzheimer's disease. All of these conditions have a peak incidence in the elderly. In addition, unprovoked seizures in the elderly frequently occur in the absence of such conditions. The total incidence of unprovoked seizures in those older than age 60 years in U.S. and in Nordic populations exceeds 100 per 100,000 population.[7, 8] In those older than age 60 years, this translates to between 45,000 and 50,000 new cases of epilepsy or first unprovoked seizure each year in the United States. As with acute symptomatic seizures, the incidence of unprovoked seizures increases with advancing age (Figure 2.3). The high incidence and increasing incidence with advancing age may be phenomena limited to Western countries. Although there are few reliable studies of incidence in developing countries, an increase in incidence in the elderly was not docu-

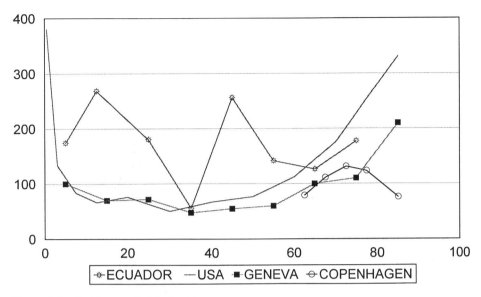

Figure 2.4   Incidence of afebrile seizures.

mented in an incidence study in Chile, where the entire pattern of incidence is at variance with that observed in studies from industrialized countries.[27] The increase in incidence was somewhat less dramatic in a study in Ecuador, which combined acute symptomatic and unprovoked seizures and is somewhat masked by higher peaks in incidence at earlier ages[28] (Figure 2.4). The findings in Ecuador contrast with findings in Geneva and in Rochester, Minnesota, when both unprovoked and acute symptomatic seizures (inclusion criteria in Ecuador) are applied.[7, 9] The study of these geographic differences in incidence in industrialized countries and developing countries may provide clues to etiology and interventions. In populations with concentrations of high-risk individuals, such as those in nursing homes, incidence of unprovoked seizures may be as high as 1% per year.[29]

Seizure Type

It is frequently assumed that virtually all new cases of epilepsy in the oldest age groups will be characterized by partial (or localization related) seizures. In epidemiologic studies, approximately 70% of newly diagnosed patients older than age 60 years will experience partial onset seizures.[7] Generalized onset seizures occur in patients with a history of anoxic insults and in association with CNS degenerative diseases such as Alzheimer's disease. Even in the absence of conditions associated with diffuse brain pathology, generalized onset seizures in the elderly are indistinguishable from generalized onset epilepsies identified in

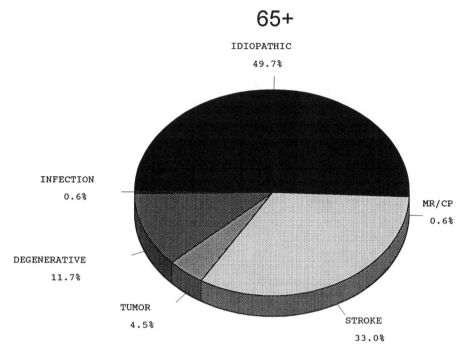

Figure 2.5 Causes of epilepsy.

younger individuals. Epileptologists assume these cases represent either misclassified partial onset seizures with rapid secondary generalization or cases of long-standing but unrecognized epilepsy of generalized onset. Nonetheless, such cases may truly represent the new onset of primary generalized epilepsy in the elderly. If the latter is the case, environmental influences must be important for the clinical manifestation of what many consider to be a predominantly genetic condition. As a corollary, genetic predisposition or a predisposition to genetically determined electroencephalographic patterns may modify risk for seizures or epilepsy in the elderly.

Etiology

In population-based series of epilepsy, a definitive cause can be identified in only about 30% of cases. Even in the oldest age groups, for whom the incidence of insults to the CNS associated with an increased risk for epilepsy in survivors is quite high, a definitive etiology can be identified in only about 50% (Figure 2.5).[6, 7] The distribution may be somewhat different if all afebrile seizures (acute symptomatic and unprovoked) are included.[30, 31] For all of these conditions, the risk for epilepsy is highest in the first year or two after the occurrence of the insult, although risk for epilepsy remains elevated for many years.

Cerebrovascular Disease

The incidence of cerebrovascular disease increases with advancing age. Individuals with cerebrovascular disease have more than a twentyfold increased risk of developing epilepsy compared with that expected in the general population.[32] In industrialized countries, cerebrovascular disease is the most frequently identified antecedent of epilepsy, and the proportion of incidence cases with epilepsy attributed to cerebrovascular disease increases with advancing age. In the oldest age groups, stroke accounts for 30–40% of all newly occurring cases of epilepsy. Approximately 15% of survivors of stroke will experience unprovoked seizures within 5 years after a first clinically identified cerebrovascular insult, although the risk of developing epilepsy remains significantly elevated above that expected for at least 20 years after the stroke. In those with a vascular insult, both early seizures and supratentorial infarction (including lacunes) are associated with an increased risk for epilepsy. Recurrent strokes are associated with an incremental increase.

Trauma

The incidence of craniocerebral trauma is highest in the adolescent and young adults, but there is an additional peak in the elderly.[16, 17] The increase in brain trauma in the elderly is primarily attributable to falls. Overall, trauma with loss of consciousness is associated with a threefold increase in risk for epilepsy in the survivors; this risk (as mortality) increases with increasing severity of injury. Unfortunately, mortality after severe trauma is quite high in the elderly (≥70%).[17] Trauma accounts for no more than 2–3% of all new cases of epilepsy in the oldest age groups.

Central Nervous System Infection

The incidence of CNS infections is highest in children, but an additional peak in incidence also occurs in the elderly. Survivors of a CNS infection have a threefold increase in risk for epilepsy.[26] This risk is independent of age at infection but does vary by type of infection. CNS infection accounts for only 2–3% of all newly identified cases in the oldest age groups.

Neoplasm

The incidence of brain tumors also increases with advancing age. Approximately 30% of patients with brain tumors will present with seizures as an initial symptom. Brain tumors as an assigned etiology account for a substantial proportion of individuals included in many epilepsy case series in the elderly, but as yet there is no quantification of risk. Whether such cases should actually be termed "epilepsy" may be questioned, as most tumors represent progressive conditions, even after operation. For most individuals with seizures caused by a primary CNS neoplasm, the diagnosis will be made at the time of first evaluation for the seizures. For tumors of glial origin, subsequent seizures are frequently related to recurrence or expansion of the original lesion and, as such, are not truly unprovoked. Because of this, tumors account for only a small proportion of cases with unprovoked seizures.

Degenerative Disease

The incidence of primary degenerative diseases of the CNS increases with advancing age[33]; these conditions account for a substantial proportion of the cases with epilepsy in the elderly. The most frequent of these conditions, Alzheimer's disease, affects 1–2% of the population older than age 60 years, and the incidence increases with advancing age. Alzheimer's disease is associated with a five- to tenfold increase in risk for epilepsy compared with that expected in the general population.[34–36] By 10 years after diagnosis, 15% or more of Alzheimer's disease survivors will have experienced unprovoked seizures. Other degenerative conditions such as Parkinson's disease may also be associated with an increase in risk for epilepsy.

Alcohol

Based on volume and frequency criteria, at least 5% of the elderly (including the oldest age groups) drink alcohol frequently and heavily. Individuals who drink heavily on a chronic basis have a risk not only for acute symptomatic seizures with abrupt reduction or discontinuation of alcohol ingestion (withdrawal seizures), but also have a threefold increased risk for epilepsy. Although chronic alcohol abuse has not been considered to be a major etiologic factor in most studies of epilepsy in the United States, a history of alcohol abuse was the sole antecedent identified in adults with newly diagnosed epilepsy in Denmark and may be an important etiology in the older population.[37, 38]

Idiopathic (Cryptogenic) Epilepsy

Despite this impressive array of factors, all of which are particularly common in the elderly, the largest group of elderly individuals with newly diagnosed epilepsy (>40%) is etiologically classified as "idiopathic" or "cryptogenic." It is frequently assumed that such individuals have "silent strokes." It is true that risk factors for stroke are also risk factors for epilepsy, even in the absence of a documented cerebrovascular insult.[39–41] Epidemiologic studies suggest that a history of asthma[42], hypertension,[38, 39] use of illicit drugs (particularly heroin),[43] depression, use of psychotropic agents, and electroconvulsive therapy[44, 45] all have been demonstrated to increase the risk for epilepsy. The process of the aging of the CNS alone may modify epileptogenesis. After controlling for known risk factors, age alone seems to be associated with an elevation of risk of about 0.3 for each decade of life after the age of 20.[46] Even so, a substantial proportion of cases of epilepsy with onset in the oldest age groups has no established etiology.[5, 7] It is clear that we have much to learn before we understand the antecedents of epilepsy in the elderly.

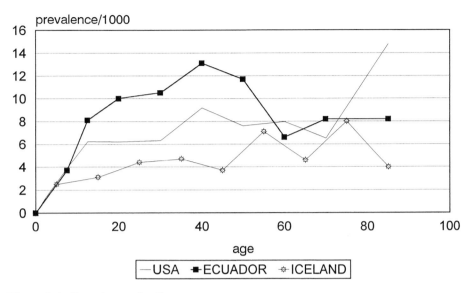

Figure 2.6 Prevalence of epilepsy.

Even though the incidence of stroke has fallen in recent years and stroke is the major identified cause of epilepsy in the elderly, there has been a substantial increase in the incidence of epilepsy in the elderly in the past three decades.[7] This seems primarily attributable to improved survivorship in people with cerebrovascular disease.[47]

PREVALENCE

The concept of prevalence is attractive for those interested in health care needs, but prevalence can contribute little to our understanding of mechanisms for the development of epilepsy. The combination of chronic epilepsy cases with a substantial influx of new cases provides an indecipherable concoction. To make matters worse, most of the many prevalence studies of epilepsy use varying methodologies and varying definitions that virtually preclude comparison. As one might predict from the incidence, which increases in the elderly, and from the mortality, which is not substantially increased among individuals with epilepsy alone, the prevalence of epilepsy also increases with advancing age in the elderly in the few large scale studies recently undertaken—at least in the United States and in Nordic countries. In those age 75 and older, the prevalence of active epilepsy (those experiencing unprovoked seizures or are taking anti-seizure medication as treatment for epilepsy) is between 1% and 1.5% (Figure 2.6).[8, 11] Contemporary prevalence studies in developing countries do not show this dramatic increase, again raising questions of geographic variation. It is difficult to understand how "lifetime prevalence" (a history of a seizure at any age) can fall with advancing age.

The prevalence of epilepsy is even higher in some highly select populations. Surveys in chronic care facilities suggest that at least 5% of residents have a diagnosis of epilepsy and that 7–10% are taking antiepileptic medication.[29, 48, 49] This high prevalence is not surprising given that the major reasons for admission to such facilities are, for the most part, neurologic conditions that are also risk factors for seizures and epilepsy. The incidence of newly diagnosed epilepsy in patients in these facilities is more than 1% per year.[29]

REFERENCES

1. Zielinski JJ. Epidemiology and Medical-Social Problems of Epilepsy in Warsaw. Warsaw: Psychoneurological Institute, 1974.
2. Hauser WA, Kurland LT. The epidemiology of epilepsy in Rochester, Minnesota, 1935–68. Epilepsia 1975;16:1.
3. Lühdorf K, Jensen LK, Plesner AM. Epilepsy in the elderly: incidence, social function, and disability. Epilepsia 1986;27:135.
4. Keränen T, Reikkinen P, Sillanpää M. Incidence and prevalence of epilepsy in adults in eastern Finland. Epilepsia 1989;30:413.
5. Forsgren L. Prospective incidence study and clinical characterization of seizures in newly referred adults. Epilepsia 1990;31:292.
6. Loiseau J, Loiseau P, Duché B, et al. A survey of epileptic disorders in southwest France: seizures in elderly patients. Ann Neurol 1990;27:232.
7. Hauser WA, Annegers JF, Kurland LT. The incidence of epilepsy in Rochester, Minnesota, 1935–84. Epilepsia 1993;34:453.
8. Ólafsson E, Hauser WA, Lúðvigsson P, Guðmundsson G. Incidence and prevalence of epilepsy in rural Iceland. Epilepsia 1994;35:151.
9. Jallon P, Morabia A. First epileptic seizures in Geneva County: incidence rate and epidemiologic classification of the risk factors. Epilepsia 1994;35(Suppl 8):110.
10. Sander JWA, Hart YM, Johnson AL, Shorvon SD. National general practice study of epilepsy: newly diagnosed epileptic seizures in a general population. Lancet 1990;336:1267.
11. Hauser WA, Annegers JF, Kurland LT. Prevalence of epilepsy in Rochester, Minnesota, 1940–1980. Epilespia 1991;32:428.
12. Commission on Epidemiology and Prognosis, International League Against Epilepsy. Guidelines for Epidemiologic Studies on Epilepsy. Epilepsia 1993;34:592.
13. Broderick JP, Phillips SJ, Whisnant JP, et al. Incidence rates of stroke in the eighties: the end of the decline in stroke? Stroke 1989;20:577.
14. Boden-Albala B, Gu Q, Kargman DE, et al. Increased stroke incidence in blacks and Hispanics: The Northern Manhattan Stroke Study. Neurology 1995;45(Suppl 4): A300.
15. Annegers JF, Grabow JD, Kurland LT, Laws ER. The incidence, causes, and secular trends of head trauma in Olmsted County, Minnesota, 1935–1974. Neurology 1980;30:912.
16. Cooper KD, Tabaddor K, Hauser WA, et al. The epidemiology of head injury in the Bronx. Neuroepidemiology 1983;2:70.
17. Nicolosi A, Hauser WA, Beghi E, Kurland LT. Epidemiology of central nervous system infections in Olmsted County, Minnesota, 1950–1981. J Infect Dis 1986;154:399.
18. So EL, Annegers JF, Hauser WA, et al. Population-based study of the risk factors of epileptic seizures following cerebral infarction. Neurology 1994;44(Suppl 2):A337.

19. Annegers JF, Hauser WA, Lee JR-J, Rocca WA. Acute symptomatic seizures in Rochester, Minnesota, 1935–1984. Epilepsia 1995;36:327.
20. Hauser WA, Cascino GD, Annegers JF, Rocca WA. Incidence of status epilepticus and associated mortality. Epilepsia 1994;35:33.
21. Kilpatrick CJ, Davis SM, Tress BM, et al. Early seizures after acute stroke. Risk of late seizures. Arch Neurol 1992;49:509.
22. So EL, Annegers JF, Hauser WA, et al. Prognosis of early seizures following cerebral infarction—functional outcome and long-term survival. Epilepsia 1994;35:91.
23. Annegers JF, Grabow JD, Groover RV, et al. Seizures after head trauma: a population study. Neurology 1980;30:683.
24. Hauser WA, Tabaddor K, Frankowski R, et al. Risk factors for early posttraumatic seizures. Neurology 1985;35:S133.
25. Salazar AM, Jabbari B, Vance SC, et al. Epilepsy after penetrating head injury. I. Clinical correlates: a report of the Vietnam Head Injury Study. Neurology 1985;35:1406.
26. Annegers JF, Nicolosi A, Beghi E, et al. The risk of unprovoked seizures after encephalitis and meningitis. Neurology 1988;38:1407.
27. Lavados J, Germain I, Morales A, et al. A descriptive study of epilepsy in the District of El Salvador, Chile 1984–1988. Acta Neurol Scand 1992;91:718.
28. Placencia M, Shorvon SD, Paredes V, et al. Epileptic seizures in an Andean region of Ecuador. Incidence and prevalence and regional variation. Brain 1992;115:771.
29. Hauser WA. The incidence and prevalence of epilepsy and antiepileptic medication use in nursing homes in the Bronx. Presented at Epilepsy International. London, 1982.
30. Lühdorf K, Jensen LK, Plesner AM. Etiology of seizures in the elderly. Epilepsia 1986;27:458.
31. Roberts MA, Godfrey JW, Caird FI. Epileptic seizures in the elderly. I. Aetiology and type of seizure. Age Ageing 1982;11:24.
32. Hauser WA, Ramirez-Lassepas M, Rosenstein R. Risk for seizures and epilepsy following cerebrovascular insults. Epilepsia 1984;25:666.
33. Kokrnen E, Chandra V, Schoenberg BS. Trends in incidence of dementing illness in Rochester, Minnesota, in three quinquannial periods 1960–1974. Neurology 1988;38:975.
34. Hauser WA, Morris ML, Hewton LL, Anderson VE. Seizures and myoclonus in patients with Alzheimer's disease. Neurology 1986;36:1226.
35. Romanelli MF, Morris JC, Ashkin K, Coben LA. Advanced Alzheimer's disease is a risk factor for late onset seizures. Arch Neurol 1990;47:847.
36. Hesdorffer DC, Hauser WA, Annegers JF, et al. Dementia and adult onset unprovoked seizures. Neurology 1996;46:727.
37. Ng SKC, Hauser WA, Brust JCM, Susser M. Alcohol consumption and the risk of new onset seizures. N Engl J Med 1988;319:666.
38. Dam AM, Fuglsang-Frederiksen A, Svarre-Olsen U, Dam M. Late-onset epilepsy: etiologies, types of seizures, and value of clinical investigation, EEG, and computerized tomography scan. Epilepsia 1985;26:227.
39. Shinton RA, Gill JS, Zezulka AV, Bevers DG. The frequency of epilepsy preceding stroke: case control study in 230 patients. Lancet 1987;i:11.
40. Ng SKC, Hauser WA, Brust JCM, Susser M. Hypertension and the risk of new onset unprovoked seizures. Neurology 1993;43:425.
41. Hesdorffer DC. Stroke risk factors as risk factors for unprovoked seizures: a case control study in an incidence cohort. Submitted in partial fulfillment of requirements for a Ph.D, Columbia University, May 1993.
42. Ng SKC, Gergen P, Hauser WA, Brust JCM. Asthma, allergies and seizures. Epilepsia 1984;25:644.
43. Ng SKC, Hauser WA, Brust JCM, Susser M. Illicit drug use and first onset seizures. Am J Epidemiol 1990;132:147.

44. Hesdorffer DC, Hauser WA, Annegers JF, Kurland LT. Psychiatric diagnoses preceding unprovoked seizures in adults: A population-based case control study. Epilepsia 1992;33(Suppl 3):16.
45. Hesdorffer DC, Hauser WA, Annegers JF, Kurland LT. Therapy for psychiatric disorders as a risk factor for unprovoked seizures in adults: a population-based case control study. Epilepsia 1992;33(Suppl 3):112.
46. Ng SKC, Hauser WA, Brust JCM, et al. Risk factors for adult-onset first seizures. Ann Neurol 1985;18:153.
47. Annegers JF, Hauser WA, Lee JR, Rocca W. Secular trends in epilepsy in Rochester, Minnesota, 1935–84. Epilepsia 1995;36:575.
48. Moseley JL, Penry JK. Antiepileptic medication in chronic care facilities. Results of a review of the medical records of 773 patients in seven nursing homes, Montgomery County, MD. Public Health Rep 1975;90(2):140.
49. Cloyd JC, Lackner TE, Leppik IE. Antiepileptics in the elderly. Pharmacoepidemiology and pharmacokinetics. Arch Fam Med 1994;3:589.

II

Pathophysiology of Aging and Its Relationship to Seizures

3

Epileptogenesis and the Aging Brain

Marc A. Dichter and Leonard M. Weinberger

INTRODUCTION

Studies of the epidemiology of epilepsy have demonstrated a second peak in incidence occurring in the elderly, following a childhood peak and a relative plateau in adulthood.[1] A large number of these patients have symptomatic epilepsy after developing cerebrovascular disease. Others have degenerative diseases, such as Alzheimer's disease, that predispose them to epilepsy. A remaining 8–25% of these cases of elderly-onset epilepsy are without a known etiology.[2, 3] In none of these patients are the mechanisms that lead to the development of epilepsy understood. Clearly, the field is ripe for investigation.

In this chapter, what is known about specific issues of epileptogenesis in the aging brain is reviewed. The chapter begins with a brief discussion of current experimental models of epileptogenesis, focusing on age-dependent or developmental aspects. A variety of studies have investigated the relationship between the maturational age of experimental animals and their propensity to develop seizures in a number of experimental paradigms such as kindling, application of excitatory amino acids, and exposure to anoxia.[4–8] These studies suggest that there are differences in seizure susceptibility, as well as in responses to insults such as hypoxia, between immature and adult animals. Recent studies that focus on synaptic reorganization in human or kindled epileptic hippocampus by the use of the Timm stain technique are also reviewed.[9–11]

Next, changes in human brain structure that occur with aging, which may have ramifications for the development of seizures, are surveyed. These include small, clinically silent infarcts, generalized and focal cortical atrophy, and amyloid deposition in cerebral microvessels. Alzheimer's disease is associated with prominent derangements of cerebral cortical and hippocampal synaptic density, connectivity, and neurochemistry,[12–15] all of which may be relevant to the increased risk of seizures in patients with this disease.[16]

Finally, the relatively limited number of experimental studies that directly examine seizure susceptibility and epileptogenesis, typically in aged rats, and the extrapolation of findings in animal models of epileptogenesis to human neuropathology are considered. As will become clear from this chapter, relatively little work has been directed at this important issue. There are a number of areas of research in epileptogenesis in the aging population that could be fruit-fully pursued and that could lead to strategies for prophylaxis.

MODELS OF EPILEPTOGENESIS

A variety of factors converge to produce epileptiform activity in nervous tissue. The abnormality seems to require a derangement in excitatory and inhibitory influences on populations of susceptible neurons, leading to hyperexcitable and hypersynchronous aggregate behavior. Thus, both the intrinsic electrophysiolog-ic properties of the individual neuron and the behavior of neuronal circuits must be relevant in the initiation of epileptic discharges.[17] For example, changes in the excitability of individual neurons within a circuit due to enhanced voltage-dependent calcium currents or diminished potassium currents could produce a state of aggregate hyperexcitability. Similarly, reduced synaptic inhibition or enhanced synaptic excitation (or both) could produce an epileptic state. In addi-tion, alterations in local circuit arrangements, such as the appearance of new recurrent excitatory connections or reduced recurrent inhibitory connections, could produce seizures. All of these mechanisms have been postulated to pro-duce epilepsy in one animal model or another, and most have also been implicat-ed in some form of human epilepsy. How any of these may specifically relate to the aging brain remains to be determined.

During the last 30 years, a number of experimental animal models of epileptogenesis have been developed. The principle of these paradigms is to deliver a specific, quantifiable insult to brain tissue that produces an enduring change in cerebral structure or function and leads to episodic self-initiating epileptic seizures. By studying the pharmacologic, electrophysiologic, neu-ropathologic, and neurochemical concomitants of these experimentally pro-duced epileptic animals, an understanding of the pathophysiology underlying spontaneous seizure generation may be achieved. Commonly used animal mod-els include kindling, application of irritative substances or excitatory amino acids to the cerebral cortex, exposure to anoxia, and genetically inbred species with a particular predisposition to seizures.

By working within these well developed paradigms, a number of investi-gators have studied the effects of varying maturational age on experimental epileptogenesis.[4–8] Significant differences have emerged between immature and mature animals. For example, Jensen et al.[5] studied the effects of acute hypoxia on long-term seizure susceptibility to flurothyl exposure in rats of varying mat-urational ages. They found increased seizure susceptibility in rats of 10 days postnatal age, compared with either 5-day-old or adult animals. This age win-dow paralleled the susceptibility to acute epileptiform activity in response to hypoxia, but, interestingly, not to long-term behavioral sequelae of the hypoxic insult. These results suggest an age-dependent gradient of seizure susceptibility that is dissociable from long-term effects on learning and memory in this experimental paradigm. Other investigators have found age-dependent susceptibilities to audiogenic seizures in DBA/2 genetically epilepsy-prone mice[6] and in rats administered the excitatory amino acids quisqualic acid and glutamate.[7]

These results suggest that variable propensities to the development of epilepsy may result more from differences in the mature and immature brain's response to a pathologic insult rather than from differences in the insult itself. What could account for these findings? In early brain development, increasing maturation is heralded by a vast increase in the number and complexity of synaptic contacts as a result of axonal and dendritic production and differentiation as well as subsequent reorganization of patterns of synaptic connectivity. There are also differences in the intrinsic neurophysiologic characteristics between mature and immature neurons. These principles are discussed further in the section on possible modes of epileptogenesis in the elderly. Suffice it to say that it seems possible that these processes can occur throughout the lifespan and that experiments similar to those described can just as easily be performed on aged, as opposed to developing, animals.

The concept that reorganization of neuronal connectivity may play a role in epileptogenesis has been given major support by recent investigations using both human epileptic tissue and experimental preparations. By the use of the Timm stain technique, mossy fiber synaptic terminals may be selectively labeled as a result of their high zinc content. Abnormally reorganized mossy fiber terminals may produce recurrent excitation of dentate granule cells, possibly leading to a recurrent excitatory circuit, which may favor the initiation of seizures.

HUMAN AGING AND ALZHEIMER'S DISEASE

A variety of changes in the human brain that occur with aging may have implications for the development of seizures and epilepsy. Processes such as cerebrovascular disease, neoplasms, or trauma, which pose obvious risks for the subsequent development of epilepsy, are not considered in detail here. Rather, the discussion focuses on alterations associated with normal aging, unrecognized pathologic processes, and degenerative diseases such as Alzheimer's disease. The structural, histologic, and neurochemical alterations accompanying normal aging have been well studied.[18] On a gross structural level, the brain shrinks with age, with a compensatory increase in ventricular size. Histologically, there is considerable neuronal dropout of unknown mechanism and remaining neurons exhibit loss of dendrites, which leads to overall synaptic loss. A number of other histologic abnormalities, including amyloid deposition in cerebral microvessels, neuritic plaques, neurofibrillary tangles (particularly in hippocampus), and deposition of lipofuscin, occur in normal elderly individuals. Alterations in neurotransmitter function have been studied as well.[6, 18–22]

These normal, age-related changes are not typically thought to be associated with an increased risk of epilepsy, but they should be considered from the standpoint of how they might alter the aging brain's ability to respond to injury or other pathologic processes. How the loss of neurons and dendrites affects neuronal plasticity, for example, is unknown.[23] Given the significant age-related changes described above, it is not unreasonable to question whether there may be differences between young and elderly individuals in their response to cerebral insults such as hypoxia or trauma, which may have implications for the subsequent development of epilepsy. How much more likely, for example, is the tangle-laden hippocampus of an elderly individual, containing scarce neurons with sparse dendritic arborizations, to respond to a hypoxic insult by becoming epileptogenic as compared with a normal structure? Or is it less likely?

Ostensibly normal elderly individuals may also have unrecognized central nervous system pathology that may contribute to epileptogenesis. Cerebral infarcts that were clinically silent during life are often discovered during autopsy examinations of elderly individuals.[18] These increase the risk of seizures (although by an as yet unknown mechanism). Given the ubiquity of cerebrovascular disease in the aging population, this factor may weigh heavily as a potential source of epilepsy in the "healthy" elderly.[24] Another possibility is that genetic factors may produce seizures in an elderly patient as their first clinical manifestation. Although this is seemingly unlikely, this would be analagous to the situation in which genetic disorders first present in adulthood as a dementing illness, a situation that may be more common than previously believed.[25] The frequency with which this may occur in the case of elderly-onset epilepsy is unknown.

Finally, Alzheimer's disease is a degenerative neurologic disease that affects large numbers of elderly individuals. Patients with this disease are 10 times more likely to have epilepsy than age-matched controls.[1, 16] The etiology of epilepsy in Alzheimer's disease is unknown. The pathologic hallmarks are neuritic plaques and neurofibrillary tangles, which occur in great numbers in entorhinal cortex, amygdala, and hippocampus.[26] Interestingly, recent quantitative anatomic studies of Alzheimer's patients' entorhinal cortex revealed preservation of synaptic density, in marked contrast with other cortical regions, possibly due to enhanced plasticity in this region.[27] How this finding relates to the mechanism of epileptogenesis in Alzheimer's disease remains to be seen. To our knowledge, no one has yet examined Alzheimer's disease hippocampi, using the Timm stain technique as described above, to determine whether similar patterns of synaptic reorganization to those seen in patients with chronic temporal lobe epilepsy are present.

AGE-RELATED EPILEPTOGENESIS

Relatively few studies have focused on mechanisms of epileptogenesis in aged experimental animals. Thompson et al.[28] studied the effects of senescence on seizure susceptibility in the genetically epilepsy-prone rat (GEPRs). They found that although there was an age-dependent effect in developing animals, there were no significant changes in either latency to seizure onset or seizure intensity in rats ages 480–540 days. They concluded that, once developed, seizure susceptibility in GEPRs is a lifelong trait.

Wozniak et al.[29] administered kainate to young (5–6 months), middle-aged (12–13 months), and senescent (22–25 months) rats in an attempt to study the neurologic toxicity of domoate, a glutamate analogue excitotoxin acting at the kainate receptor subtype. Mussels containing high concentrations of domoate have been implicated in a recent seafood poisoning incident in which victims developed a severe encephalopathy, sometimes leading to convulsions, coma, or death. They found that although low doses of kainate were nontoxic to young rats, in middle-aged and senescent rats it frequently triggered status epilepticus, resultant brain damage, and death.

Dawson et al.[30] have replicated the above findings and studied the neurochemical correlates of kainate neurotoxicity in aged rats. They found that release of aspartate in response to kainic acid, and to a lesser extent glutamate, was augmented in the aged rats compared with adult controls. They conclude that these findings lend support to the notion that the aged brain may exhibit alterations in excitatory amino acid metabolism and speculate that enhanced sensitivity to kainate-receptor–mediated excitotoxicity may play a role in age-related neuronal loss.

These preliminary findings have interesting implications. If the elderly brain is more sensitive to kainate-mediated excitotoxicity, how significant could this be in the production of epilepsy? Could there be a population of patients with elderly-onset epilepsy for whom the cause is a lifetime of exposure to environmental toxins, analogous to the hypothesis that environmental exposure is critical for the development of certain degenerative diseases such as Parkinson's disease?[31]

CONCLUSIONS

In summary, at present there are many more questions than answers regarding possible mechanisms of epileptogenesis in the elderly. It is anticipated that future research in this area will focus on the following questions:

1. Is there a subset of patients with elderly-onset epilepsy who have "idiopathic" genetic disease not otherwise manifest, or are all such cases a result of remote symptomatic injury?
2. Are there differences in the propensity to develop epilepsy, after similar brain insults, between elderly and adult individuals?
3. What differences, if any, exist between elderly and adult individuals in their response to insults such as hypoxia or trauma? Are there differences in axon sprouting or neuronal plasticity? Or does the sheer number of insults accumulating with aging explain the subsequent development of epilepsy?
4. Is it possible that, in the elderly, the pattern of response to injury itself predisposes to the development of seizures, perhaps by leading to a greater degree of excitability than would occur in younger individuals? Or is the reverse true?

5. Do the brains of elderly human beings have enhanced sensitivity to excitotoxins, and how significant is this in the production of clinical symptoms such as epilepsy?
6. Neuronal dropout occurs as a normal function of aging. Does this lead to reorganization of local hippocampal circuitry, in the absence of other insults, that may predispose to the development of seizures?
7. Do the changes in hippocampal structure associated with Alzheimer's disease lead to patterns of synaptic reorganization that are similar to those seen in patients with hippocampal epilepsy?

REFERENCES

1. Hauser WA, Hesdorffer DC. Epilepsy: Frequency, Causes and Consequences. New York: Demos, 1990.
2. Lühdorf K, Jensen LK, Piesner AM. Etiology of seizures in the elderly. Epilepsia 1986;27:458.
3. Hauser WA, Morris ML, Heston LL, Anderson VE. Seizures and myoclonus in patients with Alzheimer's disease. Neurology 1986;36:1226.
4. Swann JW, Smith KL, Brady RJ. Age-dependent alterations in the operations of hippocampal neural networks. Ann N Y Acad Sci 1991;627:264.
5. Jensen FE, Holmes GL, Lombroso CT, et al. Age-dependent changes in long-term seizure susceptibility and behavior after hypoxia in rats. Epilepsia 1992;33:971.
6. Rowley HL, Ellis Y, Davies JA. Age-related effects of NMDA-stimulated concomitant release of nitric oxide and glutamate in cortical slices prepared from DBA/2 mice. Brain Res 1993;613:49.
7. Holmes GL, Thurber SJ, Liu Z, et al. Effects of quisqualic acid and glutamate on subsequent learning, emotionality, and seizure susceptibility in the immature and mature animal. Brain Res 1993;623:325.
8. Tsuda H, Ito M, Oguro K, et al. Age- and seizure-related changes in noradrenaline and dopamine in several brain regions of epileptic El mice. Neurochem Res 1993;18:111.
9. Cavazos JE, Golarai G, Sutula TP. Mossy fiber reorganization induced by kindling: time course of development, progression, and permanence. J Neurosci 1991;11:2795.
10. Babb TL, Kupfer WR, Pretorius JK, et al. Synaptic reorganization by mossy fibers in human epileptic fascia dentata. Neuroscience 1991;42:351.
11. Isokawa M, Levesque MF, Babb TL, Engel J. Single mossy fiber axonal systems of human dentate granule cells studied in hippocampal slices from patients with temporal lobe epilepsy. J Neurosci 1993;13:1511.
12. McKee AC, Kowall NW, Kosik KS. Microtubular reorganization and dendritic growth response in Alzheimer's disease. Ann Neurol 1989;26:652.
13. Geddes JW, Ulas J, Brunner LC, et al. Hippocampal excitatory amino acid receptors in elderly, normal individuals and those with Alzheimer's disease: non-N-methyl-D-aspartate receptors. Neuroscience 1992;50:23.
14. Terry RD. Synaptic plasticity in Alzheimer's disease [editorial]. Ann Neurol 1993;34:321.
15. Hyman BT, Penney JB, Blackstone CD, Young AB. Localization of non-N-methyl-D-aspartate glutamate receptors in normal and Alzheimer hippocampal formation. Ann Neurol 1994;35:31.
16. Romanelli MF, Morris JC, Ashkin K, Cohen LA. Advanced Alzheimer's disease is a risk factor for late-onset seizures. Arch Neurol 1990;47:847.

17. Dichter M, Ayala GF. Cellular mechanisms of epilepsy: a status report. Science 1987;237:157.
18. Katzman R, Terry R. Normal Aging of the Nervous System. In R Katzman, R Terry (eds), The Neurology of Aging (Contemporary Neurology Series Vol. 22). Philadelphia: FA Davis, 1983;15.
19. Nomura Y, Kitamura Y, Kawai M, Segawa T. α_2-Adrenoceptor-GTP binding regulatory protein-adenylate cyclase system in cerebral cortical membranes of adult and senescent rats. Brain Res 1986;379:118.
20. Harik SI, McCracken KA. Age-related increase in presynaptic noradrenergic markers of the rat cerebral cortex. Brain Res 1986;381:125.
21. Tamaru M, Yoneda Y, Ogita K, et al. Age-related decreases of the N-methyl-D-aspartate receptor complex in the rat cerebral cortex and hippocampus. Brain Res 1991;542:83.
22. Meldrum M, Glenton P, Dawson R Jr. [3H] D-Aspartic acid release in brain slices of adult and aged Fischer 344 rats. Neurochem Res 1992;17:151.
23. Agnati LF, Benfenati F, Solfrini V, et al. Brain aging and neuronal plasticity. Ann N Y Acad Sci 1992;673:180.
24. Ng SKC, Hauser WA, Brust JCM, Susser M. Hypertension and the risk of new-onset unprovoked seizures. Neurology 1993;43:425.
25. Coker SB. The diagnosis of childhood neurodegenerative disorders presenting as dementia in adults. Neurology 1991;41:794.
26. Cummings JL. Cortical Dementias: Alzheimer's and Pick's Diseases. In JL Cummings, DF Benson (eds), Dementia: A Clinical Approach. Boston: Butterworth, 1983;35.
27. Scheff SW, Sparks DL, Price DA. Quantitative assessment of synaptic density in the entorhinal cortex in Alzheimer's disease. Ann Neurol 1993;34:356.
28. Thompson JL, Carl FG, Holmes GL. Effects of age on seizure susceptibility in genetically epilepsy-prone rats (GEPR-(s)). Epilepsia 1991;32:161.
29. Wozniak DF, Stewart GR, Miller JP, Olney JW. Age-related sensitivity to kainate neurotoxicity. Exp Neurol 1991;114:250.
30. Dawson R Jr, Wallace DR. Kainic acid-induced seizures in aged rats: neurochemical correlates. Brain Res Bull 1992;29:459.
31. Tanner CM, Langston JW. Do environmental toxins cause Parkinson's disease?: a critical review. Neurology 1990;40(Suppl 3)10:17.

4

Renal and Hormonal Changes Affecting Fluid and Electrolyte Balance in the Elderly

Myron Miller

It is well recognized by clinicians who are involved in the care of the elderly that disturbances of body water and electrolyte balances are common in this age group. Clinically evident entities include primary alterations of water balance that lead to either dehydration or water overload with accompanying hyper- or hyponatremia and primary alterations of sodium regulation that lead to either sodium retention or loss with accompanying edema or plasma volume depletion.

The normal aging process is associated with a number of changes in the body systems that are involved in water and electrolyte regulation (i.e., renal function, hormone secretion, and thirst perception).[1] It is these changes of normal aging that predispose the elderly to clinically significant disturbances in water and electrolyte status when they are challenged by disease, drugs, or extrinsic factors such as access to fluids or control of diet composition.

The confluence of normal aging changes, diseases common in the elderly, and the administration of many classes of drugs can lead to derangement of the already impaired homeostatic systems involved in water and sodium regulation and result in symptomatic consequences (Table 4.1). The central nervous system (CNS) is particularly sensitive to deviations in sodium and water balance; altered function may be expressed by symptoms such as confusion, coma, or seizures, which are erroneously considered to be due to primary disease of the CNS. Thus, knowledge of normal aging effects on water and sodium regulatory systems can lead to reduction in risk of derangement and to accurate diagnosis and appropriate management when alterations do occur.

RENAL CHANGES OF NORMAL AGING

Normal aging is accompanied by changes in renal anatomy and function. Kidney mass undergoes progressive decline from a normal weight of approximately 250–340 g in young adults to 180–200 g by age 80–90 years. This decline is primarily due to atrophy of the renal cortex. By the ninth decade, there is an approximately 40% loss of renal volume.[2]

29

Table 4.1 Factors influencing sodium and water handling in the elderly

1. Impaired water intake
    Decreased thirst
    Altered mental status
    Impaired mobility
2. Renal changes
    Decreased kidney mass
    Decline in renal blood flow
    Decline in glomerular filtration rate
    Distal renal tubular diluting defect
    Impaired renal concentrating capacity
    Impaired renal response to vasopressin
    Impaired sodium conservation
3. Hormonal changes
    Age-related increased vasopressin secretion
    Increased atrial natriuretic hormone
    Decreased plasma renin activity and aldosterone
4. Exogenous factors
    Secondary hyperaldosteronism of disease states
    Iatrogenic sodium retention (nonsteroidal anti-inflammatory drugs)
    Iatrogenic decline in diluting capacity (thiazides)
    Iatrogenic increase in vasopressin (chlorpropamide, fluoxetine)
    Iatrogenic sodium loss (diuretics)

Histologic examination of the aged kidney reveals a decline in the number of glomeruli as a function of increasing age, with a corresponding increase in percent of glomeruli that are hyalinized or sclerotic.[3] This process accelerates after age 40 years, and the decrease in cortical glomeruli may be as high as 30% in normal people by 70 years of age.[4] The residual glomeruli themselves also undergo changes with age. Thus, there is a decrease in effective filtering surface, an increase in number of mesangial cells, a decrease in number of epithelial cells, and a thickening of the glomerular basement membrane.[5] Along with these glomerular changes are alterations in the renal tubules as evidenced by diverticula of the distal nephron[6] and decreased proximal tubular length and volume.[7] In studies of aging animals, the amount of cholesterol in brush-border membranes on the luminal surface of proximal renal tubule cells is increased, and this change is accompanied by decreased permeability of the membranes to sodium chloride and potassium chloride.[8]

Renal vasculature undergoes changes as part of the normal aging process independent of vascular or renal disease. Atherosclerotic lesions are observed in larger renal arteries but do not lead to occlusion of these vessels. There is tapering of interlobar arteries, alterations in the arcuate arteries, and increased tortuosity of intralobular arteries. At the level of the arteriole, hyalin deposition occurs in the vessel walls, leading to atrophy of smooth muscle cells, obliteration of the arteriolar lumen, and loss of the glomerular capillary tuft. These changes take place primarily in the cortical glomeruli.[9, 10] In the juxtamedullary area, glomerular sclerosis may lead to anastomosis between afferent and efferent arterioles, with direct shunting of blood between these vessels. Blood flow to the medulla through the arteria rectae is maintained in old age.

Associated with anatomic changes in the kidney that occur with age are alterations in renal function, although a direct relationship between anatomic and functional changes is not firmly established. It is well recognized that renal blood flow declines during the course of normal aging by approximately 10% per decade after young adulthood so that by the age of 90 years the renal plasma flow is approximately 300 ml/minute—a reduction of 50% of the value found at 30 years of age.[11] The decrease in renal perfusion is most extensive in the outer cortex, with lesser impairment of inner cortex and minimal effect on the medulla.

Glomerular filtration rate (GFR) remains relatively stable until age 40, after which it undergoes decline at an annual rate of approximately 0.8 ml/minute/1.73 m². [12] There is considerable variability of this renal alteration within the elderly population, so decline in GFR is not seen in all aged individuals.[13] Estimation of GFR can be made by calculation of creatinine clearance with corrections for the sex, age, and weight of the individual through use of the Cockroft and Gault equation:

$$\text{Creatinine clearance} = \frac{(140 - \text{age}) \times \text{weight in kg}}{72 \times \text{serum creatinine in mg/dl}}$$

The value for women is derived by multiplying the result by 0.85.[14]

RENAL FACTORS PREDISPOSING TO SODIUM AND WATER RETENTION

Clinical experience suggests that normal aging changes in renal systems predispose the elderly to sodium retention and to water overload and hyponatremia. This section reviews the changes that occur as part of normal aging that can result in increased susceptibility to significant states of sodium and water excess.

Renal Sodium Retention

Several situations may lead to sodium retention in the elderly. The previously described age-related decrease in renal blood flow and glomerular filtration rate favor enhances conservation of sodium. Disease states resulting in secondary hyperaldosteronism, such as congestive heart failure, cirrhosis, or nephrotic syndrome, are common in the elderly. Finally, certain drugs such as nonsteroidal anti-inflammatory agents, which are frequently used in the elderly, may promote sodium retention.

Renal Water Excretion

There are only a few studies that have assessed free-water clearance in the senescent kidney, and these suggest that there is a modest age-related impairment in the ability to dilute the urine and excrete a water load. The ability to generate free-water is dependent on several factors, including the following: adequate delivery of solute to the diluting region (sufficient renal perfusion and glomerular filtration rate); a functional, intact distal diluting site (ascending limb of Henle's loop and the distal tubule); and suppression of antidiuretic hormone in order to escape reabsorption in the collecting duct.[15] The age-related decline in GFR is the most important factor in the aged kidney's diluting capacity. The presence of an age-related diluting defect that is independent of changes in GFR remains controversial.

Lindeman et al. in 1966 studied the diluting capacity of the aged kidney by determining the minimum urine osmolality and maximum free-water clearance after water loading in three groups of men.[16] The minimal urine osmolality in young men (mean age of 31 years) was 52 mOsm/kg, in middle-aged men (mean age of 60 years) was 74 mOsm/kg, and in the older men (mean age of 84 years) was 92 mOsm/kg. The free-water clearance was lowest in the older group. When these results were expressed as free-water clearance per ml of GFR, however, the values were not different, suggesting that the defect in diluting capacity was due to an age-related reduction in GFR. Recently, Crowe et al. carried out a similar study in which groups of six healthy elderly subjects ages 63–80 years (mean age of 72 years) and six healthy young subjects ages 21–26 years (mean age of 22 years) were given a water load.[17] The peak free-water clearance was 5.7 ml/minute in the older group and 8.4 ml/minute in the younger group. When adjustments were made for changes in creatinine clearance, however, the difference in these indices was not statistically significant.

A differing view was presented by Dontas et al., who reported a significantly lower CH_2O to creatinine ratio in 26 elderly subjects from an institutional setting, as compared with 11 healthy younger subjects.[18] The maximal urinary dilution (urinary/plasma osmolality) declined from 0.247 in younger subjects to 0.418 in the elderly. The authors concluded that the CH_2O defects persist after correction for a lower GFR. A smaller study in healthy elderly subjects came to a similar conclusion.[19]

In addition to impaired diluting capacity, the changes in renal plasma flow and GFR that occur with aging can lead to passive reabsorption of fluid, thereby increasing the risk of water overload and hyponatremia. This effect is clinically evident in elderly patients who have congestive heart failure, extracellular volume depletion, and hypoalbuminemia.

The role of diuretics, especially thiazides, in decreasing renal diluting capacity is well known.[20] In the elderly, this effect becomes important, as it is superimposed on the already diminished diluting capacity of the aged kidney. Thus, the many changes in the kidney that occur with aging can increase the elderly's risk of developing water intoxication by impairing their ability to excrete excess water promptly.

FACTORS PREDISPOSING TO RENAL SODIUM AND WATER LOSS

Age-Related Sodium Wasting

Lindeman et al. have shown that elderly individuals are more likely to develop an exaggerated natriuresis after a water load than are younger subjects.[21] In a study of 22 patients with benign hypertension, Schalekamp et al. described an excess in sodium excretion related to increased patient age.[22] Epstein et al. have shown that the response of the aged kidney to salt restriction is sluggish. In their study of the renal response to a restriction in sodium intake to 10 mmol per day, the half-time for reduction of urinary sodium excretion was 17.6 hours in young individuals and 30.9 hours in older subjects.[23] These data suggest that the aging kidney is more prone to sodium wasting. Mechanisms underlying this tendency may be multifactorial and are related to the effects of age on atrial natriuretic hormone, the renin-angiotensin-aldosterone system, and renal tubular function.

Water-Losing States

As early as 1938, Lewis and Alving observed age-related changes in renal concentrating capacity.[24] In their study of healthy men ages 40–101 years old undergoing 24 hours of water deprivation, maximum attainable urine specific gravity declined from 1.030 at age 40 years to 1.023 at age 89 years. This age-related decrease in urine concentrating ability has been confirmed by others. Lindeman et al. studied the response of hospitalized men (ages 23–72 years) to 24 hours of dehydration and demonstrated a progressive decline in maximum urine osmolality with increasing age.[25] Rowe et al. examined urine concentrating ability in 98 healthy, active, community-dwelling volunteers who participated in the Baltimore Longitudinal Study of Aging. After 12 hours of water deprivation, young subjects responded with a marked decrease in urine flow (1.2 ± 0.10 to 0.49 ± 0.03 ml/minute) and a moderate increase in urine osmolality (969 ± 41 to 1109 ± 22 mOsm/kg), whereas elderly subjects were unable to significantly alter urine flow (1.05 ± 0.15 to 1.03 ± 0.13 ml/minute) or osmolality (852 ± 64 to 882 ± 49 mOsm/kg). The effect of age persisted after correction for the age-related decrease in glomerular filtration rate.[26] Part of this effect may be due to a down-regulation of renal vasopressin (AVP) receptors secondary to chronic elevation of plasma AVP in the eldery.

The effect of age on renal responsiveness to vasopressin was first explored by Miller and Shock.[27] Renal tubular response to AVP was measured by determining the urine to plasma inulin concentration ratio in 29 males who ranged in age from 26 years to 86 years and were free of clinically demonstrable cardiovascular and renal disease. The ratio fell from 118 in young men (mean age of 35 years) to 77 in the middle-aged group (mean age of 55 years) and 45 in the older men (mean age of 73 years). Miller studied rats, 8–9 months old, that were injected daily for 28 days with 200 mU of vasopressin tannate in oil to produce a twofold increase in plasma AVP concentration. Response to water deprivation or intraperitoneal desmopressin (dDAVP) in these animals was decreased compared with controls. Cyclic adenosine monophosphate content of renal medullary slices from control animals doubled in response to exposure to dDAVP, whereas no change was observed in the group that had received chronic vasopressin injections.[28]

These data are further supported by the effect of chronically low AVP levels. Rats heterozygous for hypothalamic diabetes insipidus have half the AVP secretory capacity of normal rats and a reduced plasma AVP concentration. The decreased AVP secretion in these animals is associated with maintenance of maximal urine-concentrating capacity with age in contrast with the decline noted in aging normal rats.[28] Thus, it appears that the age-related increase in AVP secretion may result in decreased responsiveness to this hormone, perhaps through downregulation of renal AVP receptors, and serve as the basis for decreased renal concentrating capacity in the elderly.

SECRETION OF VASOPRESSIN

Basal Plasma Vasopressin Levels

There are conflicting data regarding basal concentration of AVP in the blood during normal aging. In 1972, Helderman et al. studied eight older individuals, mean age 59 years (age range of 52–66 years), and eight younger individuals, mean age 37 years, and demonstrated that under basal condition, plasma AVP levels did not change with advancing age.[29] Likewise, Chiodera et al. found similar basal AVP levels in 30 normal men ages 22–81 years who were divided into three age groups: group 1, mean age 30.6 years; group 2, mean age 52.1 years; and group 3, mean age 72.5 years.[30]

Other studies, however, have reported elevated basal AVP levels in healthy elderly as compared with younger individuals. Frolkis et al. studied healthy human subjects ages 20–80 years and observed a progressive rise in plasma AVP concentration with age that became most evident in subjects older than 60 years of age.[31] Identical studies in rats also demonstrated an increase in blood AVP levels with age.[31] In the study of Rondeau et al., it was shown that plasma AVP levels, both in normal patients and in patients with heart failure, rose steadily with increasing age and that the patients with cardiac insufficiency as a group always had higher values.[32] Kirkland et al. demonstrated that healthy older people (ages 61–82 years) have higher basal levels of AVP than younger subjects under identical conditions.[33]

A rise in basal plasma AVP with age cannot be attributed to age-related changes in vasopressin pharmacokinetics. No differences could be demonstrated between young and elderly subjects in vasopressin half-life, volume of distribution, or clearance.[34] Thus, evidence of increased basal plasma vasopressin most likely reflects age-related changes in central control systems for vasopressin release.

Vasopressin Stimulation Studies

Secretion of AVP varies in response to several regulatory stimuli: changes in blood tonicity, blood volume, and blood pressure. AVP release is also affected by other factors such as nausea, pain, emotional stress, a variety of drugs, cigarette smoking, and glucopenia.[35] In recent years, a growing body of information has emerged that suggests that normal aging affects the way these stimuli act and interact to influence AVP release.

The major physiologic stimulus for AVP secretion in humans is plasma osmolality, which is itself regulated by hypothalamic osmoreceptors.[36] Studies performed by Helderman et al. tested osmoreceptor sensitivity in the elderly.[29] The AVP response to hypertonic saline infusions in healthy elderly (ages 54–92 years) was compared with the response of younger individuals ages 21–49 years. Infusion of hypertonic saline raised plasma osmolality, with a consequent increase in plasma AVP in both groups, but the hormone concentrations in the older subjects were almost double those in the younger subjects. Thus, for any given level of osmotic stimulus there was a greater release of AVP in the elderly, suggesting that aging resulted in osmoreceptor hypersensitivity.

Studies using water deprivation as a stimulus for AVP secretion have supported the concept of an age-related enhancement in vasopressin secretion. In a study by Phillips et al., a group of seven young healthy individuals (20–31 years old) and a group of seven healthy elderly man (67–75 years old) were deprived of water for 24 hours.[37] The older individuals responded to water deprivation and hyperosmolality with higher serum concentrations of AVP than the younger individuals. Only one study has produced results that conflict with the above findings. In this study, water deprivation for 14 hours in 30 healthy subjects ages 63–87 years was reported to result in mean AVP concentrations significantly lower than those in the young control group.[38]

MODULATION OF VASOPRESSIN RELEASE

Changes in blood volume and blood pressure influence the secretion of AVP through effects on pressure-sensitive receptors in the neck, heart, and large arteries of the chest. Volume affects low pressure left atrial stretch receptors, whereas a change in blood pressure affects high pressure baroreceptors in the carotid arteries and aorta. A decrease in blood volume and blood pressure provokes the release of AVP; conversely a rise in volume and pressure inhibits it.

The sensitivity of the hypothalamic-neurohypophyseal axis to these volume and pressure stimuli was studied by Rowe et al.[39] Acute upright posture was assumed in 12 younger (ages 19–31 years) and 15 older (ages 62–80 years) subjects after overnight dehydration. In the young subjects, the expected change in pulse and blood pressure was accompanied by a more than twofold elevation in plasma AVP. In the older subjects, similar changes in pulse and blood pressure did not uniformly lead to increased vasopressin secretion, with only eight of 15 older individuals experiencing increased plasma AVP. A subsequent study by

Bevilacqua et al. produced similar findings, suggesting the presence of an age-related failure of volume and pressure mediated AVP release.[40]

Ethanol induces a water diuresis by inhibiting the secretion of AVP at a central locus. Helderman et al. studied the age-related AVP response to ethanol infusion.[29] Nine young (ages 21–49 years) and 13 older (ages 54–92 years) subjects received intravenous ethanol. The younger subjects demonstrated a sustained inhibition of AVP secretion during the infusion of ethanol. Response in the older group was paradoxical, with initial AVP inhibition followed by breakthrough secretion and rebound to twice basal levels. These findings were attributed to an age-related osmoreceptor hypersensitivity.

Metoclopramide, a known potent stimulator for aldosterone secretion, was found by Norbiato et al. to stimulate AVP secretion in man.[41] This effect on AVP release could not be attributed to changes in known mechanisms regulating vasopressin secretion, as no alterations in plasma osmolality, heart rate, or blood pressure occurred after metoclopramide administration. In addition, the mechanism could not be linked to metoclopramide's antidopaminergic properties, as other powerful dopamine antagonists did not produce any increase in AVP secretion. Studies by Steardo et al. were subsequently carried out in the rat and provided evidence that cholinergic mechanisms may be involved in metoclopramide-induced AVP release.[42]

Norbiato et al. examined the AVP response to a 20-mg metoclopramide injection in seven normal elderly subjects ages 65–80 years as compared with a group of normal young subjects ages 16–35 years.[41] They found significantly higher plasma AVP concentrations in the older group. No significant changes in plasma osmolality, blood pressure, or heart rate were observed. Thus, elderly subjects were found to have an increased sensitivity to metoclopramide, with the mechanism presumed to be through activation of cholinergic neurons regulating hypothalamic AVP release.

Recently, AVP responses to cigarette smoking and insulin-induced hypoglycemia, in addition to metoclopramide, were evaluated by Chiodera et al. in 30 male subjects ages 22–81 years.[30] Corroborating the prior findings of Norbiato et al., the AVP response to metoclopramide was significantly higher in the older group as compared with the two younger groups. The response to cigarette smoking was similarly affected: Plasma AVP concentration increased 3.25 times after smoking in the older group, as compared with 2.5 times in the two younger groups. In contrast, the AVP response during an insulin hypoglycemia test was identical in pattern and magnitude in all age groups.

In conclusion, results of stimulation studies indicate that, in aging, the AVP response to osmotic stimuli is increased owing to a hyperresponsive osmoreceptor, whereas the AVP response to upright posture is reduced owing to impaired baroreceptor function. Likewise, aging accentuates the AVP stimulatory response to metoclopramide and to cigarette smoking and reduces the suppressibility of AVP to ethanol. The AVP response to hypoglycemia, however, is not affected by aging.

EFFECT OF AGE ON THE RENIN-ANGIOTENSIN-ALDOSTERONE SYSTEM

Weidmann et al. compared 12 young healthy volunteers (ages 20–30 years old) with seven healthy older individuals (ages 62–70 years old) and described a slightly lower plasma renin activity and aldosterone concentration in the elderly group in the supine position and on a normal sodium diet.[43] Under the stimuli of upright posture and sodium depletion, consistent significant increases in circulating renin and aldosterone concentrations were observed in both age groups, but the mean values achieved were always significantly lower in the elderly than young. Differences between both groups were more pronounced when these stimuli were applied than under basal conditions.[43] The decrease in plasma renin activity in the elderly is not due to changes in plasma renin substrate concentration but to a decrease in active renin concentration.[44] The decreased conversion of inactive to active renin might be responsible in part for the reduced active renin concentration in the elderly. The decrease in aldosterone concentration with age appears to be a direct result of the age-related decrease in plasma renin activity and is not due to age changes in the adrenal gland, as aldosterone and cortisol responses to corticotropin infusion are unaltered in the elderly.[44] The age-related decrease in aldosterone concentration, as a result of decreased plasma renin activity, predisposes the elderly to renal sodium wasting.

AGE-RELATED CHANGES IN ATRIAL NATRIURETIC HORMONE SECRETION, REGULATION, AND ACTION

Atrial natriuretic hormone (ANH) is synthesized, stored, and released in the atria of the heart of humans and animals. Through its action on the kidney, ANH produces a pronounced natriuresis and diuresis; through its action on blood vessels, it produces vasodilation and, as a result, has been shown to decrease blood pressure in both normal and hypertensive individuals. Since it is an important regulator of sodium excretion, ANH may be a significant factor in mediating the altered renal sodium handling of age.

Ohashi et al. compared 19 young normal men and 31 elderly male nursing home residents and noted a fivefold increase in mean ANH levels and an exaggerated ANH response to the stimulus of saline infusion in the elderly group.[45] McKnight et al. also reported an age-related increase in basal ANH levels but no change with age in the response to saline infusion.[46] Tajima et al. compared ANH levels in eight healthy young (ages 21–28 years) and seven healthy elderly individuals (ages 62–73 years).[47] In their study, baseline ANH levels were twice as high in the elderly than in the young and ANH response to the stimulus of head-out water immersion was greater in the elderly.[47] We have studied 40 healthy male and female subjects 22–64 years of age to determine the influence of age on circulating levels of ANH both under basal conditions and after physiologic stimulation of ANH release by controlled exercise. Supine exercise using a bicycle ergometer to 80% of maximum predicted heart rate resulted in marked increases in ANH. Subjects older than age 50 years had higher baseline levels and greater response to exercise when compared with subjects younger than age 50 years. Thus, increasing age results in increased ANH basal levels and an increased ANH response to both physiologic and pharmacologic stimuli.

Heim et al. suggest that the renal effects of ANH may be exaggerated in elderly versus young individuals.[48] In their study, the natriuretic response to a bolus injection of ANH was higher in 12 older individuals (mean age 52.3 years) compared with 16 younger subjects (mean age 26 years). These findings require confirmation, since rapid intravenous infusion of ANH results in higher ANH levels in the elderly as a result of diminished ANH clearance.[49] Jansen et al. did not measure the renal action of ANH, but they noted no change with age in the blood pressure response to intravenous ANH infusion after correction for higher ANH levels in the elderly.[50]

ANH is known to interact with the renin-angiotensin-aldosterone system. Increases of ANH result in suppression of renal renin secretion, plasma renin activity, plasma angiotensin-II, and aldosterone levels, suggesting an indirect inhibition of aldosterone secretion by ANH.[51] Cuneo et al. found that minimal increases in ANH within physiologic levels, produced by slow rate ANH infusion, can inhibit angiotensin-II–induced aldosterone secretion in normal men, thus suggesting an additional direct inhibitory effect of ANH on aldosterone release.[52] Clinkingbeard et al. have confirmed that ANH can suppress aldosterone in humans through both direct and indirect actions.[53] Thus, ANH may further promote renal sodium loss through inhibition of aldosterone release.

In summary, ANH may be an important mediator of age-related renal sodium loss. This effect may be the consequence of increased basal ANH levels, increased ANH response to stimuli, increased renal sensitivity to ANH, and ANH-induced suppression of adrenal sodium–retaining hormones.

FLUID INTAKE

The ingestion of appropriate quantities of fluid to maintain a normal state of fluid balance requires that thirst perception be present, that a suitable source of fluid be available, and that the individual be physically capable of obtaining and consuming the fluid. Evidence has been generated that indicates that a decline in thirst perception is an accompaniment of normal aging. In normal individuals, thirst becomes evident when plasma osmolality rises to values of more than 292 mOsm/kg.[54] Study of healthy older people (ages 67–75 years) has demonstrated that prolonged water deprivation capable of raising plasma osmolality to more than 296 mOsm/kg is accompanied by diminished subjective awareness of thirst. Thus, when these individuals are subsequently presented with water, they consume significantly less than young subjects whose plasma osmolality rose to a lesser level (mean 290 mOsm/kg) after the same period of water deprivation.[37] Other studies of elderly patients with cerebrovascular accidents have similarly documented impaired thirst perception in the face of volume depletion and hyperosmolality, both normally being potent stimuli for thirst.[55] The common occurrence of cognitive impairment in the elderly can lead to failure of water-seeking behavior in the presence of major physiologic stimuli for thirst. Further confounding the ability of the elderly to ingest adequate amounts of fluid is the frequent presence of physical disability (e.g., blindness, arthritis, stroke) and impaired mobility, thus limiting the capacity of the patient to gain access to fluids.

HYPERNATREMIA AND HYPONATREMIA

The above described alterations in renal, hormonal, and fluid intake regulatory systems predispose the elderly person to clinically important alterations in water and sodium balance. The most common expression of these alterations is in the concentration of sodium in the blood, reflected by hypernatremia and hyponatremia.

Prevalence of Hypernatremia

A number of studies support the clinical impression that aging is associated with an increased risk of development of hypernatremia. Hypernatremia can be considered to be present when the serum sodium concentration is more than 146 mmol/liter. In a study of 15,187 hospitalized patients older than age 60 years, an incidence of approximately 1% has been reported. The mean serum sodium concentration in the hypernatremic patients was 154 mmol/liter, and the disorder was accompanied by depression of sensorium and high mortality.[56] Similarly, a study of elderly residents of a long-term–care institution disclosed an incidence of 1%, but the prevalence of hypernatremia in this population increased to 18% when the patients were monitored during a 12-month period.[57] Of 264 nursing home patients who developed acute illness requiring hospitalization, 34% became markedly hypernatremic, with serum sodium concentrations of more than 150 mmol/liter.[58]

Prevalence of Hyponatremia

Hyponatremia, defined as a serum sodium concentration of less than 136 mmol/liter, is a common finding in elderly individuals. Analysis of plasma electrolyte values for healthy individuals indicates an age-related decrease of approximately 1 mmol/liter per decade from a mean value of 141 ± 4 mmol/liter in young subjects.[59] In a population of people older than age 65 years who were living at home and who were without acute illness, a 7% incidence of serum sodium concentration of 137 mmol/liter or less has been observed.[60] In hospitalized patients, hyponatremia is even more common. Thus, an analysis of 5,000 consecutive sets of plasma electrolytes from a hospital population (mean age of 54 years) revealed a mean serum sodium of 134 ± 6 mmol/liter, with the values skewed toward the hyponatremic end of the distribution curve.[59] A high prevalence of hyponatremia has been found in patients hospitalized for a variety of acute illnesses, with the risk being greater with increasing age of the patient.[61-64]

Elderly residents of long-term–care institutions appear to be especially prone to develop hyponatremia. A study of 160 patients with a mean age of 72 years who resided in a chronic disease hospital disclosed 22.5% to have repeated serum sodium determinations of less than 135 mmol/liter.[65] In patients admitted to an acute geriatric unit, 11.3% were found to have serum sodium concentrations of 130 mmol/liter or less.[66] A survey of nursing home residents older than age 60 years has revealed a cross-sectional incidence of 18% with serum sodium less than 136 mmol/liter. When this population was followed on a longitudinal basis during a 12-month period, 53% were observed to experience one or more episodes of hyponatremia.[57] A recent study by the author has confirmed the high prevalence of hyponatremia (44%) in nursing home residents evaluated on a longitudinal basis.

Clinical Consequences of Hypernatremia and Hyponatremia

Both hypernatremia and hyponatremia are capable of producing significant clinical symptoms, the most important being the result of effects on CNS function. This is especially likely to be the case in the elderly, who may already have an underlying CNS disease, so that the interaction of disease and electrolyte disturbance can cause major clinical consequences such as delirium, confusion, stupor, coma, and convulsions.

Awareness of the physiologic alterations that place the elderly person at increased risk for disturbance of sodium and water balance, as well as the disease processes and drugs that may lead to clinically significant further alterations and symptomatic consequences, will allow the physician to anticipate and recognize the presence of such disturbances. Understanding of the mechanisms involved can lead to appropriate therapeutic intervention and management.

REFERENCES

1. Miller M, Gold GC, Friedlander DA. Physiological changes of aging affecting salt and water balance. Rev Clin Gerontol 1991;1:215.
2. McLachlan M, Wasserman P. Changes in size and distensibility of the aging kidney. Br J Radiol 1981;54:488.
3. Kaplan C, Pasternack B, Shah H, Gallo G. Age-related incidence of sclerotic glomeruli in human kidneys. Am J Pathol 1975;80:227.
4. Kappel B, Olsen S. Cortical interstitial tissue and sclerosed glomeruli in the normal human kidney, related to age and sex. Virchows Arch 1980;387:271.
5. Taylor SA, Price RG. Age-related changes in rat glomerular basement membrane. Int J Biochem 1982;14:201.
6. Darmady EM, Offer J, Woodhouse MS. The parameters of the aging kidney. J Pathol 1973;109:195.
7. Goyal VK. Changes with age in the human kidney. Exp Gerontol 1982;17:321.
8. Pratz J, Ripoche P, Corman B. Cholesterol content and water and solute permeabilities of kidney membranes from aging rats. Am J Physiol 1987; 253:R8.

9. Takazakura E, Wasabu N, Handa A, et al. Intrarenal vascular changes with age and diseases. Kidney Int 1972;2:224.
10. Ljungqvist A, Lagergren C. Normal intrarenal arterial pattern in adult and aging human kidney. J Anat 1962;96:285.
11. Davies DF, Shock NW. Age changes in glomerular filtration, effective renal plasma flow and tubular excretory capacity in adult males. J Clin Invest 1950;29:496.
12. Rowe JW, Andres RA, Tobin JD, et al. The effect of age on creatinine clearance in man: a cross-sectional and longitudinal study. J Gerontol 1976;31:155.
13. Lindeman RD, Tobin JD, Shock NW. Longitudinal studies on the rate of decline in renal function with age. J Am Geriatr Soc 1985;33:278.
14. Cockroft DW, Gault MH. Prediction of creatinine clearance from serum creatinine. Nephron 1976;16:31.
15. Sica DA, Hartford A. Sodium and Water Disorders in the Elderly. In ET Zawade Jr, DA Sica (eds), Geriatric Nephrology and Urology. Littleton, MA: PSG, 1985;127.
16. Lindeman RD, Lee DT, Yiengst MJ, Shock NW. Influence of age, renal disease, hypertension, diuretics and calcium on the antidiuretic responses to suboptimal infusions of vasopressin. J Lab Clin Med 1966;68:202.
17. Crowe MJ, Forsling ML, Rolls BJ, et al. Altered water excretion in health elderly men. Age Ageing 1987;16:285.
18. Dontas AS, Karkenos S, Papanayioutou P. Mechanisms of renal tubular defects in old age. Postgrad Med J 1972;48:295.
19. Lye M. Electrolyte Disorders in the Elderly. In DB Morgan (ed), Clinics in Endocrinology and Metabolism. Philadelphia: Saunders, 1984:377.
20. Zanuszewicz W, Heinemann H, Demartini F, et al. A clinical study of effects of hydrochlorothiazide on renal excretion of electrolyte and free water. N Engl J Med 1959;261:264.
21. Lindeman RD, Adler S, Yiengst MJ, Beard ES. Natriuresis and carbohydrate-induced antinatriuresis after overnight fast and hydration. Nephron 1970;7:289.
22. Schalekamp MA, Krauss XH, Schalekamp-Kuyken MP, et al. Studies on the mechanisms of hypernatriuresis in essential hypertension in relation to measurements of plasma renin concentration, body fluid compartments and renal function. Clin Sci 1971;41:219.
23. Epstein M, Hollenberg NK. Age as a determinant of renal sodium conservation in normal man. J Lab Clin Med 1976;87:411.
24. Lewis WH, Alving AS. Changes with age in the renal function in adult men. Am J Physiol 1938;123:500.
25. Lindeman RD, Van Buren C, Raisz LG. Osmolar renal concentrating ability in health young men and hospitalized patients without renal disease. N Engl J Med 1960;262:1306.
26. Rowe JW, Shock NW, DeFronzo RA. The influence of age on the renal response to water deprivation in man. Nephron 1976;17:270.
27. Miller JH, Shock NW. Age differences in the renal tubular response to antidiuretic hormone. J Gerontol 1953;8:446.
28. Miller M. Influence of Aging on Vasopressin Secretion and Water Regulation. In RW Schrier (ed), Vasopressin. New York: Raven, 1985;249.
29. Helderman JH, Vestal RE, Rowe JW, et al. The response of arginine vasopressin to intravenous ethanol and hypertonic saline in man. The impact of aging. J Gerontol 1978;33:39.
30. Chiodera P, Capretti L, Marches M. Abnormal arginine vasopressin response to cigarette smoking and metoclopramide (but not to insulin-induced hypoglycemia) in elderly subjects. J Gerontol 1991;46:M6.
31. Frolkis VV, Golovchenko SF, Medved VI, Frolkis RA. Vasopressin and cardiovascular system in aging. Gerontology 1982;28:290.

32. Rondeau E, Delima J, Caillens H, et al. High plasma anti-diuretic hormone in patients with cardiac failure. Influence of age. Mineral Electrolyte Metab 1982;8:267.
33. Kirkland J, Lye M, Goddard C, et al. Plasma arginine vasopressin in dehydrated elderly patients. Clin Endocrinol (Oxf) 1984;20:451.
34. Engel PA, Rowe JW, Minaker KL, Robertson GL. Stimulation of vasopressin release by exogenous vasopressin: effect of sodium intake and age. Am J Physiol 1984;246:E202.
35. Robertson GL, Rowe JW. The effect of aging on neurohypophysial function. Peptides 1980;1(Suppl 1):159.
36. Robertson GL, Shelton RL, Athar J. The osmoregulation of vasopressin. Kidney Int 1976;10:25.
37. Phillips PA, Rolls BJ, Ledingham JGG, et al. Reduced thirst after water deprivation in healthy elderly men. N Engl J Med 1984;311:753.
38. Li CH, Hsieh SM, Nagai I. The response of plasma arginine vasopressin to 14 h. water deprivation in the elderly. Acta Endocrinol 1984;105:314.
39. Rowe JW, Minaker KL, Robertson GL. Age-related failure of volume pressure mediated vasopressin release in man. J Clin Endocrinol Metab 1982;54:661.
40. Bevilacqua M, Norbiato G, Chebat E, et al. Osmotic and nonosmotic control of vasopressin release in the elderly: effect of metroclopramide. J Clin Endocrinol Metab 1987;65:1243.
41. Norbiato G, Bevilacqua M, Chebat E, et al. Metoclopramide increases vasopressin secretion. J Clin Endocrinol Metab 1986;G3:747.
42. Steardo L, Iovino M, Monteleone P, et al. Evidence that cholinergic receptors of muscarinic type may modulate vasopressin release induced by metoclopramide. J Neural Transm 1990;82:213.
43. Weidmann P, De Myttenaere-Bursztein S, Maxwell MH, De Lima J. Effect of aging on plasma renin and aldosterone in normal man. Kidney Int 1975;8:325.
44. Tsunoda K, Abe K, Goto T, et al. Effect of age on the renin-angiotensin-aldosterone system in normal subjects: simultaneous measurement of active and inactive renin, renin substrate, and aldosterone in plasma. J Clin Endocrinol Metab 1986;62:384.
45. Ohashi M, Fujio N, Nawata H, et al. High plasma concentrations of human atrial natriuretic polypeptide in aged men. J Clin Endocrinol Metab 1987;64:81.
46. McKnight JA, Roberts G, Sheridan B, Brew Atkinson A. Relationship between basal and sodium stimulated plasma atrial natriuretic factor, age, sex and blood pressure in normal man. J Human Hypertens 1989;3:157.
47. Tajima F, Sagawa S, Iwamoto J, et al. Renal and endocrine responses in the elderly during headout water immersion. Am J Physiol 1988;254:R977.
48. Heim JM, Gottmann JW, Strom TM, Gerzer R. Effects of a bolus dose of atrial natriuretic factor in young and elderly volunteers. Eur J Clin Invest 1989;19:265.
49. Ohashi M, Fugio N, Nawata H, et al. Pharmacokinetics of synthetic alpha-human atrial natriuretic polypeptide in normal men; effect of aging. Regul Pept 1987;19:265.
50. Jansen TL, Tan AC, Smits P, et al. Hemodynamic effects of atrial natriuretic factor in young and elderly subjects. Clin Pharmacol Ther 1990;48:179.
51. Genest J, Larochelle P, Cusson JR, et al. The atrial natriuretic factor in hypertension: state of the art lecture. Hypertension 1988;11(Suppl 1):13.
52. Cuneo RC, Espiner EA, Nicholls MG, et al. Effect of physiological levels of atrial natriuretic peptide on hormone secretion: inhibition of angiotensin-induced aldosterone secretion and renin release in normal man. J Clin Endocrinol Metab 1987;65:765.
53. Clinkingbeard C, Sessions C, Shenker Y. The physiological role of atrial natriuretic hormone in the regulation of aldosterone and salt and water metabolism. J Clin Endocrinol Metab 1990;70:582.

54. Robertson GL. Thirst and vasopressin function in normal and disordered states of water balance. J Lab Clin Med 1983;101:351.
55. Miller PD, Krebs RA, Neal BJ, McIntyre DO. Hypodipsia in geriatric patients. Am J Med 1982;73:354.
56. Snyder NA, Feigal DW, Arieff AI. Hypernatremia in elderly patients. A heterogenous, morbid, and iatrogenic entity. Ann Intern Med 1987;107:309.
57. Miller M, Morley JE, Rubenstein LA, et al. Hyponatremia in a nursing home population. Gerontologist 1985;25:11.
58. Lavizo-Mourey R, Johnson J, Stolley P. Risk factors for dehydration among elderly nursing home residents. J Am Geriatr Soc 1988;36:213.
59. Owen JA, Campbell DG. A comparison of plasma electrolyte and urea values in healthy persons and in hospital patients. Clin Chem Acta 1968;22:611.
60. Caird FI, Andrews GR, Kennedy RD. Effect of posture on blood pressure in the elderly. Br Heart J 1973;35:527.
61. Anderson RJ, Chung H, Kluge R, Schrier RW. Hyponatremia: prospective analysis of its epidemiology and the pathogenetic role of vasopressin. Ann Intern Med 1985;102:164.
62. Hochman I, Cabili S, Peer G. Hyponatremia in internal medicine ward patients: causes, treatment and prognosis. Isr J Med Sci 1989;25:73.
63. Kennedy PGE, Mitchell DM, Hoffbrand BI. Severe hyponatremia in hospital inpatients. BMJ 1978;2:1251.
64. Tierney WM, Martin DK, Greenlee MC, et al. The prognosis of hyponatremia at hospital admission. J Gen Intern Med 1986;1:380.
65. Kleinfeld M, Casimir M, Borra S. Hyponatremia as observed in a chronic disease facility. J Am Geriatr Soc 1979;27:156.
66. Sunderam SG, Mankikar GD. Hyponatremia in the elderly. Age Ageing 1983;12:77.

5

Endocrinologic Changes in the Elderly Predisposing to Seizures: Hypoglycemia

Kenneth L. Minaker and Linda Ann Morrow

INTRODUCTION

Although epilepsy has its greatest incidence in infancy, it increases in incidence substantially in those older than age 60 years. Overall, epilepsy has an incidence of 48 per 100,000 population, but in those older than age 60 years the rate is 82 per 100,000 per year.[1] Epilepsy, which implies chronic recurrent seizures, usually has a primary basis in a chronic cerebral abnormality that may be fixed or progressive over time. The appearance of epilepsy in an older individual should be considered secondary to some underlying cause rather than the result of idiopathic or genetic factors. In a large study of a geriatric Scandinavian population, 75% of patients had an identifiable cause for their seizures, with previous cerebral infarct causing 32% and tumors causing 14%. Other causes included prior head trauma; alcohol and drug abuse; dementing illnesses; and metabolic disorders, including hypoglycemia and hyponatremia. Other studies have confirmed these observations.[2–4]

The dominant metabolic or endocrine cause of seizures is hypoglycemia, the focus of this chapter.[5] Initially, the regulation of glucose homeostasis in the elderly is reviewed, differentiating normal physiologic control of glucose homeostasis from that of the disease condition highly prevalent in the elderly, diabetes mellitus. The counterregulation of lowered blood glucose is emphasized. Next, the differential diagnosis of hypoglycemia is reviewed, emphasizing not only the metabolic but also the pharmacologic causes of hypoglycemia. Finally, the approach to treatment of hypoglycemia is discussed.

GLUCOSE HOMEOSTASIS

An age-related impairment in the capacity to maintain carbohydrate homeostasis after glucose challenge has been recognized for more than 60 years. In the last two decades, gerontologists have focused their attention on the elucidation of the mechanisms underlying this aged-related impairment in carbohydrate economy, and a general consensus is now emerging.[6] Many clinical studies indicate a very slight age-related increase after maturity in fasting blood glucose levels in healthy humans that approaches 1 mg/dl per decade. This change is not affected by sex and is only slightly enhanced by cortisol administration. This modest age-related increase in fasting blood glucose levels is accompanied by rather striking increases in blood sugar after oral or intravenous glucose challenge. Lack of consideration of the age effect on glucose tolerance testing has resulted in an erroneous diagnosis of impaired carbohydrate tolerance or diabetes in many healthy elderly. In an extensive review of the English literature, Davidson found that the average blood glucose increase with advancing age was 9.5 mg/dl per decade at 1 hour after an oral glucose load and 5.3 mg/dl per decade at 2 hours.[7] These higher postprandial glucose levels seen with aging are also reflected in increased levels of glycosylated hemoglobin.

The physiologic mechanism underlying these changes has been the subject of extensive investigation. Alterations in glucose absorption associated with aging are unlikely to play an important role in these findings. Recent study has shown that during a 2-hour period after oral glucose intake, total posthepatic glucose delivery was comparable in young and older men, with younger individuals showing greater posthepatic glucose delivery of glucose in the first hour and a reversal of the phenomenon during the second hour.[8] These studies reinforce the role of impaired peripheral use as the primary mechanism for glucose intolerance of aging.[9] Distribution of blood glucose levels at 1 and 2 hours after glucose challenge in older people is unimodal, which suggests that the change does not reflect the increase in prevalence of a second population of diabetics who are skewing the data. Evidence that age-associated changes in body composition may play an important role in determining age effects in carbohydrate metabolism, even under basal conditions, has been established in a study of fasting levels of glucose, insulin, glucagon, and growth hormone in normal male volunteers ranging in age from 23 years to 93 years. In these studies, obesity was associated with increases in basal insulin, glucagon, and fasting glucose, whereas basal levels of these main glucoregulatory hormones were not influenced by aging.[10]

Substantial literature is now available that evaluates the effect of age on the molecular species of circulating insulin, the amount of insulin released from the pancreas in response to glucose or amino acid stimulation, the clearance of insulin from plasma, and insulin action on the liver and peripheral tissues. As similar circulating proportions of pro-insulin and total insulin in older and younger adults are seen after oral glucose challenge, there appears to be no deficit in the conversion of the former to the latter. Insulin release with advancing age has been studied with care. Aging in the rat is associated with an increase in the number of large islets.[11] In spite of the greater beta-cell mass, however, investigators have demonstrated an age-related decrease in glucose- or leucine-stimulated insulin secretion per beta cell of collagenase-isolated islets. The number of beta cells per islet increases in the older rodent, suggesting that the impaired capacity of individual beta cells to secrete insulin with advancing age is compensated for by an increase in numbers of beta cells in an effort to maintain normal carbohydrate homeostasis. Numerous studies have evaluated circulating insulin levels in individuals across the adult age range, but perhaps the most elegant have been those studies employing the hyperglycemic glucose clamp technique. Plasma insulin levels during steady-state hyperglycemia appear to be relatively well preserved in the aged, with suggestions of a slight insulin secretory defect being counterbalanced by an age-related decline in insulin clearance.[12] These latter observations may reconcile the discrepancy between the lack of the effect on age on circulating insulin levels in most studies and in vitro studies showing impaired pancreatic insulin release with advancing age.

Studies in humans have shown no effect of age on basal hepatic glucose production or any alterations in response to high physiologic and superphysiologic levels of hyperinsulinemia. Hepatic glucose output is rapidly and almost completely suppressed in both young and elderly individuals during conditions of hyperinsulinemia. The sensitivity of peripheral tissues to insulin has been evaluated in humans using several techniques. Several studies employing the insulin clamp technique to evaluate glucose disposal have been performed in young and elderly individuals over a range of circulating steady-state insulin levels. These studies have demonstrated that aging, in active nonobese healthy men with normal glucose tolerance on normal diets, is associated with marked insulin resistance. Rowe and his colleagues found that maximal insulin-induced glucose disposal rates were the same in the young and the older patients but that the dose response curve was substantially shifted to the right in the older subjects.[13] The insulin level at which half maximal glucose uptake was reached was 64 ± 14 µIU/ml in the young and 113 ± 11 µIU/ml in the older subjects. Correction of glucose metabolism rate for lean body mass had no effect on comparisons between these groups. These data have been interpreted as indicating an age-associated decline in sensitivity of peripheral tissues to insulin without a change in maximal tissue responsiveness.

The overwhelming bulk of available data indicates that normal aging is not associated with a change in insulin receptor number or infinity in rodents or humans. Thus, most of the insulin resistance observed must occur at early postreceptor intracellular events. Several studies have evaluated the influence of aging on the release and response to glucagon in men.[14] In general, fasting levels of glucagon are not influenced by age, nor is the post–glucose-induced suppression of glucagon release. In addition, glucose release in response to alanine or arginine and glucagon kinetics is not impaired with aging.

Thus, blood glucose levels with advancing age show a number of characteristic changes, but the overall blood glucose level under fasting conditions is well preserved. The physiology of aging promotes, if anything, a tendency for relative hyperglycemia to occur under usual physiologic conditions. As is discussed in the section on comorbid illness and clinical hypoglycemia and the elderly patient, comorbid diseases and nutritional impairment make the elderly prone to hypoglycemia from a variety of causes.

Table 5.1 Glycemic thresholds

Response	Blood Glucose (mg/dl)
Decline in insulin secretion	83
Counterregulatory hormone secretion	
Epinephrine	69
Glucagon	68
Growth hormone	66
Cortisol	58
Hypoglycemic symptoms	53
Impaired cognition	49
Seizures	<25

COUNTERREGULATION OF HYPOGLYCEMIA

Glucose and oxygen are the predominant metabolic fuels of the brain. Neither can be synthesized or stored for more than a few minutes; thus, numerous physiologic mechanisms maintain a continuous supply of both oxygen and glucose from the circulation. A variety of physiologic mechanisms have evolved to prevent or correct hypoglycemia. Declines in plasma glucose normally trigger a sequence of responses (Table 5.1) that occur at differing blood glucose levels.[15]

Initially, insulin secretion decreases when blood glucose falls below approximately 80 mg/dl. Glucose levels just below the physiologic range cause increases in secretion of epinephrine, glucagon, growth hormone, and cortisol. These appear to be released between 50 mg/dl and 60 mg/dl of glucose. These responses to changing plasma glucose concentrations occur at glucose levels well above those that produce symptoms of hypoglycemia, and these responses usually delay or prevent hypoglycemia from becoming clinically evident.[16] Symptoms of hypoglycemia do develop below 50 mg/dl and are classically divided into signs and symptoms of autonomic (neurogenic) and neuroglycopenic arousal (Table 5.2).

Autonomic symptoms are by and large peripheral warnings of developing hypoglycemia, and neuroglycopenic symptoms are the result of brain dysfunction caused by deprivation of glucose. Autonomic symptomatology includes sweating, pounding heart, trembling, hunger, and anxiety. Neuroglycopenic symptoms include confusion, odd behavior, inability to concentrate, and difficulty in speaking. Incoordination and difficulty walking, blurred vision, and tingling around the mouth are less reliably reported.

Although not well studied, clinical reports suggest that the levels of glucose resulting in seizure activity are substantially below those producing neuroglycopenic symptomatology. A number of case reports suggest that levels are 25 mg/dl or lower when seizures occur.[17, 18]

The counterregulatory responses to insulin-induced glucose reduction in the elderly have been studied by several investigators. Prior studies suggested

Table 5.2 Hypoglycemic symptoms

Autonomic symptoms
   Sweating
   Pounding heart
   Trembling
   Hunger
   Anxiety
Neuroglycopenic symptoms
   Confusion, odd behavior, poor concentration
   Incoordination, impaired gait
   Blurred vision
   Perioral tingling
Other
   Headache, weakness, nausea, dry mouth

that basal levels of counterregulatory hormones do not change with age, and in response to profound hypoglycemia, cortisol and growth hormone responses are normal or slightly diminished. In a study by Meneilly et al., elderly individuals were subjected to moderate reductions in blood glucose, and the impact of age on glucagon and epinephrine responses, the most important counterregulatory hormones, was described.[19] The study employed constant infusions of insulin in normal young and elderly subjects to gradually reduce blood glucose and examine counterregulatory hormone responses. Basal whole blood glucose levels were similar in the young and older subjects at 88 mg/dl, and blood glucose declined 37 mg/dl in both groups. There was no difference between groups in the rate or magnitude of the decline in glucose or the rate of recovery from glucose reduction. The data demonstrated that glucagon, cortisol, growth hormone, and adrenal medullary responses to this stimulus are preserved during aging.

Previous studies revealed glucagon as the primary hormone responsible for hypoglycemic counterregulation in young subjects, and the study by Meneilly and colleagues demonstrated that the glucagon responses in the elderly subjects are preserved.[19] Two other studies that produced greater degrees of hypoglycemia than the Meneilly study did show some impairment in glucagon response. Marker et al.[20] found diminished absolute glucagon levels and attenuated glucose recovery, whereas Lenters et al.[21] found no decrement in absolute glucagon levels but a time delay in glucagon secretion. These differing results are likely due to differences in study protocol and the magnitude of hypoglycemia. There were few differences between young and elderly subjects in the other counterregulatory hormones in all three studies. Epinephrine, which plays a minor role in glucose counterregulation under normal conditions, is of paramount importance when glucagon is deficient. This is frequently the case in long-standing diabetes mellitus, in which glucagon release has been shown to be impaired. Basal levels of epinephrine were similar in young and aged groups, and the increases in epinephrine in response to reductions in blood glucose were similar and modest in young and aged subjects. As recent studies have indicated that epinephrine clearance is on the order of two times greater in the elderly, these results suggest that epinephrine responses to induced hypoglycemia may be enhanced with age. Plasma norepinephrine response to reduced blood glucose was maintained with age. Adrenalectomized patients with intact sympathetic nervous systems do not demonstrate increases in norepinephrine in response to hypoglycemia; thus, an increase in norepinephrine in these studies is probably due to adrenal norepinephrine secretion. The cortisol response to moderate blood glucose reduction was minimal in these studies and was preserved with age, a finding consistent with previous studies. Growth hormone does not play a critical role in short-term glucose counterregulation, and previous studies in the aged showed a normal or diminished growth hormone response to profound hypoglycemia. These studies demonstrated that counterregulatory responses are largely intact in healthy elderly subjects in response to moderate insulin-induced reductions in blood glucose.

The counterregulatory response of elderly individuals with diabetes mellitus, a group at relatively high risk of hypoglycemia, has been little studied. One preliminary report[22] suggests that counterregulatory responses of elderly diabetic individuals during insulin-induced hypoglycemia are intact and may occur at higher glucose levels than in age-matched nondiabetic elderly individuals. This result may be related to previous diabetic control. It is important to note that all of the elderly subjects had symptoms with their episode of hypoglycemia, suggesting that elderly individuals are capable of sensing hypoglycemia.

COMORBID ILLNESS AND CLINICAL HYPOGLYCEMIA AND THE ELDERLY PATIENT

Although there is a broad differential diagnosis for severe hypoglycemia, medications are the most common cause. Insulin or sulfonylureas used to treat diabetes are the most common agents. In general, recurrent drug-induced hypoglycemia in patients with diabetes becomes greater over time as their physiologic defenses against hypoglycemia are progressively compromised. Known risk factors for sulfonylurea-induced hypoglycemia include advanced age and suboptimal nutrition. Nutritional impairment is a clear risk factor for increased hospitalization and death in patients admitted to acute care facilities, and hypoglycemia is an important contributing factor.[23] The agents most likely to induce hypoglycemia are longer acting agents such as chlorpropamide or glyburide. New agents expected to appear include metformin, which helps produce gluconeogenic substrate including lactate and is much less likely to produce drug-induced hypoglycemia.

After insulin or sulfonylurea ingestion, alcohol is a relatively common cause of emergency admissions with severe hypoglycemia. Alcohol inhibits gluconeogenesis but not the breakdown of glycogen. As a result, alcoholic hypoglycemia occurs in the setting of starvation, which has resulted in the depletion of glycogen stored in the liver. This commonly occurs after a several-day binge during which no food

Table 5.3   Drugs that cause hypoglycemia

Alcohol
Analgesics
Phenylbutazone, aspirin, acetaminophen, dextropropoxyphene
Antibiotics
Sulfa drugs, chloramphenicol, oxytetracycline, pentamidine
Quinine
Anticoagulants
Dicumarol
Hypoglycemic agents
Cardiac agents
Propranolol, disopyramide
Psychiatric agents
Monoamine oxidase inhibitors, phenothiazines, haloperidol, amphetamine, lithium
Others
Halofenate, orphenadrine, manganese, hypoglycin, onion extract, kerola, ethylenedi aminetetraacetic acid (EDTA)

has been ingested. Other drugs that frequently produce hypoglycemia include pentamidine and quinine, which are used to treat malaria. Hypoglycemia can be a rare complication of commonly used medications, including aspirin and sulfonamides.

Several major illnesses that are increasingly prevalent in the elderly can predispose to hypoglycemia. Severe organ failure involving the liver, kidney, or heart, as well as sepsis or severe nutritional impairment, can result in hypoglycemia. As the liver is the only endogenous source of glucose release into the bloodstream, the mechanism for fasting hypoglycemia in a patient with hepatic necrosis is clear. Mechanisms for renal- and cardiac failure–induced hypoglycemia are less clear. Hypoglycemia can occur in Addison's disease, perhaps as a result of malnutrition. Other rare causes of severe hypoglycemia and seizures in the elderly include certain extrapancreatic tumors that produce of insulin-like growth factors or insulin. Even more rare in older individuals are the autoimmune hypoglycemias. Surgical illnesses can produce alimentary hypoglycemia in which rapid absorption of glucose results in high insulin levels and a delayed hyperinsulinemia without the availability of glucose substrate.

A list of medications associated with hypoglycemia is listed in Table 5.3. To be added to this list, but rarely seen in older individuals as drug-induced causes of hypoglycemia, are the narcotic analgesics commonly used by drug addicts.

INVESTIGATION AND TREATMENT

Once an individual presents with seizures and associated hypoglycemia, the initial response is to increase the plasma glucose level by intravenous infusion of 50% dextrose and water. Depending on the cause, repeated infusions may be required to maintain the blood glucose level. Such patients should be hospitalized until a diagnosis is made and appropriate treatment initiated. In the elderly population, hypoglycemia is usually medication-related, and this should be the focus of the initial review and discussion of diagnosis. Treatment will thus involve removal of the offending agent or modification of nutrition or drug intake patterns to prevent further episodes of hypoglycemia.

RELATIONSHIP OF SEIZURES TO THE DEGREE OF HYPOGLYCEMIA AND THE ELDERLY PATIENT

The relationship of seizure threshold to the degree of hypoglycemia in the elderly patient is largely unresearched and anecdotal. There is no literature to support an age-related change in threshold to hypoglycemia-induced seizures; case reports are not detailed enough to permit a linkage among age, severity of hypoglycemia, and the appearance of seizures. Similarly, although we can speculate that advancing age leads to a diminished behavioral response to the early autonomic symptoms of hypoglycemia, no data exist that support such a relationship. It certainly must be the case, however, that frail, older individuals with cognitive impairment or mobility disorders who have nutritional impairment may find it very difficult to respond to a hypoglycemic threat; they thus would seem more likely to suffer the consequences of hypoglycemia, including seizures. In particular, this appears to be the case with the diabetic patient who has deficient glucagon responses required to prevent severe degrees of hypoglycemia. The concomitant administration of beta-adrenergic blocking agents, which may suppress the early warning signs of hypoglycemia, is a potential confounding factor in many individuals. Also unclear in the literature is the level of glucose at which seizures may appear. Current literature supports the fact that seizure activity occurs at very low levels of ambient blood glucose, but there is no systematic study that examines seizure threshold risk in individuals with normal brains and those who have a lowered seizure threshold from intrinsic brain injury or structural lesions. It is possible that a primary seizure focus may become more excitable during episodes of hypoglycemia, but this remains unclear at the present time.

REFERENCES

1. Hauser WA, Kurland LT. The epidemiology of epilepsy in Rochester, Minnesota, 1935 through 1967. Epilepsia 1975;16:1.
2. Lühdorf K, Jensen LK, Plesner AM. Etiology of seizures in the elderly. Epilepsia 1986;27:458.
3. Roberts MA, Godfrey JW, Caird FI. Epileptic seizures in the elderly. I. Aetiology and type of seizure. Age Ageing 1982;11:24.
4. Lopez JLP, et al. Late onset epileptic seizures: a retrospective study of 250 patients. Acta Neurol Scand 1985;72:380.
5. Miller JW, Ferrendelli JA, Hazzard WR (eds), Principles of Geriatrics and Gerontology (3rd ed). New York: McGraw-Hill, 1994;1089.

6. Minaker KL, Meneilly GS, Rowe JW. Endocrine Systems. In C Finch, E Schneider (eds), Book of the Biology of Aging (2nd ed). New York: Van Nostrand Reinholt, 1985;433.
7. Davidson MB. The effect of aging on carbohydrate metabolism: a review of the english literature and a practical approach to the diagnosis of diabetes mellitus in the elderly. Metabolism 1979;28:688.
8. Tonino RP, Minaker KL, Rowe JW. Effect of age on systemic delivery of oral glucose in men. Diabetes Care 1989;12:394.
9. Meneilly GS, Minaker KL, Elahi D, Rowe JW. Insulin action in aging man: evidence for tissue specific differences at low physiologic insulin levels. J Gerontol 1987;1402:196.
10. Elahi D, Muller DC, Tzankoff SP, et al. Effect of age and obesity on fasting levels of glucose, insulin, glucagon, and growth hormone in man. J Gerontol 1982;37:385.
11. Reaven EP, Wright E, Mondon CE, et al. Effect of age and diet on insulin secretion and insulin action in the rat. Diabetes 1983;32:175.
12. Minaker KL, Rowe JW, PalloKa JA, Sparrow D. Clearance of insulin: influence of steady state insulin level and age. Diabetes 1982;31:132.
13. Rowe JW, Minaker KL, Pallotta JA, Flier JS. Characterization of the insulin resistance of aging. J Clin Invest 1983;71:1581.
14. Dudl RJ, Ensinck JW. Insulin and glucose relationships during aging in man. Metabolism 1977;26:33.
15. Cryer PE. Hypoglycemia of obscure cause. Hosp Pract (Off Ed) 1992;27:119.
16. Cryer PE. Glucose Homeostasis and Hypoglycemia. In JD Wilson, DW Foster (eds), Williams Textbook of Endocrinology (8th ed). Philadelphia: Saunders, 1992;1223.
17. Malouf R, Brust JCM. Hypoglycemia: causes, neurologic manifestations, and outcomes. Ann Neurol 1985;17:421.
18. Wijdicks EFM, Sharbrough FW. New onset seizures in critically ill patients. Neurology 1993;43:1042.
19. Meneilly GS, Minaker KL, Young JB, et al. Counterregulatory responses to insulin-induced glucose reduction in the elderly. J Clin Endocrinol Metab 1985;61:178.
20. Marker JC, Cryer PE, Clutter WE. Attenuated glucose recovery from hypoglycemia in the elderly. Diabetes 1992;41:671.
21. Lenters KM, Ortiz FJ, Herman WH, et al. Impaired glucose counterregulation in response to insulin-induced hypoglycemia in the elderly [abstract]. Clin Res 1990;38:270A.
22. Morrow LA, Herman WH, Silberg E, et al. Altered hormone responses and symptoms during hypoglycemia in older adults with diabetes mellitus [abstract]. J Am Geriatr Soc 1991;39:A19.
23. Herrmann FR, Safran C, Levkoff SE, Minaker KL. Serum albumin on admission as a predictor of death, length of stay, and readmission. Arch Intern Med 1992;152:125.

6

Age-Related Changes in Drug Metabolism and Action

Judith C. Ahronheim

Physiologic and pathologic changes that occur in late life may have a significant effect on the body's ability to handle drugs ("pharmacokinetics"). The most consistent change is an age-related decline in renal function, which leads to a reduced ability to handle drugs eliminated by the kidney. Glomerular filtration rate (GFR) declines, on average, by approximately 50% between the third and eighth decade of life.[1] Longitudinal study indicates, however, that approximately one-third of aged individuals may fail to experience this decline.[2] Furthermore, the serum creatinine level does not decline in parallel with declining GFR because muscle mass, the source of serum creatinine, declines with age. Thus, it is difficult to predict actual renal function in a given geriatric patient. Predictive formulas have been validated in certain patient groups[3] but are unreliable in chronically ill, debilitated patients[4] and in the dynamic setting of acute illness. Their validity in healthy elderly individuals has also been questioned.[5] In the presence of impaired renal function, drugs that are eliminated by the kidney may increase to toxic levels with repeated administration unless the dose is adjusted according to actual renal function. This is most important for drugs with a narrow therapeutic index (ratio of dose producing desired effect to dose producing toxic effects). Great caution must be exercised when renally excreted drugs with a narrow therapeutic index are given to elderly patients. Examples of such drugs are given in Table 6.1.

Age-related hepatic changes are complex, and their impact on drug metabolism in the elderly is variable. Hepatic metabolism depends on nonhepatic factors such as exogenous agents (enzyme "inducers" and "inhibitors"), sex differences, and genetic variables. In addition, the limited correlation between biological and chronologic age leads to an increased physiologic heterogeneity of population groups with advancing age.

Most studies have shown that liver size and blood flow decline in late life,[6, 7] so drugs with a high hepatic extraction ratio, such as lidocaine and imipramine, are generally eliminated more slowly. Some but not all studies have also demonstrated a decline in hepatic oxidative processes ("phase I metabolism").[8] In contrast, there is general agreement that hepatic conjugation ("phase II metabolism") does not decline with advancing age.

It is not surprising that there are no generalizable results of hepatic oxidation studies. Age-related decline in hepatic oxidation may be limited to a few

Table 6.1 Drugs with narrow therapeutic index and potential for accumulation in the presence of diminished renal function

Antimicrobial agents
   Aminoglycosides
   Imipenem
   Pyrazinamide
   Vancomycin
Benzodiazepines with active metabolites
   Chlorazepate
   Chlordiazepoxide
   Diazepam
   Flurazepam
Digoxin
Hypoglycemic agents with active metabolites
   Chlorpropamide
   Acetohexamide
Lithium
Normeperidine (active metabolite of meperidine)
N-acetyl procainamide (active metabolite of procainamide)
Salicylates

Source: Adapted from JC Ahronheim, MA Howland. Geriatric Principles. In L Goldfrank et al. Toxicologic Emergencies (5th ed). Norwalk, CT: Appleton & Lange. 1994;448.

specific enzymes in the cytochrome P450 (CP450) system, but much further study will be needed to elucidate this complex issue. The CP450 system is a family of enzymes, each the product of a specific gene and each with different substrate specificities. Owing to genetic variability, each enzyme does not exist in every person. The system is further modified by exogenous factors, such as drugs, alcohol, and cigarette smoke, that can stimulate or inhibit members of this family of enzymes by a variety of complex mechanisms. The physiologic heterogeneity of the geriatric population, genetic and sex differences in drug metabolism, environmental influences, and the presence of other drugs make it extraordinarily difficult to identify a "pure" sample of subjects to study or to draw precise conclusions about drug metabolism related to aging.

Racemic compounds may undergo stereoselective metabolism, with one enantiomer metabolized more slowly in the elderly and the other without age-dependent metabolism. This has been demonstrated for hexobarbital[9] and mephobarbital.[10] In the case of mephobarbital, there may also be exaggerated sex differences in metabolism in the elderly[10]; this interplay between sex and age, although not fully explained, could theoretically be related to changes in the hormonal milieu that occur with advancing age.[11] Some CP450 enzymes may have significant activity only in males, so, along with age-related declines in androgenic hormones, the metabolic capacity for certain drugs in men might more closely resemble that of women. The clinical implications of age-related stereoselective metabolism require further study.

There is controversy over whether there are any age-related changes in the inducibility or suppression of enzyme activity. Although it is likely that many gene products within the CP450 system have not yet been identified, a number of studies have failed to demonstrate that advanced age hampers the induction[12, 13] and inhibition[13, 14] of these enzymes to a significant degree. A recent study, however, suggested significantly less induction of hexobarbital metabolism by rifampin in elderly as compared with young subjects; the age difference was stereoselective, suggesting that some but not all processes are affected by age.[15]

More study is needed to elucidate the effects of advanced age on the very complex process of hepatic drug metabolism. Drug interactions with hepatically active agents, such as phenytoin, phenobarbital, cimetidine, and others, have been reported in all age groups, and a prescriber should assume that these are possible in any elderly patient. Geriatric patients take larger numbers of prescription medications at a time than any other age group.[16] The more drugs in a regimen, the more likely the patient will experience a significant drug-drug interaction.[17]

There is an increase in the body's fat-to-lean ratio with age.[18] This can affect the volume of distribution (VD) of many drugs. Water-soluble drugs tend to have a decreased VD and may have an earlier onset of action in the elderly. In contrast, fat-soluble drugs tend to have an increased VD, and steady-state concentrations after regular dosing are reached later. Drugs that undergo phase I metabolism often yield renally excreted metabolites with significant pharmacologic activity. If such a drug also has an increased VD, half-life may be markedly prolonged in a geriatric patient, and steady state reached much later than expected after repeated dosing. In this situation, toxicity may occur in a delayed fashion and may be mistaken for a nondrug effect. First-generation benzodiazepines, such as diazepam and flurazepam, are examples of such drugs.[19, 20]

Drug binding to serum proteins, such as albumin and alpha-1 acid glycoprotein (AAG), can be affected by many factors in late life. Protein synthesis may be impaired, and there is diminished reserve when dietary intake is marginal.[21, 22] Thus, although serum albumin remains normal in healthy elderly,[23] albumin levels may decline rapidly in illness. In contrast, serum levels of AAG, an acute phase reactant, may increase in late life.[24] Changes in drug binding to albumin and to AAG may have little or no direct clinical impact on the patient but may affect interpretation of therapeutic drug levels of highly protein bound drugs, including many anticonvulsants.

Despite the high prevalence of gastric mucosal atrophy and hypoacidity in late life, gastrointestinal absorption of drugs (most of which occurs in the small intestine) is generally adequate.[8]

Important pharmacodynamic changes may occur with advancing age. *Pharmacodynamics* refers to the actual effect of the drug at the tissue level. The effect may be decreased, altered, or enhanced. Most frequently, enhanced pharmacodynamic effects have been described.[8, 25] It is not always possible to determine whether an enhanced effect is actually related to altered pharmacodynamics or merely altered pharmacokinetics. Medications with sedating properties are more likely to cause unwanted side effects in the elderly than in younger adults,[26, 27] but elimination of many of these may be prolonged and higher levels attained with ordinary doses. For example, a given dose of the short-acting second-generation benzodiazepine triazolam is more likely to produce sedation and impaired psychomotor performance in elderly than in younger adults, but the same dose produces higher drug levels in the elderly, therefore suggesting a mechanism independent of age-related sensitivity.[26] In contrast, an infusion of midazolam produces a greater magnitude of electroencephalographic changes in elderly than in younger adult subjects, independent of plasma levels attained.[27] Pharmacodynamic alterations may be noted in the target tissue or a nontarget organ. The frequency of enhanced effects in the central nervous system (CNS) is presumably due to the high prevalence of CNS disease in geriatric patients. Therapeutic drug use is an important cause of reversible confusion in the elderly.[28, 29] Drug-induced acute and subacute confusional states presumably represent worsening of underlying dementia or unmasking of preclinical dementia.[28] Confusion due to anticholinergic drugs may be related to age- and disease-related diminished "cholinergic reserve." Although there is considerable disagreement over the extent of cholinergic deficits in the normal aged brain[30], cholinergic deficits are profound in Alzheimer's disease[31], and drug-related cognitive impairment is more likely to occur in patients with the disease, compared with age-matched controls.[32] It is possible that less severe cholinergic deficits are present to a greater or lesser degree in some overtly normal elderly, representing subclinical Alzheimer's disease. Objective evidence confirming this supposition is lacking, however.

The elderly are also theoretically more prone to drug-induced seizures because of delayed elimination of many "proconvulsive" drugs; a propensity to develop hypoalbuminemia, leading to enhanced delivery of drug to the CNS; and the presence of subclinical or overt CNS lesions, in particular those due to cerebrovascular disease. The purported mechanisms responsible for drug-induced seizures have been reviewed elsewhere for a variety of drugs.[33] There are no data confirming an age-associated proclivity to drug-induced seizures, however. Some drugs that can produce seizures are given in Table 6.2.

Enhanced drug effects may show up in non–target organs. Metoclopramide, a central dopamine antagonist, is used therapeutically to enhance gastric motility and prevent nausea, but it may produce neurologic side effects. The spectrum of metoclopramide-induced reactions appears to vary with age. Tremor, rigidity, tardive dyskinesia, and related symptoms generally appear in elderly patients, and acute dystonic reactions in younger ones.[34, 35] This suggests an unmasking of Parkinson's disease in the former group and an independent mechanism in the latter. Tricyclic antidepressants and other agents with anticholinergic activity may not only produce confusion, as noted earlier, but also other anticholinergic effects, such as urinary retention. Anticholinergic agents reduce the activity of the bladder detrusor muscle. Drug-induced urinary retention, generally a problem of late life, occurs more commonly in men than in women, presumably because of a potential bladder outlet obstruction due to prostatic hyperplasia.

Table 6.2   Some drugs that can produce seizures

Bupropion
Imipenem
Isoniazid
Lidocaine
Noreperidine (active metabolite of meperidine)
Penicillins
Psychostimulants
Theophylline
Tricyclic antidepressants
Any drug producing metabolic derangements, particularly hyponatremia or
   hypoglycemia

Drug side effects may be altered rather than enhanced. For example, vasodilators such as hydralazine or nifedipine commonly produce reflex tachycardia, an undesired consequence of the desired effect of blood pressure lowering. These drugs, however, may fail to produce reflex tachycardia in the elderly. Failure to mount a reflex tachycardia could be related to underlying sinus node disease, but the net effect might be seen as desirable.

Pharmacodynamic action may also be blunted. For example, there is evidence that alpha- and beta-adrenergic receptor sensitivity declines with age.[36] Although some studies suggest that older patients treated with beta blockers tend to achieve blood pressure lowering less often than younger adults,[37] there is little or no evidence from clinical trials that these drugs are ineffective in that age group. In fact, older patients (roughly 65–80 years old) treated with beta blockers after having myocardial infarction may achieve significantly improved survival compared with patients younger than 60 years of age,[38] an outcome believed to be mediated by suppression of beta-adrenergic actions on the heart. Although this discrepancy could be theoretically explained by prolonged elimination of beta blockers in the elderly or by other independent effects of beta blockers, ischemia may enhance beta receptor density or even reverse beta desensitization.[39] Also, since the oldest patients have the highest mortality rate after having a myocardial infarction,[40] any small reduction in mortality magnifies the apparent effect in the more vulnerable population group.

Although many aspects of pharmacology are not generalizable to all elderly, it is important to recognize that the incidence of adverse drug side effects increases with age. In older patients, side effects are more likely to be serious, leading to hospitalization or even death.[16] This vulnerability can be reduced with physician recognition of age-related changes in drug metabolism and action. There are, however, a number of practical problems that can influence the patient's clinical outcome. A complex drug regimen makes noncompliance highly likely and increases the possibility of drug-drug interactions. Visual and hearing deficits increase the likelihood that the patient will misunderstand the treatment regimen, and dementia (even when mild) makes this a virtual certainty. Impaired manual dexterity may limit the patient's access to prescribed medications, especially when they are packaged in "childproof" or tamper-proof containers. Last, but not least, patients often visit more than one physician, who may prescribe conflicting medications, resulting in a serious drug-drug interaction. Strategies to improve compliance and reduce adverse outcomes have been reviewed.[41, 42]

REFERENCES

1. Rowe JW, Andres RA, Tobin JD, et al. The effect of age in creatinine clearance in man: a cross sectional and longitudinal study. J Gerontol 1976;31:155.
2. Lindeman RD, Tobin J, Shock NW. Longitudinal studies on the rate of decline in renal function with age. J Am Geriatr Soc 1985;33:278.
3. Cockcroft DW, Gault M. Prediction of creatinine clearance from serum creatinine. Nephron 1976;16:31.
4. Drusano GL, Muncie HL, Hoopes JM, et al. Commonly used methods of estimating creatinine clearance are inadequate for elderly debilitated nursing homes patients. J Am Geriatr Soc 1988;36:437.
5. Malmrose LC, Gray SL, Pieper CF, et al. Measured versus estimated creatinine clearance in a high-functioning elderly sample: MacArthur Foundation Study of Successful Aging. J Am Geriatr Soc 1993;41:715.
6. Woodhouse KW, Wynne HA. Age-related changes in liver size and hepatic blood flow. The influence on drug metabolism in the elderly. Clin Pharmacokinet 1988;15:287.
7. Wynne HA, Cope LH, Mutch E, et al. The effect of age upon liver volume and apparent liver blood flow in healthy man. Hepatology 1989;9:297.
8. Vestal RE, Cusack BJ. Pharmacology and Aging. In EL Schneider, JW Rowe (eds), Handbook of the Biology of Aging (3rd ed). San Diego: Academic Press, 1990;349.
9. Chandler MHH, Scott SR, Blouin RA. Age-associated stereoselective alterations in hexobarbital metabolism. Clin Pharmacol Ther 1988;43:436.
10. Hooper WD, Qing MS. The influence of age and gender on the stereoselective metabolism and pharmacokinetics of mephobarbital in humans. Clin Pharmacol Ther 1990;48:633.
11. Fujita S, Chiba M, Ohta M, et al. Alteration of plasma sex hormone levels associated with old age and its effect on hepatic drug metabolism in rats. J Pharmacol Exp Ther 1990;253:369.
12. Crowley JJ, Cusack BJ, Jue SG, et al. Aging and drug interactions. II. Effect of phenytoin and smoking on the oxidation of theophylline and cortisol in healthy men. J Pharmacol Exp Ther 1988;245:513.
13. Vestal RE, Cusack BJ, Mercer GD, et al. Aging and drug interactions. I. Effect of cimetidine and smoking on the oxidation of theophylline and cortisol in healthy men. J Pharmacol Exp Ther 1987;241:488.
14. Wynne HA, Mutch E, Williams FM, et al. The relation of age to the acute effects of ethanol on acetanilide disposition. Age Ageing 1989;18:123.
15. Smith DA, Chandler MHH, Shedlofsky SI, et al. Age-dependent stereoselective increase in the oral clearance of hexobarbitone isomers caused by rifampicin. Br J Clin Pharmacol 1991;32:735.
16. Burke LB, Jolson HM, Goetsch RA, Ahronheim JC. Geriatric drug use and adverse drug event reporting in 1990: a descriptive analysis of two national data bases. Annu Rev Gerontol Geriatr 1992;12:1.
17. May EE, Stewart RB, Cluff LE. Drug interactions and multiple drug administration. Clin Pharmacol Ther 1977;22:322.

18. Novak LP. Aging, total body potassium, fat free mass and cell mass in males and females between the ages 18 and 85 years. J Gerontol 1972;27:438.
19. Salzman C, Shader RI, Greenblatt, DJ, et al. Long versus short half-life benzodiazepines in the elderly: kinetics and clinical effects of diazepam and oxazepam. Arch Gen Psychiatry 1983;40:293.
20. Greenblatt DJ, Divoll M, Harmatz JS, et al. Kinetics and clinical effects of flurazepam in young and elderly noninsommniacs. Clin Pharmacol Ther 1981;30:475.
21. Gersovitz M, Munro HN, Udall J, Young VR. Albumin synthesis in young and elderly subjects using a new stable isotope methodology: response to level of protein intake. Metabolism 1980;29:1075.
22. Young VR. Amino acids and proteins in relation to the nutrition of elderly people. Age Ageing 1990;10(Suppl):S10.
23. Campion EW, deLabry LO, Glynn RJ. The effect of age on serum albumin in healthy males: report from the normative aging study. J Gerontol 1988;43:M18.
24. Verbeeck RK, Cardinal JA, Wallace SM. Effect of age and sex on the plasma binding of acidic and basic drugs. Eur J Clin Pharmacol 1987;27:91.
25. Feely J, Coakley D. Altered pharmacodynamics in the elderly. Clin Geriatr Med 1990;6:269.
26. Greenblatt DJ, Harmatz JS, Shapiro L, et al. Sensitivity to triazolam in the elderly. N Engl J Med 1991;324:1691.
27. Greenblatt DJ, Ehrenberg BL, Scavone JM, et al. Increased sensitivity to midazolam in the elderly [abstract]. Clin Pharmacol Ther 1990;47:210.
28. Larson EB, Kukull WA, Buchner D, Reifler BV. Adverse drug reactions associated with global cognitive impairment in elderly persons. Ann Intern Med 1987;107:169.
29. Francis J, Martin D, Kapoor WN. A prospective study of delirium in hospitalized elderly. JAMA 1990;263:1097.
30. Creasey H, Rapoport SI. The aging human brain. Ann Neurol 1985;17:2.
31. Bartus RT, Dean RL, Beer B, Lippa AS. The cholinergic hypothesis of geriatric memory dysfunction. Science 1982;217:408.
32. Sunderland T, Tariot PN, Cohen RM, et al. Anticholinergic sensitivity in patients with dementia of the Alzheimer type and age-matched controls. Arch Gen Psychiatry 1987;44:418.
33. Zaccara G, Muscas GC, Messori A. Clinical features, pathogenesis and management of drug-induced seizures. Drug Saf 1990;5:109.
34. Miller LG, Jankovic J. Metoclopramide-induced movement disorders. Arch Intern Med 1989;149:2486.
35. Grimes JD, Hassan MN, Preston DN. Adverse neurologic effects of metoclopramide. Can Med Assoc J 1982;126:23.
36. Vestal RE, Wood AJJ, Shand DG. Reduced beta-adrenoceptor sensitivity in the elderly. Clin Pharmacol Ther 1979;26:181.
37. Wallin JD, Shah SV. Beta-adrenergic blocking agents in the treatment of hypertension. Arch Intern Med 1987;147:654.
38. Olsson G, Rehnqvist N, Sjogren A, et al. Long-term treatment with metoprolol after myocardial infarction: effect on 3 year mortality and morbidity. J Am Coll Cardiol 1985;5:1428.
39. Strasser RH, Krimmer J, Marquetant R. Regulation of beta-adrenergic receptors: impaired desensitization in myocardial ischemia. J Cardiovasc Pharmacol 1988;12:S15.
40. Rich MW, Bosner MS, Chung MK, et al. Is age an independent predictor of early and late mortality in patients with acute myocardial infarction? Am J Med 1992;92:7.
41. Ahronheim JC. Handbook of Prescribing Medications for Geriatric Patients. Boston: Little, Brown, 1992;1.
42. Rowe JW, Ahronheim JC (eds). Focus on Medications and the Elderly. New York: Springer, 1992.

7

Pathologic Processes in the Elderly and Their Association with Seizures

Pierre Loiseau

INTRODUCTION

To understand the relationship between seizures and their underlying pathologic processes, the distinction between seizures and epilepsy should be clarified. A *seizure* is the "clinical manifestation of an abnormal and excessive discharge of a set of neurons of the brain, including cortical cells."[1] An *unprovoked seizure* is a seizure that occurs without an identified precipitant. An *acute symptomatic (provoked) seizure* is a seizure that occurs in close temporal association with an acute insult to the central nervous system (CNS) or in association with a generalized systemic, metabolic disturbance. "*Epilepsy* is defined as a condition characterized by recurrent unprovoked seizures."[1]

The causes of seizures and the causes of epilepsy are not identical. Many factors provoke epileptic seizures without causing epilepsy. On the other hand, recurrent unprovoked seizures do not necessarily follow acute symptomatic seizures. Thus, seizures associated with pathologic processes in the elderly may belong to two groups: (1) acute symptomatic seizures, or situation-related seizures, according to the International Classification of Epilepsies and Epileptic Syndromes,[2] and (2) symptomatic epilepsies, considered the consequence of a known or suspected disorder of the CNS.[2] The Guidelines for Epidemiologic Studies on Epilepsy[3] subdivide the symptomatic epilepsies into remote symptomatic epilepsies secondary to static encephalopathies and into and symptomatic epilepsies caused by progressive disorders of the CNS.

Many systemic disorders and nearly all local pathologic processes that involve the brain may precipitate seizures. Systemic factors include abnormalities in body fluids and electrolytes, various other metabolic disturbances, and toxic mechanisms.

By convention, structural lesions are defined as those observed on standard anatomic neuroimaging techniques, presumed to be irreversible, and later detectable on autopsy. The advent of new imaging techniques, however, may lead to a redefinition of structural lesions. In fact, the borderline between symptomatic and cryptogenic epilepsies[2] has become blurred, and the number of cryptogenic cases of epilepsy has declined. Cerebral metabolic studies using positron emission tomography or cerebral blood flow estimation with single photon emission computed tomography (CT) have revealed defects undetectable by other neuroimaging techniques such as radiographs, CT scans, and even magnetic resonance imaging (MRI). The time of testing is a critical factor in detecting lesions because abnormalities may change over time. A single early examination may miss late-evolving lesions, such as cerebral infarcts. A late CT scan will miss reversible lesions. These limitations explain in part a certain arbitrariness that exists in the definition.

After a declining incidence of *remote symptomatic epilepsies* during the first part of adult life, there is an increase after the age of 60 and especially over 70 years. In these age groups, symptomatic epilepsies are the largest category of spontaneous seizures. In an epidemiologic survey conducted in southwest France,[4] they represented two-thirds of all spontaneous seizures, either isolated or recurrent.[4] Similarly, *acute symptomatic seizures* are far more numerous in the elderly than in younger adults.

Estimation of the respective importance of pathologic processes responsible for seizures or epilepsies in the elderly is difficult for many reasons.

1. *Deficiency in patient reporting.* Some patients never seek medical attention. This is probably more common in the elderly than in younger patients. Others do not pay attention to seizures when they are only part of a disease picture and often only a minor part. Physicians may share the same attitude. "Epilepsy is often lost in the rather noisy background of changes due to aging and diseases that occur more commonly with advancing age...So much is going wrong anyway that the odd fit or two hardly counts."[5]

2. *Deficiencies in the diagnosis of seizures.* The diagnosis of epileptic seizures is mainly based on the description of the episode. An incomplete history is rather common in elderly patients with aged relatives. Syncope has been considered much more frequent.[6] Cerebral anoxia often associated with syncope may itself cause muscular jerks, increasing the difficulty. Many elderly patients referred to an epilepsy clinic are found to have cardiac arrhythmias on 24-hour electrocardiographic monitoring,[7] but the significance of such abnormalities in such subjects is very difficult to establish.[8] They may have no relation at all to an individual patient's clinical problems. Another common problem is that postictal confusional states and postictal paresis may mimic strokes.

3. *Deficiencies in case-ascertainment methods and selection bias in the patient population chosen for study.* This may occur, for example, when patients with clear metabolic causes of seizures are not referred for further investigation in neurologic centers because the underlying disease is the dominant clinical feature. "It seems that the 'fit fitters' go to the neurologists and the 'ill fitters' to the geriatricians."[9]

4. *Differing definitions and classifications of epileptic events*, for example, patients presenting with acute symptomatic seizures and symptomatic epilepsies gathered under the same etiologic heading.
5. *Pathologic processes are obviously age-dependent conditions, even in the elderly group.* A patient in his or her 60s does not have the same risk factors as a patient in his or her 70s, as demonstrated by epidemiologic surveys.[10]
6. *The relationship between a lesion and seizures is not always simple*, for similar pathology may be seen in patients who are not epileptic. The significance of old lesions commonly associated with cerebrovascular disease, such as lacunae and perivascular lucencies, is controversial.
7. *Seizures are quite often associated with several risk factors*, and it may be difficult to determine which one is primarily responsible for the seizures. Many patients present with metabolic disturbances superimposed on structural lesions. More than one metabolic disorder may be present, for instance, both renal and respiratory insufficiency. The role of genetic factors must be taken into consideration, as suggested by one study of 13 patients with stroke and early seizures in which six were found to have had seizures previously.[11] "The patient who has developed an epileptogenic lesion in the brain is more likely to have seizures if there is a strong genetic background."[12]

In the literature, the percentage of elderly patients with a particular causative factor for epilepsy has varied greatly for all the reasons indicated above. The data given in Table 7.1 come from a few selected studies listed below.

The medical records of 50 previously healthy patients, ages 69 years and older, who were admitted for seizures of recent onset to the Denver General Hospital Neurology Service, were reviewed. Acute and remote symptomatic seizures were included.[13]

Between October, 1972, and September, 1980, 81 patients were seen in the University Department of Geriatric Medicine at Glasgow for seizures beginning after the age of 60.[14] Thirty-one were older than 75 years of age. CT scan was performed in 60 patients. Easily recognized provoked seizures were likely to have been underrepresented, as patients were admitted for diagnostic investigation.

Gupta[15] studied the records of 74 patients older than age 69 years, with a mean age of 75 years, who had been examined in the general medical or geriatric departments of a hospital in London during a 3-year period. CT scan was performed in 12 patients. No patient was found to have a brain tumor.

Epileptic seizures in people ages 60 years and older were investigated during the 5-year period from 1979 to 1983 in a Danish urban area.[16] Patients were identified from diagnostic registers in two hospitals that received virtually all the patients from the region, both as inpatients and outpatients. The authors assume that nearly all the elderly with seizures were diagnosed. Two hundred fifty-one patients were included, 151 with a first seizure, 88 with established epilepsy at

Table 7.1 Cause of first seizure in individuals older than age 60 years (%)

Reference Number	13	14	15	16	17	18	19	20	4	23
Stroke	30	44	31	32	38	22	39	30	47	32.4
Neoplastic	2	12	0	14	5.9	24	11	18	8.8	2.7
Post-traumatic	8	6	4	6	9.8	6	21	9	3.2	3.3
Toxic-metabolic	10	11	0	18	—	4	10	7	18	18
Infection	—	—	—	—	—	—	4	4	1.8	0.5
Dementia	8	2	6.9	11	3	—	4	5.6	11.5	—
Unknown	50	16	28	25	20	34	11	7	13.4	48.9

the time of admission, and 12 with previously untreated seizures and new epileptic events during the study period. Only the first group is considered in Table 7.1. Neuroimaging was variable, and acute symptomatic and unprovoked seizures were not separated.

Of 317 patients admitted to hospital a few hours after a first seizure, 102 were 60 years or older.[17] All the patients in this study underwent a CT scan. Provoked and unprovoked seizures were included.

Sixty-seven consecutive, unselected patients with seizure onset after the age of 60 years were studied prospectively in a tertiary care general hospital in Saskatchewan, Canada, between January 1, 1984, and June 30, 1985.[18] Investigation in most cases included CT scan.

A series of 342 patients whose seizures occurred after the age of 60 years in a period from 1981 to 1986 and who were admitted to the department of neurology of the main hospital in Taiwan has been published.[19] A CT scan was mandatory for inclusion. Seizures were carefully looked for in the medical records of patients who were hospitalized for reasons other than epilepsy. Provoked and unprovoked seizures were included. The authors note that their hospital-based study was biased toward the more severely ill patients.

Another retrospective study of 100 inpatients with onset of epileptic seizures after the age of 60 was carried out in Switzerland.[20] Acute symptomatic seizures and symptomatic epilepsies were included. Ninety-six patients were investigated by CT scan.

During the period of March 1, 1984, to February 28, 1985, all the neurologists and electroencephalographers of an administrative district in southwest France prospectively collected data on people who experienced a first epileptic seizure.[4, 21] In a 1982 census, there were 1,128,164 residents, 223,224 of whom were 60 years or older. A special effort was made to find patients presenting with acute symptomatic seizures in departments of internal medicine. Of the 804 patients considered as having had a first afebrile seizure during the recording period, 284 were 60 years or older. Symptomatic epilepsies were diagnosed in 74 patients, and acute symptomatic (situation-related) seizures in 172 patients.

CEREBROVASCULAR DISEASE AS A CAUSE OF SEIZURES AND EPILEPSY IN ELDERLY PATIENTS

Cerebrovascular disease is by far the main cause of seizures in the elderly. The occurrence of stroke is age related; thus, with an increasing elderly population, which during the early part of the next century will probably reach 20% of the population in some countries, the frequency of stroke and related seizures is certain to increase.

Definitions

In the past, estimates of the importance of vascular disease as a cause of seizures or of epilepsy have varied because of lack of uniformity in definition. Many authors have had a very broad concept of vascular epilepsy, leading to an overestimation of vascular epilepsy in elderly patients. They considered that systemic or extracranial atheromatous disease, or hypertensive disease, could generate epileptic seizures. However, "coexistence does not necessarily imply causation."[24] The assumption that systemic vascular disease is associated with cerebrovascular disease has never has been convincingly demonstrated. Furthermore, a lack of relationship between vascular risk factors and seizures has been documented in several studies. Clinical features of systemic vascular and cardiac disease in patients older than 40 years old with an apparently cryptogenic epilepsy did not differ from controls. In both groups, the incidence of these abnormalities in those older than age 60 years was more than double that found in younger patients.[25] Shapiro et al.[26] analyzed risk factors such as arterial hypertension, coronary artery disease, peripheral arteriopathy, diabetes mellitus, and smoking in 50 patients older than 50 years of age presenting with cryptogenic epilepsy. The study group was compared with three control groups matched for age and sex: (1) poststroke epilepsy, (2) previous stroke without epilepsy, and (3) normal subjects. Vascular risk factors were similar in subjects with cryptogenic epilepsy and in normal subjects; they were higher in patients with cerebrovascular disease, with or without seizures.

Modern authors accept as seizures of vascular origin only those related to an obvious cerebrovascular lesion. Clinically, a stroke is defined as an acute neurologic dysfunction of vascular origin with sudden or rapid occurrence of symptoms and signs corresponding to the involvement of focal areas of the brain. Transient ischemic attacks (TIAs) are a variety of the stroke syndrome, perhaps corresponding to a brief period of cerebral ischemia without cerebral infarction or to small brain infarction with rapid and complete clinical recovery. Strokes can be divided into two broad categories according to the nature of the cerebral lesion: infarcts and hemorrhages. A cerebral infarct is the result of temporary or permanent occlusion of a feeding artery, or of venous thrombosis. A spontaneous cerebral hemorrhage is due to the rupture of an abnormal artery (aneurysm or arteriovenous malformation) or arteriole in the brain parenchyma. Often it is difficult to distinguish between cerebral infarction and cerebral hemorrhage on clinical grounds.[27]

These definitions raise two questions: (1) the importance of TIAs and of silent infarcts in vascular seizures; and (2) the epileptogenic risk of ischemic and hemorrhagic insults. Seizures occurring in the acute phase of a cerebral infarct or hemorrhage are known as *early seizures*. Such seizures may be self-limited or recurrent over time. Other seizures may begin long after the insult and are termed *late unprovoked seizures* or *poststroke epilepsy*. Even in recent papers, distinction is not always made between early and late seizures. In the elderly, cerebrovascular disease is more likely to be a cause of early than of late seizures. In the French survey, it was associated with 37% of all unprovoked seizures and 55% of remote symptomatic epilepsies. All included patients had unequivocal evidence of a prior vascular event. In this survey, 54% of the acute symptomatic seizures were attributed to a vascular cause. Two forms of seizures of acute vascular origin were accepted: seizures at the onset of a stroke, and seizures occurring during severe hemodynamic disturbances.

TEMPORAL RELATIONSHIP OF SEIZURES TO STROKES

Early Seizures

Incidence

The incidence of epileptic seizures complicating acute stroke is rather low, ranging from 5.6%[28] to 15%.[29] In a series of 230 patients with a mean age of 60 years admitted to hospital with a stroke, 13 (5.7%), suffered single or multiple seizures.[11] It is interesting to note that eight of 13 were 60 years of age or older. One thousand consecutive patients with acute stroke or TIA were included in a prospective study.[30] The patients' age was not given and individuals younger than 60 were included. The figures, however, are very interesting. The incidence of early seizures (within 2 weeks of stroke onset) in each type of stroke and TIA was evaluated. On the whole, early seizures were documented in 4.4% of the patients. Significant differences were noted. Seizures occurred in 6.5% of patients with carotid territory cortical infarction, 15.4% of patients with supratentorial lobar or extensive hemorrhage, 8.5% of patients with subarachnoid hemorrhage, and 3.7% of patients with hemispheric TIA. In many studies, underreporting is likely—a single partial motor seizure in a hemiplegic or comatose patient may easily be ignored.

Time of Occurrence

Usually, seizures are in close temporal relationship with the onset of stroke. In two studies, they were the presenting sign in 6.7%[31] and 13%[32] of cases. In most cases, they occur at or shortly after stroke onset: 90% within 24 hours[30] or within the first 2 days after the stroke.[33] In a personal unpublished series of 60 patients,

55 seized the first day, two the second day, and three the third day. In a selected series of patients needing ambulatory rehabilitation, and thus excluding the mildest and the more severe cases, 12% had their first seizure during the first poststroke week.[34]

Type of Seizures

Two-thirds of seizures after stroke are focal motor events, one-quarter of which evolve to secondary generalization. Tonic–clonic seizures, apparently generalized from the onset, are also observed. In our series of 60 patients, the distribution was as follows: 41 had focal motor seizures, 13 of which were secondarily generalized; nine had sensory or sensorimotor seizures; and seven had generalized tonic-clonic seizures.

Seizure Frequency

Twenty-two of our 60 patients experienced a single epileptic event, 14 had sporadic seizures, three had numerous seizures, and 15 had status epilepticus. This proportion of status is higher than usual estimations: 9%,[30] 8%.[33] Most were motor focal status epilepticus, often termed epilepsia partialis continua.

Electroencephalographic Findings

The record can be normal (five out of 44 in Kilpatrick's study,[30] five out of 60 in our study). Epileptiform abnormalities are rare. Focal slowing is more frequent. The most interesting pattern is the occurrence of periodic lateralized epileptiform discharges (PLEDs). They consist of epileptiform abnormalities that repeat periodically or quasi-periodically at rates generally close to one per second. Since their initial description by Chatrian et al.,[35] PLEDs have been the subject of numerous reports. They are often associated with an ipsilateral hemispheric structural lesion and are more frequent in acute cerebral infarction than in any other condition such as brain tumor, intracerebral hemorrhage, encephalitis, or cerebral abscess. Their duration ranges from some hours to 3 weeks, with variation from record to record.[36] They are always accompanied by seizures without a clear relation to the seizure pattern, which ranges from a single seizure to epilepsia partialis continua. The seizures tend to remit over several days. They may, however, prove extremely difficult to control, even with a high dose of anticonvulsants. The pathophysiology of PLEDs remains unsolved. Raroque et al.[37] conducted a retrospective study of neuroimaging in relation to other clinical and electroencephalographic (EEG) findings in patients with PLEDs to determine the comparative roles of structural lesions and metabolic abnormalities in its pathogenesis. Their data support a primary role for structural abnormalities but cannot exclude an additional role for metabolic abnormalities, which may lower the convulsant threshold. This dual mechanism was suggested by Chatrian et al. 30 years ago.[35]

All surviving patients with PLEDs are likely to exhibit late recurrent seizures.[33]

Outcome

Mortality. Some authors have found no difference between patients with or without early seizures.[30, 38] In other studies, mortality in patients with poststroke seizures was significantly higher than expected, with death occurring predominantly during the first 2 days according to one group[11] or the first 2 years according to another.[20, 39] These last authors report a mortality rate of 13% in patients with seizures versus 5.9% in those without. Large infarcts or hemorrhages that involve cortical and subcortical regions also are considered poor prognostic factors.[28]

Recurrent Unprovoked Seizures. According to several authors, occurrence of early seizures infrequently leads to late unprovoked seizures.[11, 32, 40, 41] Prevalence of epilepsy was 13% in 30-day to 2-year survivors and 6.5% in 2- to 5-year survivors.[32] Other studies, however, indicate that early seizures are indeed a risk factor.[29] Lühdorf et al.,[16] for example, reported recurrent seizures in 12 of 20 patients who had seizures during the first week after stroke.

Therapy

Correction of metabolic derangements is the major therapeutic measure. The prophylactic use of anticonvulsant drugs in patients who present with an acute stroke is not justified because of the low overall rate of early attacks. Furthermore, the first epileptic event usually occurs too early to be prevented with loading doses of antiepileptic drugs.[42] The indication for anticonvulsant drugs in patients with early seizures is controversial. Because these drugs are not without risk in elderly patients, their prophylactic use should be based on a substantial likelihood that seizures will recur. In this situation, they may be prescribed for a restricted time. Repeated CT may be useful in the follow-up of patients at risk. In patients with early seizures after cerebral hemorrhage who subsequently develop recurrent seizures, the hemorrhage evolves to a hypodense appearance. After 4 months, when the hematoma appears isodense, seizures are unlikely to develop.[43]

Transient Ischemic Attacks

Partial seizures as a possible consequence of transient cerebral ischemia have been reported.[44] In this study, patients with seizures also had histories of classic TIA or angiographic findings of cerebral arterial occlusive disease. It was noteworthy that the results of CT scans performed in two patients were normal.

Late Seizures in Vascular Epilepsy

Vascular epilepsy is diagnosed in patients with a history of stroke and in patients whose CT scans show evidence of old silent cerebral infarcts.

Incidence

The reported incidence of unprovoked seizures after stroke ranges from 4% to 15%.

Incubation Period

The incubation period of poststroke epilepsy is usually short. In most cases, it ranges from 3 months to 1 year. In two reports, seizure onset was not observed after 2 years[34] or after 3 years.[32, 45] In a series of 66 cases, 36 began in the first year, 22 before the end of the second year, and only two later.[15] The mean delay was 12 months in one study, ranging from 2.5 months to 3.75 years.[46] In the rare patient, it may exceed 5 years. In two patients, we observed an onset 12 and 14 years, respectively, after stroke. In another report, 10% experienced seizure onset beyond the third year.[47]

Types of Seizures

Partial and generalized seizures are reported. Early-onset seizures are more likely to be partial (focal) than those of late onset.[33, 40] The great majority of partial seizures are motor, whereas partial complex seizures are rarely reported. They could be underestimated because of the patients' age or condition. Another explanation would be that most vascular insults involve the frontal, central, and parietal regions. In our opinion, all seizures of vascular origin are of focal onset, the clinical signs depending on the spread of the epileptic discharge. When limited, simple focal motor seizures occur. When more extensive spread occurs, secondary generalization is observed. With rapid spread, the seizure may appear to be generalized from the onset. Sometimes, seizures are followed by transient worsening of the motor deficit or of aphasia that lasts from a few minutes to 2 or 3 days. This Todd's paresis is, in our opinion, more frequent in poststroke epilepsy than in other symptomatic epilepsies.

Electroencephalographic Findings

The EEG in vascular epilepsy may be normal.[48] More commonly, continuous or discontinuous lateralized or focal slow waves, sometimes associated with sharp waves, are recorded. These abnormalities, however, are similar to those observed in nonepileptic stroke patients. Paroxysmal abnormalities have been alleged to be even more frequent in nonepileptic patients.[16]

Seizure Frequency, Outcome, and Therapy

The frequency of seizures is quite variable. Usually, they tend not to be frequent and are easily controlled by anticonvulsant drugs. In one study, 88% of 90 patients were managed with monotherapy.[33] Poor compliance was the most frequent precipitating factor in patients with recurrent seizures.[33] In four patients, we have observed partial motor status epilepticus 5 months to 13 years after a stroke without an immediate precipitant. Chronic anticonvulsant therapy is recommended, even after a first seizure, because of a high risk of recurrence and the possibility of injuries in these elderly individuals.

Persistent worsening of a neurologic deficit after the occurrence of a seizure in patients with previous stroke is possible, especially if the seizure is prolonged. This may be due to a direct effect of the seizure itself on the infarcted area.[49]

SILENT STROKES

Cerebrovascular disease may be clinically silent or subtle in its manifestations. Several studies have documented the epileptogenic role of silent infarcts. In five of a group of 20 patients with proven cerebral infarcts at autopsy, seizures were the only clinical expression of the stroke.[50]

Epilepsy preceding stroke may be related to undetectable cerebrovascular disease. Barolin and colleagues[51] proposed naming these cases vascular precursor epilepsy or precursive epilepsy. In a case-control study of 176 consecutive patients younger than age 70 years (median age 60 years) admitted to hospitals with a first acute stroke, eight (4.5%) were epileptic, compared with one of the matched controls.[52] Not all the case reports are convincing (e.g., generalized seizures starting at age 18 and infarct at age 56), but some are (e.g., right partial motor seizures starting at age 64 and subsequent infarct at age 66, causing right hemiplegia).

The CT scans of 132 patients with late-onset epilepsy (older than age 40 years) were compared with those of an age- and sex-matched group for evidence of cerebrovascular disease.[25] Fifteen of the patients with epilepsy and only two controls had infarcts on their CT scans. Fourteen of the 15 patients were older than age 60 years. In nine patients, only lacunar infarcts (discrete, deeply situated, low-density lesions <1 cm in diameter) were present. In seven patients, CT scan provided the only evidence of underlying vascular disease. It is likely that the lacunar infarcts were not directly responsible, but rather indicative of more widespread cerebral vascular disease. On follow-up examination, appearances consistent with earlier scans were found in nine patients, whereas in four the infarct disappeared. In these patients, however, MRI showed abnormalities consistent with infarction at the site of the original lesion.

In summary, either early or late epileptic seizures can be associated with overt stroke. Furthermore, seizures can be the only sign of stroke, as a rare form of TIA or as a late sequela of a clinically silent stroke. Neuroimaging techniques are mandatory for diagnosis. Because of possible transient abnormalities on radiographic CT scan, MRI scan is superior.

PATHOPHYSIOLOGY

Potential mechanisms underlying seizures in patients with stroke are many. Their relative importance remains controversial.

Early Seizures

In early seizures, dynamic factors are first-line causes. They may be listed as follows: effects of hypoperfusion and reperfusion,[53] local acidosis, edema, cytotoxic metabolites, changes in cerebral blood flow due to hypertensive episodes or periods of cardiac failure, respiratory distress leading to hypoxia, and metabolic disturbances due to renal insufficiency.[50] The presence of blood in the cerebral parenchyma is another factor. Early seizures are more common with hemorrhage than with cortical infarction.[30]

Early seizures are considered by some to be more common with embolic infarcts than with thrombotic infarcts.[24] This finding is doubtful. "There was no significant difference in the incidence of early seizures in cortical infarcts due to cardiac embolism compared with cortical infarcts due to extracranial large-vessel atherosclerotic disease."[30] It is often difficult to clinically distinguish embolic infarcts from thrombotic infarcts. It can be difficult even pathologically.[54] The likelihood of angiographic confirmation of embolization is dependent on the timing of the study after the stroke.[24] Even when evaluations can demonstrate specific cardiac sources for embolisms, patients may be atheromatosclerotic and prone to artery-to-artery embolism.

Late Seizures

The development of epileptic changes in cortical neurons, their connections, and their environment has been advocated, with different weight given to various factors. It was formerly estimated that cerebral infarcts were responsible for vascular seizures more often than intracerebral hemorrhage.[54] The data of pre-CT studies are probably biased. It is not possible to distinguish reliably a cerebral hemorrhage from a cerebral infarction on clinical grounds alone. These studies probably excluded small parenchymal brain hemorrhages that are reliably detected by CT scan. In CT-documented studies, seizure frequency has varied from 15% to 28% of hemorrhagic patients.[32, 43] As previously noted, however, many studies did not separate early and late seizures. Kotila and Waltimo[34] found the incidence of seizures to be 14% in ischemic brain infarction and 15% in intracerebral hemorrhage. Experimental studies have shown the causative role of blood components in the development of a chronic epileptogenic focus.[55] It was hypothesized that, as reported for post-traumatic epilepsy, postischemic epilepsy may be an "iron epilepsy."[45] If the incidence of postinfarction epilepsy is higher in middle cerebral artery occlusion than in carotid artery occlusion, it may be due to the fact that the former are frequently of embolic origin and most embolic infarcts are at least minimally hemorrhagic.

In cerebral infarcts, the site of the occlusion has been considered as a possible risk factor. The occurrence of seizures was investigated in 141 patients with angiographically proven carotid or middle cerebral artery occlusive disease.[31] Seizures were noted "some time during the clinical course of the disease" in 17.3% of carotid patients and 10.8% of middle cerebral artery patients. The difference was not significant. On the other hand, clinical data were collected retrospectively on 68 consecutive patients with angiographically proven internal carotid occlusion and on 56 patients with middle cerebral artery occlusion.[45] Epileptic seizures occurred during a 1- to 5-year follow-up in 9% of the carotid artery group and in 21.4% of the middle cerebral artery group, a statistically significant difference. In the carotid group, 100% of seizures occurred from 3 to

6 months after the stroke; in the middle cerebral artery group, 41% occurred during the first year.

Some authors believe there is no relationship between the size of a hemorrhagic lesion and the risk of seizures.[30, 38] Others contend that epilepsy is probably more frequent with large lesions involving cortical and subcortical structures.[28, 33]

The location of the lesion, either ischemic or hemorrhagic, is considered to be an important causative factor. An association between cortical involvement and seizures was noted by most investigators.[30] Both early and late seizures were significantly associated with cortical and corticosubcortical lesions.[33] Early seizures that occurred after intracerebral hemorrhage were significantly associated (more than eight times as likely when hemorrhage involved the cerebral cortex than when blood was restricted to subcortical regions) with extension of blood to the cerebral cortex.[38] The highest incidence of seizures, however, was found in patients with lobar hematomas. The total incidence of seizures was 54%, and, in the nonoperated patients, the incidence was 39%. Bleeding in the temporal or parietal region was more likely to produce seizures than bleeding in the frontal region. Six of a group of 36 (17%) patients with basal ganglionic bleeding had a seizure. Within the basal ganglia, caudate involvement predicted seizures. There were no seizures in patients with thalamic hemorrhages.[32] Lobar hemorrhages in the frontal, temporal, or parietal regions were more commonly associated with seizures, whereas occipital hemorrhages were not.[43] Occasional seizures were reported with deep lesions alone.[11, 56]

In summary, the occurrence of early and late epileptic seizures in cerebrovascular disease is associated with various vascular risk factors. The type of stroke probably influences the risk of epilepsy, seeming to occur more frequently in hemorrhagic than in ischemic strokes. It has been speculated that a higher incidence of seizures may be explained by the deposition of iron in the brain tissue. Classically, cortical involvement by the stroke is the most significant risk factor for the development of epilepsy. Patients with lobar hematomas, however, have a high incidence of epilepsy. The presence of early seizures represents a risk factor for the development of epilepsy. A genetic propensity for seizures is likely. A multifactorial origin is also likely: "It is our impression that cerebral infarcts act only as a *locus minoris resistentiae* and that additional local or more generalized factors are involved in the pathogenesis of vascular epilepsy."[50]

Cerebral amyloid angiopathy (CAA) deserves a special mention because it is a disease of the elderly. A prospective population-based survey of cerebrovascular disease was conducted in Japan.[57] Causes of death were verified by autopsy in more than 80% of the deceased. The incidence of CAA increased dramatically with age: 0 in patients 40–49 years of age, 18.3% in men and 23.3% in women ages 70–79 years, and 42.8% in men and 45.8% in women age 90 years or older. It may be at present an underestimated cause of epilepsy in this age group. It is likely to increase in relative significance as the proportion of elderly patients in the population rises. This condition is characterized by amyloid deposition in the media and adventitia of leptomeningeal, cortical, and subcortical arteries and arterioles. It does not correlate with blood pressure or with the severity of cerebral atherosclerosis, even if many patients present with both CAA and other cardiovascular diseases. In the past a difficulty in the diagnosis of CAA was the lack of definitive diagnostic criteria short of biopsy or postmortem examination. Neuroimaging techniques, in particular a distinctive MRI appearance, may prove important in the clinical diagnosis. CAA is a common cause of spontaneous intracerebral hemorrhage and usually presents as recurrent large cerebral lobar hemorrhages. With rare exceptions, the hemorrhages involve the cortex and subcortical white matter.[58] CAA also may present without major lobar hemorrhage and can cause ischemic strokes and TIA.[59] Neuropathologic findings are petechial hemorrhages, scattered cortical microinfarctions, meningeal and subpial hemosiderosis from repeated episodes of bleeding, and white matter lesions. Seizures of various types have been reported and can be a presenting feature of CAA. They also occur shortly before or during the cognitive decline.[60]

HEAD TRAUMA

Head trauma may be associated with both acute symptomatic seizures and epilepsy. Acute symptomatic seizures are epileptic events that occur within 7 days of a head injury or while the patient is still suffering from the direct effects of the injury. Post-traumatic epilepsy is defined as unprovoked seizures that occur more than 1 week after medical stabilization subsequent to significant head injury.[1] Head trauma is a rare cause of epilepsy with a very late onset, accounting for 2–10% of the cases.

CEREBRAL ATROPHY

More or less localized cerebral atrophy may be the consequence of any type of cerebral insult and is found in symptomatic epilepsies. Its cause, and not the atrophy per se, is a risk factor in late-onset epilepsy. For some authors, a striking CT feature of late-onset epilepsy is the frequent occurrence of diffuse cerebral atrophy.[61, 62] It may result from defined pathologic conditions, but nearly 50% of cases have no identifiable causative factor. Diffuse cryptogenic cerebral atrophy may be a causative factor of late epilepsy with a relatively early onset,[63] but not in the elderly patient. We agree with Shorvon,[64] who found that cerebral atrophy is not significantly different in epileptic and nonepileptic patients.

PROGRESSIVE SYMPTOMATIC EPILEPSIES

Brain Tumors

Brain tumors are the second most frequent cause of symptomatic seizures in the elderly. Carney et al.[65] noted an incidence of brain tumor as the cause of epilepsy in 22% in a group of 92 patients older than age 60 years with new-onset seizures. It reached 28% in the seventh decade. Whereas some studies report lower percentages, this figure is in keeping with more recent publications, at least for elderly patients investigated in neurologic departments: 24%[18] and 18%.[20] An overestimation is likely for patients who have been sent to neurologic or neurosurgical hospital services. In our prospective semipopulation survey, 8.8% of all seizures in patients 60 years of age or older were associated with brain tumors. Of first unprovoked seizures, 24.5% had a similar association.[21]

Eighteen of 20 patients in the series of Carney et al.[65] had high-grade gliomas or metastatic brain tumors, and two had meningiomas. In our survey as in others, most of the tumors found in the elderly were high-grade gliomas or metastases.[9, 41] Lühdorf et al.[16] stated that metastatic brain tumors were the most common (15 patients), followed by malignant gliomas (five patients). Some authors, however, found gliomas, meningiomata, and metastases in the same proportion.[17, 18, 20] Usually, patients with slowly growing tumors develop seizures more often than those with rapidly invading tumors. This appears to be less constant in elderly patients.

In the study of Carney et al.,[65] all lesions were supratentorial. Whatever the age, tumors are more likely to be associated with seizures when they are situated in the cerebral hemispheres than when they lie in the posterior fossa. Within the hemispheres, the tumor's position and its proximity to the cortex are important. Superficial cortical tumors and tumors in the region of the central sulcus bear the highest incidence of associated epilepsy.[66]

Seizures were the presenting sign in nearly half of the patients in this study, as well as in the Danish survey.[16] The question of long-standing epilepsy in the presence of brain tumors is obsolete. In fact, these seizures may inappropriately be termed *epilepsy*, when epilepsy is defined as unprovoked recurrent seizures.

Seizures are sometimes associated with a primary CNS lymphoma. Lymphoma may be monofocal or multifocal and infiltrating with a predilection for the frontal lobes.[67] Even though the tumors are usually located in the white matter and not in the gray matter, seizures are probably facilitated by the associated frontal circuitry.

Other tumors that infiltrate the subfrontal, basal-ganglia, and mesencephalic regions may present as diffuse encephalopathy with behavioral and mental changes, and seizures. Gliomatosis cerebri is characterized by extensive infiltration of the brain by neoplastic glial cells. The cerebral structures are enlarged, although their general configuration is preserved.[68] Malignant angioendotheliomatosis or intravascular lymphomatosis is a systemic intravascular neoplasm resulting in ischemic necrosis of multiple areas of the cerebral white matter.[69]

Dementia

Dementia as a cause of seizures is not fully characterized and is not a trendy topic. Studies are limited by several factors. Seizures may be underreported. Unless they are observed directly, generalized tonic-clonic seizures as well as partial seizures may remain unrecognized, given that complex partial seizures and postictal confusion may not differ greatly differ from the interictal state. Sample size has usually been relatively small, and the period under observation variable.

Senile Dementia of the Alzheimer's Type

Variations in the patient population under study explain figures of seizure incidence ranging from less than 2% to 16% (see Table 7.1).[41] Hauser et al.[70] reviewed 81 patients with dementia and autopsy findings of Alzheimer's disease without other neuropathologic findings. The incidence of unprovoked seizures was 10 times more than expected in a reference population. Five patients experienced recurrent seizures, and three only one seizure. The mean age at onset of dementia and the mean duration of illness were not different in patients with and without seizures. All seizures were apparently generalized from onset.

Romanelli et al.[71] compared development of seizures in 44 patients (mean age of 71 years) with mild senile dementia of Alzheimer's type (SDAT) with healthy control subjects during a period of 90 months. During the course of the study, seven (16%) of the 44 patients with SDAT developed at least one documented seizure. It was a single event in five patients, and two experienced a second seizure. No further seizures occurred after therapy was initiated. At the time of the first seizure, all patients were severely demented. The authors draw attention to the fact that, in their series as in others, seizures are associated with the advanced stages of disease.

Of 208 inpatients older than age 55 years on the Dundee Psychiatric Service with dementia, 19 (9%) were diagnosed as having epileptic seizures.[72] They were classified as major in three-fourths of the cases. Nine patients had both major and minor seizures; three had minor seizures only. Patients with epilepsy were significantly younger than a control group of dementia inpatients and were probably more cognitively impaired.

Neuropathologic changes in presenile Alzheimer's disease and senile dementia are identical. It has been suggested that these two conditions constitute a single entity. A study was designed to test the validity of this hypothesis.[73] Thirty-six demented patients with an onset of symptoms before the age of 65 were compared with 35 patients with onset after age 65. Four patients (11%) in the presenile group and two (6%) in the senile group suffered from epileptic seizures during the course of the disease.

The underlying pathology of Alzheimer's disease may be responsible for an increased risk of developing seizures in these patients. The pathophysiology of Alzheimer's disease includes alterations of neurons and glia in hippocampal and neocortical areas. A higher frequency of epilepsy in presenile than in senile dementia would support this hypothesis. Demented patients, however, are at risk for added complications, for example, nutritional, metabolic, or toxic complications, which by themselves can probably produce seizures.[65] This might explain in part why seizures mainly occur in advanced stages of the disease.

Whatever their pathophysiology, seizures in association with SDAT do not constitute a major problem: rare patients with rare seizures that are easily controlled.

Subcortical Arteriosclerotic Encephalopathy

Subcortical arteriosclerotic encephalopathy, or Binswanger's disease, is a progressive form of vascular dementia that results from diffuse and multifocal ischemic damage to subcortical white matter.[74] It is an illness of elderly hypertensive patients. A survey of 83 of such patients in their sixth or seventh decade showed that onset of symptoms began with an acute, focal neurologic deficit consistent with a stroke in one-third of cases. The subsequent course of illness was usually a gradual progression of disorders of memory, cognition, and mood, exacerbated by acute focal deficits, leading to dementia with pyramidal and pseudobulbar dysfunction. The CT and MRI changes reflecting the white matter injury are suggestive but alone do not permit an unequivocal diagnosis. Seizures are not infrequent and have been observed in 18% of 47 pathologically verified cases.[74] They were either unprovoked generalized tonic-clonic seizures, focal seizures, or situation-related seizures. They seem referable to the gray matter lesions. One patient, however, presented first with a stroke and later with seizures, with evidence of intellectual deterioration. Postmortem findings showed pathologic changes of the type typically seen in Binswanger's disease—gliosis and demyelinization of the deep white matter that spared the subcortical arcuate fibers, with no evidence of alteration of the neocortex.[75]

Other Progressive Associated Conditions

In *sarcoidosis* affecting the nervous system, granulomata form in the perivascular spaces and walls of small penetrating arteries and veins of the meninges and parenchyma.[76] Seizures in neurologic sarcoidosis occur in 5–18% of cases. Occurrence of both seizures and dementia implies a poor prognosis; the average mean survival was only 9 months in Delaney's study.[77] MRI scans show periventricular and multifocal white matter lesions.

Several types of *vasculitis* result in neurologic dysfunction by causing tissue ischemia. Lymphomatoid granulomatosis is a lymphoreticular proliferative disorder characterized by vascular cellular infiltrates. The CNS is involved in 20% of cases.[78] The manifestations at the time of presentation include headaches, confusion, various focal signs, and seizures. Polyarteritis nodosa, a systemic necrotizing vasculitis, and granulomatous angiitis of the CNS, a disease limited to the vessels within the CNS, share the same common presentation. In these rare conditions, too, focal or generalized seizures may occur.[79]

METABOLIC AND TOXIC CAUSES

Acute symptomatic seizures are very frequent in the elderly. In the French epidemiologic survey, of 284 patients 60 years or older when experiencing a first seizure, 172 (60%) were classified into this group. They are often, but not necessarily, isolated epileptic events. Some patients present with several seizures during a unique acute illness or present with repeated seizures, each related to a recurrent acute situation.

The proportion of seizures due to metabolic or toxic factors is not easy to determine. Patients with clearly metabolic causes of seizures are not referred for further investigation in neurologic centers because the underlying disease is the dominant clinical feature.[9] In our epidemiologic survey, an effort was made to detect them by carefully checking the departments of internal medicine. Of 172 patients with acute symptomatic seizures, 15.1% had a metabolic and 14.5% a toxic origin.

In patients with *diabetes mellitus* receiving sulfonamides, especially long-acting ones, an imbalance between the amounts of drug and food ingested results in hypoglycemic episodes. They are responsible for coma, confusional states, transient hemiparesis, and generalized or focal seizures.

The syndrome of *nonketotic hyperglycemic coma* results in a mortality of 30–60%.[80] The survival rate is better with an early diagnosis. In quite a few cases, the patient is not known to have been diabetic. Neurologic manifestations are often the presenting sign. They can manifest as stupor, coma, and focal deficits.[81] Seizures have been observed in approximately 25% of cases and are a prominent feature of the presenting symptomatology. They are resistant to antiepileptic drugs and controlled only by correction of the metabolic disorder. Generalized seizures are uncommon. Focal motor seizures are the rule, with two suggestive patterns: epilepsia partialis continua and reflex seizures. In a series of 21 patients, epilepsia partialis continua occurred during the initial phase of nonketotic hyperglycemia and persisted for an average of 8 days. Increasing severity of hyperglycemia led to coma and cessation of seizures.[80] Movement-induced seizures[82] are so characteristic that reflex epilepsy and nonketotic hyperglycemia in the elderly has been proposed as a specific neuroendocrine syndrome.[83] Realization that the seizures are movement-induced is the critical diagnostic clue. As with other partial seizures, they are an early manifestation of the disorder. Most authors attribute the focal seizures to a preexisting structural lesion, activated by hyperglycemia, mild hyperosmolarity, hyponatremia, and lack of ketoacidosis. Focal cortical venous sludging or thrombosis could be also be a consequence of the metabolic derangment.[84] The association of intravascular thrombosis with nonketotic hyperglycemia is well documented. A small cerebral infarct created by such thrombosis could be triggered by hyperglycemia and provoke seizures.

Hyponatremia is common in elderly patients taking diuretics, and a clear risk factor.

Alcohol abuse and withdrawal are seldom toxic precipitants. Uremia is usually accompanied by other metabolic imbalances.

The use of *medication* that lowers the seizure threshold is an important cause of acute symptomatic seizures. Drugs such as phenothiazines and other neuroleptics, tricyclic antidepressants, and CNS stimulants such as theophylline and aminophylline enter in this category.[85–88]

An abrupt discontinuation of sedative and anxiolytic drugs is probably a prominent cause of accidental seizures in the elderly. All barbiturates and all benzodiazepines present a risk of withdrawal seizures.

Generalized tonic-clonic seizures are not the only form of seizures related to an acute metabolic or toxic insult; partial seizures are also possible. Systemic factors elicit epileptic activity in a cortex rendered susceptible by some local pathologic process. Vascular insufficiency or local disturbance of function may render a localized area of cortex more susceptible to an acute metabolic imbalance.

The implication of a single factor in the pathogenesis of acute symptomatic seizures is not tenable. It would appear that a variety of factors act simultaneously in an additive fashion.

A large body of literature attests to increased interest in *nonconvulsive status epilepticus*. Confusional status is a heterogeneous epileptic condition. It may be subdivided into generalized status, with continuous, bilaterally synchronous and symmetric spike-wave discharges,[89] and into complex partial status, in which a focality could be shown on the EEG, even if the initial focal discharges rapidly become generalized from a temporal or frontal origin.[90, 91] A clinical heterogeneity exists. Clinical manifestations include a spectrum of impaired consciousness ranging from normal or subjective impairment to coma. Other behavioral manifestations include lack of initiative, inability to plan, disorientation, inappropriate behavior, fugue, hallucinations, and clumsy motor performance.[92] Nonconvulsive status epilepticus in later life seems to be an entity distinct from absence (petit mal) status of early onset. When it occurs de novo in elderly subjects with no previous history of epilepsy, it may be due to metabolic or toxic factors or to either excessive amounts or withdrawal of psychotropic drugs. Mild hyponatremia, lithium carbonate therapy, polydipsia with electrolyte imbalance,[93] antidepressant drugs,[94, 95] metrizamide myelography,[95, 96] cerebral angiography with iothalamate meglumine,[97] and benzodiazepine withdrawal[98, 99] have also been implicated.

CONCLUSION

Some aging changes in brain cells and nervous tissue might be significant in epileptogenesis. Pathologic vascular changes that occur in the brain with age are hyalinization of small blood vessels with perivascular gliosis, and incrustation with iron in the walls of blood vessels. Increasing age alone is a significant factor in the commonly observed widespread decrease in the number of nerve cells. The literature indicates numerous structural alterations in the remaining neurons, particularly in their membranes, which regulate all events at intra- and intercellular interfaces. This leads to an impaired capacity to maintain cellular equilibrium. In addition, "Aging is associated with a narrowing of homeostatic reserves. This change in homeostasis with the passage of time, aging, has been termed homeostenosis."[100]

Exposed to the same condition, in this case aging, some individuals will develop seizures; others will not. The reason was given by Tissot, a Swiss neurologist, two centuries ago: "To produce epilepsy, two conditions are necessary:

(a) a tendency for the brain to fall into spasm more readily than during health, and (b) a source of irritation that can precipitate this tendency."[101] In other words, the importance of an association of genetic and acquired factors has long been recognized.[101]

REFERENCES

1. Hauser WA, Annegers JF, Kurland LT. Prevalence of epilepsy in Rochester, Minnesota, 1940–1980. Epilepsia 1991;32:429.
2. Commission on Classification and Terminology of the International League Against Epilepsy. Proposal for revised classification of epilepsies and epileptic syndromes. Epilepsia 1989;30:389.
3. Commission on Epidemiology and Prognosis, International League Against Epilepsy. Guidelines for epidemiologic studies on epilepsy. Epilepsia 1993;34:592.
4. Loiseau J, Loiseau P, Guyot M, et al. A survey of seizure disorders in the French Southwest. I: incidence of epileptic syndromes. Epilepsia 1990;31:391.
5. Tallis R. Epilepsy in the Elderly. In D Chadwick (ed), Fourth International Symposium on Sodium Valproate and Epilepsy. Royal Society of Medicine Services International Congress and Symposium. No. 152. London: Royal Society of Medicine Services. 1989;125.
6. Gastaut H, Gastaut JL, Michel B. L'epilepsie du vieillard. Revue Med Interne 1982;23 and 24:1263.
7. Schott GD, McLeod AA, Jewitt DE. Cardiac arrythmias that masquerade as epilepsy. BMJ 1977;1:1454.
8. Camm AJ, Evans KE, Ward DE, Martin A. The rhythm of the heart in active elderly subjects. Am Heart J 1980;99:518.
9. Hildick-Smith M. Epilepsy in the elderly. Age Ageing 1974;3:203.
10. Hauser WA, Annegers JF, Kurland LK. Incidence of epilepsy and unprovoked seizures in Rochester, Minnesota, 1935–1984. Epilepsia 1993;34:453.
11. Shinton RA, Gill JS, Melnick SC, et al. The frequency, characteristics and prognosis of epileptic seizures at the onset of stroke. J Neurol Neurosurg Psychiatry 1988;51:273.
12. Robb P, McNaughton F. Etiology of Epilepsy. Introduction. In PJ Vinken, GW Bruyn (eds), Handbook of Clinical Neurology. Vol. 15, The Epilepsies. Amsterdam: North Holland Publishing Company 1974;271.
13. Schold C, Yarnell PR, Earnest MP. Origin of seizures in the elderly patients. JAMA 1977;238:1177.
14. Roberts MA, Godfrey JW, Caird FI. Epileptic seizures in the elderly: aetiology and type of seizure. Age Ageing 1982;11:24.
15. Gupta K. Epilepsy in the elderly: how far to investigate. Br J Clin Pract 1983;37:249.
16. Lüdhorf K, Jensen LK, Plesner AM. Etiology of seizures in the elderly. Epilepsia 1986;27:458.
17. Delangre T, Mihout B, Proust B, et al. Causes des premières crises convulsives de l'adulte en fonction de l'âge et du sexe. Presse Med 1989;18:1014.
18. Sundaram MBM. Etiology and patterns of seizures in the elderly. Neuroepidemiology 1989;8:234.
19. Sung CY, Chu NS. Epileptic seizures in elderly people: aetiology and seizure type. Age Ageing 1990;19:25.
20. Henny C, Despland PA, Regli F. Première crise épileptique après l'âge de 60 ans: étiologie, présentation clinique et EEG. Schweiz Med Wochenschr 1990;120:787.

21. Loiseau J, Loiseau P, Duché B, et al. A survey of epileptic disorders in southwest France: seizures in elderly patients. Ann Neurol 1990;27:232.
22. Hauser WA, Kurland LT. The epidemiology of epilepsy in Rochester, Minnesota, 1935 through 1967. Epilepsia 1975;16:1.
23. Hauser WA. Seizure disorders: the changes with age. Epilepsia 1992;33(Suppl 4):S6.
24. Lesser RP, Lüders H, Dinner DS, Morris HH. Epileptic seizures due to thrombotic and embolic cerebrovascular disease in older patients. Epilepsia 1985;26:622.
25. Roberts RC, Shorvon S, Cox TCS, Gilliatt RW. Clinically unsuspected cerebral infarction revelated by computed tomography scanning in late onset epilepsy. Epilepsia 1988;29:190.
26. Shapiro M, Neufeld MY, Korczyn AD. Seizures of unknown origin after the age of 50: vascular risk factor. Acta Neurol Scand 1990;82:78.
27. WHO Task Force on Stroke and Other Cerebrovascular Disorders. Recommendations on stroke prevention, diagnosis, and therapy. Stroke 1989;20:1407.
28. Davalos A, Cendra E, Genis D, Lopez-Pousa S. The frequency, characteristics and prognosis of epileptic seizures at the onset of stroke. J Neurol Neurosurg Psychiatry 1988;51:464.
29. Hauser WA, Ramirez-Lassepas M, Rosenstein R. Risk for seizures and epilepsy following cerebrovascular insults [abstract]. Epilepsia 1984;25:666.
30. Kilpatrick CJ, Davis SM, Tress BM, et al. Epileptic seizures in acute stroke. Arch Neurol 1990;47:157.
31. Cocito L, Favale E, Reni L. Epileptic seizures in cerebral arterial occlusive disease. Stroke 1982;13:189.
32. Faught E, Peters D, Bartolucci A, et al. Seizures after primary intracerebral hemorrhage. Neurology 1989;39:1089.
33. Gupta SR, Naheedy MH, Elias D, Rubino FA. Postinfarction seizures. A clinical study. Stroke 1988;19:1477.
34. Kotila M, Waltimo O. Epilepsy after stroke. Epilepsia 1992;33:495.
35. Chatrian GE, Shaw CM, Leffman H. The significance of periodic lateralized epileptiform discharges in EEG: an electrographic, clinical and pathological study. Electroencephalogr Clin Neurophysiol 1964;17:177.
36. Erkulvrawatr S. Occurence, evolution and prognosis of periodic lateralized epileptiform discharges in EEG. Clin Electroencephalogr 1977;8:89.
37. Raroque HG, Gonzales PCW, Jhaveri HS, et al. Defining the role of structural lesions and metabolic abnormalities in periodic lateralized epileptiform discharges. Epilepsia 1993;34:279.
38. Berger AR, Lipton RB, Lesser ML, et al. Early seizures following intracerebral hemorrhage: implications for therapy. Neurology 1988;38:1363.
39. Lüdhorf K, Jensen LK, Plesner AM. Epilepsy in the elderly: life expectancy and causes of death. Acta Neurol Scand 1987;76:183.
40. Louis S, McDowell F. Epileptic seizures in non-embolic cerebral infarction. Arch Neurol 1967;17:414.
41. Sung CY, Chu NS. Epileptic seizures in intracerebral haemorrhage. J Neurol Neurosurg Psychiatry. 1989;52:1273.
42. Asconape JJ, Penry JK. Poststroke seizures in the elderly. Clin Geriatr Med 1991;7:483.
43. Weisberg LA, Shamsnia M, Elliott D. Seizures caused by nontraumatic parenchymal brain hemorrhages. Neurology 1991;41:1197.
44. Cocito L, Loeb C. Focal epilepsy as a possible sign of transient subclinical ischemia. Eur Neurol 1989;29:339.
45. De Carolis P, D'Alessandro R, Ferrara R, et al. Late seizures in patients with internal carotid and middle cerebral artery occlusive disease following ischaemic events. J Neurol Neurosurg Psychiatry 1984;47:1345.

46. Burri H, Schaffler L, Karbowski K. Epileptische anfalle bei patienten mit zere-brovaskularen insulten. Schweiz Med Wochenschr 1989;119:500.
47. Milandre L, Broca P, Sambuc R, Khalil R. Les crises épileptiques au cours et au décours des accidents cérébro-vasculaires. Analyse clinique de 78 cas. Rev Neurol (Paris) 1992;148:767.
48. Holmes GL. The electroencephalogram as a predictor of seizures following cerebral infarction. Clin Electroencephalogr 1980;11:83.
49. Bogousslavsky J, Martin R, Regli F, et al. Persistent worsening of stroke sequelae after delayed seizures. Arch Neurol 1992;49:385.
50. De Reuck JL. Neuropathology of Epilepsy Resulting from Cerebrovascular Disorders. In M Parsonage, RHE Grant, AG Craig, AA Ward Jr (eds). Advances in Epileptology: The XIVth Epilepsy International Symposium. New York: Raven, 1983;95.
51. Barolin GS, Scherzer E, Schnaberth G. Epileptische Manifestationen als Vorboten von Schalganfällen: "Vaskuläre Präkursiv-Epilepsie." Fortschr Neurol Psychiatr 1971;39:199.
52. Shinton RA, Gill JS, Zezulka AV, Beevers DG. The frequency of epilepsy preceding stroke. Case-control study in 230 patients. Lancet 1987;i:11.
53. Armon C, Radtke RA, Massey EW. Therapy of seizures associated with stroke. Clin Neuropharmacol 1991;14:17.
54. Richardson EP, Dodge PR. Epilepsy in cerebrovascular disease. Epilepsia 1954;3:49.
55. Willmore SL. Post-traumatic epilepsy: cellular mechanisms and implications for treatment. Epilepsia 1990;31(Suppl 3):S67.
56. Olsen TS, Hogenhaven H, Thage O. Epilepsy after stroke. Neurology 1987;37:1209.
57. Masuda J, Tanaka K, Ueda K, Omae T. Autopsy study of incidence and distribution of cerebral amyloid angiopathy in Hisayama, Japan. Stroke 1988;19:205.
58. Vinters HV. Cerebral amyloid angiopathy. A critical review. Stroke 1987;18:311.
59. Smith DB, Hitchcock M, Philpott PJ. Cerebral amyloid angiopathy presenting as transient ischemic attacks. J Neurosurg 1985;63:963.
60. Greenberg SM, Vonsattel JPG, Stakes JW, et al. The clinical spectrum of cerebral amyloid angiopathy: presentations without lobar hemorrhage. Neurology 1993;43:2073.
61. Gastaut H, Michel B, Gastaut JL, Cerda M. A propos d'une eventuelle épilepsie généralisée tardive. Apport de la scannographie cérébrale. Rev Electroencephalogr Neurophysiol Clin 1980;3:276.
62. Daras M, Tuchman AJ, Strobos RJ. Computed tomography in adult-onset epileptic seizures in a city hospital population. Epilepsia 1987;28:915.
63. Regesta G, Tanganelli P. Late-onset epilepsy and diffuse cryptogenous cerebral atrophy. Epilepsia 1992;33:821.
64. Shorvon S. Imaging in the Investigation of Epilepsy. In A Hopkins (ed), Epilepsy. London: Chapman and Hall, 1987;201.
65. Carney LR, Hudgins RL, Espinosa RE, Klass DW. Seizures beginning after the age of 60. Arch Intern Med 1969;124:707.
66. Le Blanc FE, Rasmussen T. Cerebral Seizures and Brain Tumors. In PJ Vinken, GW Bruyn (eds), Handbook of Clinical Neurology. Vol. 15, The Epilepsies. Amsterdam: North Holland Publishing Company 1974;295.
67. Schwaighofer BW, Hesselink JR, Press GA, et al. Primary intracranial CNS lymphoma: MR manifestations. AJNR Am J Neuroradiol 1989;10:725.
68. Artigas J, Cervos-Navarro J, Iglesias JR, Ebhardt G. Gliomatosis cerebri: clinical and histological findings. Clin Neuropathol 1985;4:135.
69. Ferry JA, Harris NL, Picker LJ, et al. Intravascular lymphomatosis (malignant angioendotheliomatosis): a B-cell neoplasm expressing surface homing receptors. Mod Pathol 1988;1:444.
70. Hauser WA, Morris ML, Heston LL, Anderson VE. Seizures and myoclonus in Alzheimer's disease. Neurology 1986;36:1226.

71. Romanelli MF, Morris JC, Ashkin K, Coben LA. Advanced Alzheimer's disease is a risk factor for late-onset seizures. Arch Neurol 1990;47:847.
72. McAreavey MJ, Ballinger BR, Fenton GW. Epileptic seizures in elderly patients with dementia. Epilepsia 1992;33:657.
73. Sulkava R. Alzheimer's disease and senile dementia of Alzheimer type. Acta Neurol Scand 1982;65:636.
74. Babikian V, Ropper AH. Binswanger's disease: a review. Stroke 1987;18:2.
75. Mayer SA, Tatemichi TK, Hair LS, et al. Hemineglect and seizures in Binswanger's disease: clinical-pathological report. J Neurol Neurosurg Psychiatry 1993;56:816.
76. Heck AW, Phillips LH II. Sarcoidosis and the central nervous system. Neurol Clin 1989;7:641.
77. Delaney P. Seizures in sarcoidosis: a poor prognosis. Ann Neurol 1980;7:494.
78. Hogan PJ, Greenberg MK, McCarthy GE. Neurological complications of lymphomatoid granulomatosis. Neurology 1981;31:619.
79. Moore PM, Cupps RT. Neurological complications of vasculitis. Ann Neurol 1983;14:155.
80. Singh BM, Strobos RJ. Epilepsia partialis continua associated with nonketotic hyperglycemia: clinical and biochemical profile of 21 patients. Ann Neurol 1980;8:155.
81. Maccario M. Neurological dysfunction associated with nonketotic hyperglycemia. Arch Neurol 1968;19:525.
82. Aquino A, Gabor AJ. Movement-induced seizures in nonketotic hyperglycemia. Neurology 1980;30:600.
83. Brick JF, Gutrecht JA, Ringel RA. Reflex epilepsy and nonketotic hyperglycemia in the elderly: a specific neuroendocrine syndrome. Neurology 1989;39:394.
84. Stahlman GC, Auerbah PS, Strickland WG. Neurologic manifestations of non-ketotic hyperglycemia. J Tenn Med Assoc 1988;81:77.
85. Remick RA, Fine SH. Antipsychotic drugs and seizures. J Clin Psychiatry 1979;40:78.
86. Messing RO, Closson RG, Simon RP. Drug-induced seizures: a 10-year experience. Neurology 1984;34:1582.
87. Zaccara G, Muscas GC, Messori A. Clinical features, pathogenesis and management of drug-induced seizures. Drug Saf 1990;5:109.
88. Cold JA, Wells BG, Froemming JH. Seizure activity associated with antipsychotic therapy. DICP 1990;24:601.
89. Rohr Le Floch J, Gauthier G, Beaumanoir A. Etats confusionnels d'origine épileptique. Intérêt de l'EEG fait en urgence. Rev Neurol (Paris) 1988;144:425.
90. Aguglia U, Tinuper P, Farnarier G. Etat confusionnel critique prolongé à point de départ frontal chez un sujet âgé. Rev EEG Neurophysiol Clin 1983;13:174.
91. Tomson T, Svanborg E, Wedlund JE. Nonconvulsive status epilepticus: high incidence of complex partial status. Epilepsia 1986;27:276.
92. Andermann F, Robb MP. Absence status. Epilepsia 1972;13:177.
93. Lee SI. Non convulsive status epilepticus: ictal confusion in later life. Arch Neurol 1985;42:778.
94. van Sweden B. Toxic ictal confusion in middle age: treatment with benzodiazepines. J Neurol Neurosurg Psychiatry 1985;48:472.
95. Bourrat Ch, Garde P, Boucher M, Fournet A. Etats d'absence prolongée chez des patients âgés sans antécédents épileptiques. Rev Neurol (Paris) 1986;142:696.
96. Obeid T, Yaqub B, Panayiotopoulos C, et al. Absence status epilepticus with computed tomographic brain changes following metrizamide myelography. Ann Neurol 1988;24:582.
97. Vickrey BG, Bahls FH. Nonconvulsive status epilepticus following cerebral angiography. Ann Neurol 1989;25:199.
98. Thomas P, Beaumanoir A, Genton P, et al. De novo absence status. Report of 11 cases. Neurology 1992;47:104.

99. Thomas P, Lebrun C, Chatel M. De novo absence status epilepticus as a benzodiazepine withdrawal syndrome. Epilepsia 1993;34:355.
100. Weksler ME. The Cellular Pathology of the Diseases of Aging. In M Bergener, M Erminy, HB Stähelin (eds), Crossroads in Aging. London: Academic, 1988;97.
101. Tissot SA. Traité de l'Épilepsie, Faisant le Tome Troisième du Traité des Nerfs et de Leurs Maladies. Paris: Didot, 1770.

8

Falls in the Elderly

Rein Tideiksaar and Howard Fillit

INTRODUCTION

Falls in the elderly represent a major health problem. Approximately one-third of those age 65 years and older who live at home sustain one or more falls each year.[1] The extent of falls is equally problematic among the elderly in institutional settings. Within the acute hospital, elderly patients have the highest rates of falls, averaging 1.5 falls per bed annually.[2] Approximately 50% of nursing home residents fall every year, and up to 40% have recurrent falls.[2] The risk of falling increases with advanced age and reaches a prevalence of approximately 50% in those age 85 years and older.[3] Women generally fall two to three times more frequently than men.[3] The discrepancy in fall rates between females and males, however, begins to disappear and approaches unity with increasing age.[4]

The purpose of this chapter is to acquaint clinicians with the consequences of falls, the conditions under which falls and injury occur, and the factors associated with their risk. An approach to the clinical assessment of falls and fall risk and intervention strategies to reduce both also is presented.

CONSEQUENCES

Falls in the elderly are associated with significant mortality and morbidity. Falls represent a leading cause of death, accounting for up to 9,500 fatalities annually in the United States.[5] Approximately 25% of elderly people who are hospitalized for falls die within 1 year of the event.[6] These figures probably represent an underestimation, since falls as a cause of death are often unreported on death certificates. In those who survive, falls are associated with a myriad of morbid complications. Physical injury is the most serious consequence of falling. Approximately 10% of falls result in injury (e.g., fractures, soft-tissue trauma, sprains, and dislocations).[5]

The most common fractures consist of distal forearm and hip fractures.[5] Distal forearm fractures result from a fall onto an outstretched arm and hyperextended wrist that routinely follows a trip or stumble, whereas hip fractures are associated with slip-related falls in the side or backward direction that directly impact the hip. Although accounting for only 1% of fall-related injuries, hip fractures have the greatest impact. Up to 27% of elderly individuals with a hip fracture are dead 1 year after the injury.[7] Of those who survive, approximately 60% experience problems with ambulation and require either a mechanical aid (cane, walker) or human assistance for mobility.[8] Many falls also are associated with increased lie times on the ground (the person is unable to rise up without assistance). Prolonged postfall lie times can result in dehydration, malnutrition, rhabdomyolysis (i.e., pressure necrosis of muscles) and, during winter months, hypothermia.

Although the majority of falls do not cause physical injury, they are by no means benign. Many of these events are associated with significant psychological and social sequelae. Falls represent unpleasant and frightening experiences. They can cause elderly individuals to lose confidence in their ability to function safely and result in a fear of further falls. Up to 50% of elderly individuals with multiple falling episodes admit to restricting everyday activities because they fear additional falls and injury.[9] Any restriction of activities that occurs as a result can lead to periods of immobility and, subsequently, the risk of physical complications such as osteoporosis, muscle weakness, pressure sores, and joint contractions. Any resulting loss of mobility places the elderly at risk for further falls. As well, loss of mobility is emotionally devastating and can lead to depression that, in turn, can lead to isolation and decreased socialization. Eventually, the elderly person may become permanently homebound.

Family members of elderly people who fall are affected as well. Family members are often concerned about whether individuals who fall can live alone and remain safe. If they are unable to, families pursue alternatives such as having the elderly person move in with them; if this is not feasible, many consider nursing home placement. Falls and immobility account for up to one-third of all nursing home admissions.[5]

CAUSES OF FALLING

In 1960, Sheldon,[10] a noted British geriatrician, stated that the "liability of older people to tumble and often to injure themselves is such a commonplace of experience that it has been tacitly accepted as an inevitable aspect of aging and thereby deprived of the exercise of curiosity." Since then, however, interest in and research on the subject of falling have changed clinical perception of these events. Falls in the elderly are now no longer considered inevitable aspects of the aging process but, rather, as predictable occurrences that stem from a multitude of identifiable host-related and environmental factors.

The risk of falling occurs when a person engages in an activity that results in a loss of balance and the body mechanisms responsible for compensation or stability fail. Although the chances of balance loss are increased during activities that greatly exceed the limits of stability (standing on a chair seat to change a light bulb or grasp objects from shelf heights that are difficult to reach), these activities account for a small number of falls. In comparison, the risk of balance loss and the majority of falls experienced by elderly individuals take place during commonplace, everyday activities, such as walking; descending and climbing stairs; transferring on and off chairs, beds, and toilets; getting in and out of bathtubs and shower stalls; and reaching or bending to retrieve and place objects from a standing position.

Any subsequent fall should be viewed as a sign or symptom of an underlying problem, typically indicative of intrinsic factors (age-related changes, disease states, and medication effects) or extrinsic factors (environmental hazards and obstacles interfering with mobility). In general, the etiology of falls in the elderly is multifactorial, due to a combination of both intrinsic and extrinsic factors, as the following case illustrates.

> *E.L. is an 80-year-old female who experienced two falls at home. She stated that one fall occurred shortly after she got up from her bed. The other fall took place in a dimly lit room, the result of tripping over a rug edge. Her medical history consisted of hypertension treated with a thiazide diuretic. On evaluation, E.L. was dehydrated and, as a result, had orthostatic hypotension. As well, it was discovered that her vision was impaired. This patient's falls were due to both intrinsic and extrinsic factors. The bedroom fall was the result of diuretic-induced hypotension. Her tripping fall was caused by a combination of visual dysfunction and low illumination, which resulted in the failure to recognize and visualize an upended rug edge.*

AGE-RELATED CHANGES

With advancing age, several physiologic changes take place and contribute to fall risk. The most significant occur in the visual and neuromuscular systems and influence balance and gait.

Vision

The ability of the eye to adjust to various environmental stimuli diminishes with age. The response to varying levels of light and darkness is reduced.[11] As a result, the elderly require more time to adapt to lighting changes, such as walking from a well lit area to one of relatively low illumination and the reverse. Dark adaptation, the capability of the eye to adjust to low levels of illumination, is particularly affected by age.[10] This change is associated with an increased risk of falls, as the elderly person's ability to view environmental surroundings and potential trip and slip hazards under conditions of low illumination is compromised. Bright lighting may produce similar problems. With age, pupillary response and accommodation decline.[12] As a consequence, excessive illumination may lead to momentary visual impairment until the eyes are able to adjust fully.

As well, the elderly have a decreased resistance to glare (a dazzling effect associated with an intense source of illumination).[11] Glare sensitivity is attributed to age-related changes in the lens that cause a scattering of stray light over the retina. Common sources of glare include sunlight and unshielded light bulbs. These sources produce glare either directly, emitting a flood of light shining straight into the eyes, or indirectly, giving off reflected glare from window panes or polished floor surfaces. The net result is a diminished ability to see potential ground hazards (rug edges, door thresholds, wet surfaces) that can lead to trips and slips. Also, elderly people may perceive glare-producing floor surfaces as slippery. In an effort to compensate, they may alter their gait (walk slower, flat-footed, and with a wide base of support). This gait change may, however, in some instances be hazardous and lead to unsteady balance and falls.

A decline in depth perception occurs with age.[11] This can interfere with the visual detection and interpretation of ground surfaces of low contrast such as carpet and step edges or door thresholds that are indistinguishable from their background. Linoleum tile and carpet designs that are patterned, checkered, or floral may appear as either ground elevations or depressions, which can induce hazardous gaits.

Other age-related changes in visual function that may increase the risk of falls include a deterioration of dynamic visual acuity, a constriction of visual fields, a decline in contrast sensitivity, a decrease in color vision (a diminished ability to discriminate subtle differences in the blue-green range), and a reduced speed of visual processing.[13]

Balance

Balance is a complex function. The ability to maintain an upright posture during standing and walking is dependent on the operation and integrity of vision, vestibular input, proprioceptive feedback, muscular strength, and joint flexibility. Working in unison, these components culminate in postural sway, an anteroposterior and lateral motion or movement of the body that counters the effects of gravity and controls upright posture. In the standing position, balance is achieved by the body's constant positioning of its center of gravity (COG) over a base of support (BOS), the area surrounding the borders of the feet (Figure 8.1). During ambulation, the COG extends beyond the BOS and stretches the limits of stability (Figure 8.2). This instability is detected by the visual, proprioceptive, and vestibular systems and transmits a number of signals to stretch receptors located in joints and muscles of the lower extremities. In turn, these messages initiate a set of coordinated body movements, or stepping strategy (e.g., a rapid forward or backward shifting of the feet), that readjusts the body's COG in alignment with the BOS. An inability to initiate or complete this strategy results in balance loss and fall risk.

Age-related changes can affect any of these components of balance and increase the risk of postural instability. The proprioceptive system, located in joint mechanoreceptors of the spine and extremities, supplies the body with kinesthetic information, or feedback, on the surrounding environment. With respect to ambulation, proprioception provides a person with proper orientation to ground conditions. With advanced age, proprioceptive feedback declines and

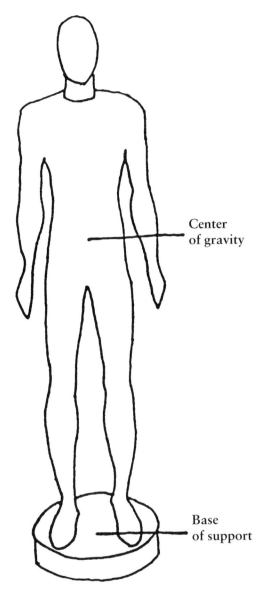

Center
of gravity

Base
of support

Figure 8.1 The center of gravity in relationship to the base of support.

leads to increased postural sway.[14] Vision can augment proprioception or provide a substitute for its loss. This can be observed by having elderly individuals with proprioceptive loss ambulate. They walk by viewing the location of their feet on the ground to ensure proper placement. If visual input is decreased, maintaining balance becomes difficult. When elderly individuals are asked to stand with their eyes closed or walk in a dark room, they typically demonstrate

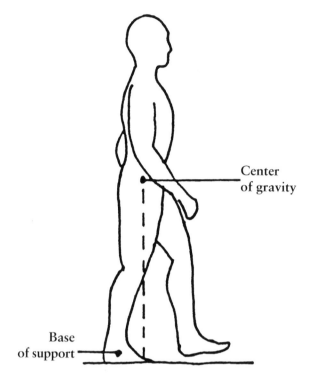

Figure 8.2 The center of gravity in relationship to the base of support during ambulation.

increased sway and unsteady balance. Postural sway has been shown to increase with advanced age, and is more marked in females than in males at all ages.[15] The reason for this sex difference is unknown.

The vestibular system helps a person achieve balance by maintaining visual perception and body orientation during movement about the environment. During periods of balance loss or body displacement, vestibular receptors located in the ear (semicircular canals and otoliths) initiate a series of compensatory limb, trunk, and head movements that serve to control postural sway and stability. This body-orientating response, or righting reflex, diminishes with age.[16] As a result, if an elderly person trips or slips (i.e., balance displacement) the chances of regaining stability and avoiding a fall decline.

In addition, certain musculoskeletal changes occur with age that influence balance. The elderly tend to display a slight curvature or kyphosis of the spine. This occurs as a consequence of either vertebral osteopenia and collapse or a need by the person with poor balance to maintain a low COG in relation to his or her BOS. In response, this forward, or stooped, posture may alter the balance threshold, as the COG is shifted forward beyond the BOS or critical point of stability. Subsequently, it becomes more difficult to thrust the foot forward (i.e., stepping strategy) fast enough to preserve stability during balance displacements. Also, there is an age-associated decline in proximal and distal muscle strength and ankle function.[17, 18] These changes may complicate the execution of a stepping strategy, making it difficult to adjust the COG in line with the BOS rapidly enough to avoid a fall. As well, the ability of an elderly person to transfer on and off furnishings and toilets or to get in and out of bathtubs safely and maintain balance is affected by a decline in muscle strength and joint function.

Normally, there is some redundancy in the sensory information needed to maintain balance. The failure of one source of input (e.g., a loss of proprioception) can be compensated for by another system, such as that derived from visual feedback. Dysfunction in more than one system, however, is likely to result in balance problems and an increased risk of falls. Studies of the elderly have shown that postural sway or unsteadiness is significantly greater in fallers than in nonfallers.[15] Moreover, there is an appreciable reduction in muscle strength and joint function in fallers compared with nonfallers.[3]

Gait

Gait, the manner of walking, consists of two phases: stance and swing. The stance phase occurs when one leg is in contact with the ground, and the swing phase occurs when the other leg advances forward to take the next step. Walking is accomplished by a series of reciprocal leg movements alternating between stance and swing (Figure 8.3): pushing off on the leg in stance, while at the same time swinging the other leg forward. To allow for adequate ground clearance during the swing phase, the leg is flexed at the knee and dorsiflexed at the ankle. When the heel of the swing leg strikes the ground (a return to the stance phase), the knee extends, and the foot plantar flexes to provide sufficient ground support.

Compared with younger individuals, elderly individuals experience a number of alterations in gait. The speed of walking, stride length (the distance the foot travels during the swing phase), heel lift (the level of ground clearance by the foot during swing phase), and ankle dorsiflexion decline with age.[19] Elderly women develop a narrow standing and walking base, often take small steps, and exhibit a pelvic waddle during ambulation. Conversely, elderly men tend to adopt a wide standing and walking base.

Whether these gait changes represent a decline in neuromuscular function or, in part, are attributable to environmental influences (e.g., the type and condition of shoes worn and ground surfaces walked on) remains speculative. In addition, their role in causing falls is not well understood. The gait of elderly individuals who fall, however, is often more compromised than the gait of elderly nonfallers and, to a certain degree, influences fall susceptibility. When the swing phase is interrupted, either because the foot fails adequately to clear the ground or because it encounters an irregularity on the floor (i.e., curled-up carpet or tile edge), a trip is likely to occur. When a bare foot bottom either encounters a surface of low frictional resistance (a wet floor, sliding rug) or approaches the ground with a change in stride length, a slip can occur. Whether

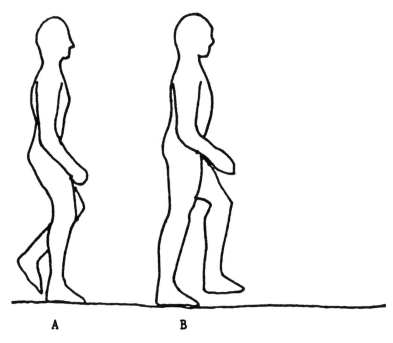

Figure 8.3 The stance (A) and swing (B) phase of gait.

a trip or slip results in a fall depends on a person's the ability to initiate and execute maneuvers that correct balance.

Diseases

Disease processes and the impairments that result play a more decisive role in fall causation than age-related physiologic changes occurring alone. Evidence indicates that elderly people who fall tend to have more medical diagnoses than elderly nonfallers.[1] Both acute and chronic conditions are often factors.

A fall may either be premonitory, in that the event represents the initial presentation of an underlying acute disease, or may follow the onset of illness. Acute disease processes most often identified as contributing to falls are those that interfere with postural stability. These include syncope, hypovolemia (dehydration, blood loss), cardiac arrhythmias, electrolyte disturbances, seizures, stroke, febrile conditions (e.g., urinary tract infections, pneumonias), and acute exacerbations of chronic diseases such as congestive heart failure and obstructive pulmonary disease.

Chronic disease processes that predispose to falling include any condition that interferes with mobility. The most common originate in the sensory and neuromuscular systems. For example, diseases of the eye (e.g., cataracts, macular degeneration, and glaucoma) adversely affect visual perception, acuity, dark adaptation, and contrast sensitivity. When combined with low illumination, these alterations in vision can interfere in the recognition of ground hazards (upended floor tiles and carpet edges, wet surfaces, and low-lying furnishings) and predispose to trips and slips. Parkinsonism affects postural control. The disease is associated with a loss of autonomic postural reflexes, leading to both propulsion and retropulsion. In addition, those with parkinsonism exhibit gait changes (short and shuffling steps, and poor initiation and freezing of gait) and cognitive impairments (characterized by a degree of depression, apathy, inertia, and an inflexibility of thought processes). Such abnormalities can lead to balance problems and difficulties with the recognition of environmental hazards. Dementia, particularly of the Alzheimer's type, is associated with gait ataxia and apraxia, proprioceptive loss, visual-spatial problems, agnosia, and decline in judgment. These deficits lead to a likelihood of falls due to misinterpretations of safe versus hazardous environmental conditions.

Neuropathy secondary to conditions such as diabetes, vitamin B_{12} deficiency, and cervical spondylosis is associated with lower-extremity weakness and altered proprioception. Proximal muscle weakness of the lower extremities, concomitant with conditions such as osteomalacia, thyroid disease, polymyalgia rheumatica, or deconditioning, can lead to a waddling, or a "penguin's gait," and balance loss (gluteal muscle weakness results in exaggerated lateral trunk movements). Lower-extremity hemiplegia or paresis results in decreased ankle dorsiflexion on foot clearance in walking and places a person at risk for tripping.

Osteoarthritis of the hips and knees can lead to a decrease in single-limb support due to pain and stiff or inflexible joints. Both can interfere with foot-ground clearance and maintaining stability during ambulation. Foot disorders (uncut nails, bunions, callouses) can lead to mechanical gait disorders.

Medications

Any drug that interferes with postural control and cognitive function may influence gait and balance and thereby place elderly people at fall risk. Common offenders include sedatives, antipsychotics, antihypertensives, and antidepressants.[9] Alcohol deserves special mention because most studies have failed to demonstrate an association between alcohol and an increase in falls.[20] Commonsense dictates otherwise, however. Alcohol is a central nervous system depressant and, as such, may adversely affect gait, balance, cognition, and increase risk-taking behavior. Also, given equal intake, blood alcohol levels in the elderly tend to be higher than those in younger subjects. Even small amounts of alcohol, particularly in those with existing physical frailty, can increase the risk of falling. As well, alcohol may have osteoporotic effects that can increase the risk of fall-related fractures.

In general, the risk of drug-related falls is increased with medications that have extended half-lives and with the number of medications taken simultaneously, as the chances of drug-drug interactions are greater.

Environmental Factors

The overwhelming majority of falls experienced by community-residing elderly individuals occur in the home setting.[21] This may be a reflection of the increased time that elderly people at risk spend at home. Most falls take place in the bedroom, bathroom, living room, and on stairways.[21] Within acute-care hospitals and nursing homes, the majority of falls occur in the bedroom and bathroom.[21] Environmental factors have been implicated as a contributing factor in one-third to one-half of all falls.[1, 2, 20] Several environmental obstacles and design features, in conjunction with host-initiated mobility activities, are associated with falling. These consist of low or elevated bed heights; unstable, low-seated, armless chairs; low toilet seats that lack grab bar support; getting in and out of bathtubs and stepping on wet or low frictional ground surfaces; walking in poorly illuminated areas; tripping over elevated floor coverings (thick pile carpets, unsecured rug edges, door thresholds); slipping on polished or wet ground surfaces and sliding rugs; climbing and descending stairs that lack handrail support and sufficient lighting; and reaching up to place or retrieve objects from excessively high shelves.[21] The likelihood of the environment contributing to fall risk is greatest in those with impaired mobility, as the environment and its design may interfere with the person's level of competence.

Assistive devices (canes, walkers) that support mobility can contribute to falls, particularly if they are used improperly, are in poor repair (worn rubber tips, structural defects), or are not easy to use because of space limitations in the home. Improper footwear can lead to gait and balance problems. Wearing high-heeled shoes narrows one's standing and walking BOS, decreases stride length, and causes one to assume a forward leaning posture. Poorly fitting shoes, particularly when loose, can alter the gait pattern. In an effort to keep their feet in the shoes, an elderly person may assume a shuffling type of gait. Wearing leather-soled shoes or socks promotes slipping. Rubber crepe soles, often prescribed for the elderly because they are slip-resistant, may stick to linoleum or carpet surfaces. In those with decreased foot-ground clearance, rubber-soled footwear can lead to immediate an halting gait and the risk of balance loss and falls. Thick-soled footwear (running shoes, tennis sneakers) may be overly absorptive and decrease proprioceptive feedback (gained from the foot striking the ground), thus contributing to balance loss.

Fall Risk Factors

A host of intrinsic factors are strongly associated with the risk of falls in the elderly. These include previous falls and stumbles, postural hypotension, reduced lower-extremity strength and sensory impairment, decreased vision, altered cognition, urinary dysfunction (incontinence, nocturia), and polypharmacy.[1, 2, 9] The risk of falling increases with the number of intrinsic factors present.[1] Environmental hazards can exacerbate the risk of falls, particularly in those with decreased mobility. Psychological and behavioral factors that influence how an elderly person perceives and adapts to dynamic changes in their capabilities are potential fall risk factors.

Injury Risk Factors

As stated previously, falls are associated with both physical and psychological injury. For anyone, the risk of sustaining a hip fracture is dependent on a number of interacting factors.[22] These include the height of the fall, the ability to exhibit protective reflexes, the presence of shock absorbers (to cushion the impact of a fall), bone strength, and the type of impact surface. A fall from a standing or walking height, particularly when unexpected, is more likely to result in injury than a fall from a relatively low height, such as from a toilet or chair. The initiation of protective reflexes—extending the arm outward (the righting reflex) to grasp an environmental structure (e.g., chair back, wall surface) and shifting the feet quickly to regain a BOS—may avert a fall in progress or minimize the force of impact on the ground. Conversely, the presence of neuromuscular dysfunction or medications that interfere with reaction time and the ability to display a protective response increases both the force or impact of falling and the risk of injury. Increased fat and muscle bulk surrounding the hip area may absorb the impact of a fall. In those who have decreased fat padding or muscle atrophy, injury after a fall to the ground is more likely to occur. A loss of bone strength due to osteoporosis may result in "spontaneous" hip fractures during weight-bearing or a fracture even with minimal ground impact. And lastly, falls against a hard, nonabsorptive floor surface are more likely to result in injury than falls onto absorptive surfaces such as carpets. Interventions that attenuate the force of impact of the fall, such as the wearing of hip pads or absorbent floor surfaces, may help decrease the risk of hip fractures.[23]

The risk of developing a fear of falling is greatest in those who have an underlying gait or balance impairment, recurrent falls occurring over a short time period, and sustaining, as a result, physical injury or functional loss. Living alone (lack of others to provide activities of daily living assistance) and suffering prolonged postfall lie times are associated with a fear of falling. The use of emergency alarm response systems (such as a pendent device, which is activated by a fall) may reduce lie times and the fear of falling.

INTERVENTIONS

The overall goal of fall prevention is to minimize fall risk by ameliorating or eliminating contributing factors while at the same time maintaining or improving the patient's mobility and autonomy. Potential interventions are based on known risk factors and postulated causes of falls and consist of medical, rehabilitative, and environmental strategies.

Medical Strategies

Medical interventions aimed at fall prevention consist of ruling out contributing acute or chronic pathologic conditions and adverse effects associated with medications as well as instituting appropriate treatment when necessary. After an episode

Table 8.1   Clinical evaluation of falls and fall risk

Step 1: Has the person fallen? If yes, proceed to Step 2. If no falls have occurred, proceed to Step 3 and assess fall risk.
Step 2: After evaluating and treating for physical injury, obtain a fall history.
Step 3: Review medical and medication history.
Step 4: Obtain performance-oriented mobility screen.
Step 5: Perform physical examination.
Step 6: Obtain laboratory studies and diagnostic testing.
Step 7: List differential diagnosis of fall(s) or identified fall risk factors.
Step 8: Implement interventions to reduce fall risk.
Step 9: Follow up to determine success of interventions.
Step 10: Repeat evaluation if the patient continues to fall. Repeat fall risk assessment on a regular basis.

of falling, depending on the time interval between the episode and patient examination, evaluate and treat any life-threatening medical conditions that may have precipitated the event and any physical injury that may have occurred. Once the person is medically stable, a focused clinical evaluation should be performed. The intent of the evaluation of those with a history of falls is to discover the causative factors, and in those without falls, to identify the presence of fall risk factors. Second, based on the factors found, targeted interventions to minimize the risk of falling should be initiated. The components of the clinical evaluation of falls and fall risk are listed in Table 8.1. This stepped approach is applicable for both the community- and institutional-residing populations.

Fall History

The purpose of the fall history is to ascertain the possible factors involved. It consists of inquiring about the circumstances surrounding the fall. Ask about any symptoms preceding or associated with the fall, the location of the fall, the activity engaged in at the time, the time of the fall, and the consequences of the fall (injury, prolonged postfall lie time, fear of falling). Inquire about previous falls and their circumstances. This may help to establish a pattern of falling and determine an etiology. Many repeat falls occurring over a short time period have a solitary cause. A convenient acronym to help remember and record the components of the fall history is SPLATT: Symptoms, Previous falls, Location, Activity, Time, and Trauma (the physical and psychological consequences). Information acquired from a fall history will usually provide important clues to the diagnosis of falling and its effect on the patient. The following case study illustrates this point.

M.B. is an 82-year-old female with a history of five falls. Her medical history was remarkable for osteoarthritis of the knees, treated with a non-

Table 8.2 Fall diary

Falling down is not a normal part of growing old. There are many causes of falls that can be treated. In order to prevent falls, we need to know as much about your falls as possible. This diary will help you remember the times when you fall. Each time you fall, write down the date of the fall, time of day when you fall, where you fall (location), what you were doing at the time (activity), and how you felt (symptoms). Below we have listed two examples:

Date	April 8
Time	8 A.M.
Location	Bedroom
Activity	Getting out of bed
Symptoms	I felt dizzy.
Date	May 1
Time	10 P.M.
Location	Bathroom
Activity	Slipped while walking
Symptoms	None

steroidal anti-inflammatory drug (NSAID). During questioning, M.B. stated that all her falls occurred in the bedroom while getting out of bed in the morning and were accompanied by symptoms of "dizziness." She also expressed a fear of falling and sustaining a hip fracture. The circumstances surrounding M.B.'s falls suggested a differential diagnosis of postural hypotension. An evaluation revealed the presence of orthostatic hypotension and an iron-deficiency anemia. Further diagnostic studies uncovered gastrointestinal bleeding secondary to the use of NSAIDs. Her orthostasis, falls, and, eventually, her fear of falls subsided after treatment of the anemia and discontinuation of the NSAIDs.

Although some elderly people give a clear account of their falls, others, because of memory problems, may not be able to recall accurately the number or circumstances of the occurrences. This is a common problem in the community, as it may be weeks to months before an elderly person is questioned about falling episodes. A fall diary (Table 8.2) used to record the circumstances of further falls may be helpful. Others, out of embarrassment or a fear of being viewed as frail and dependent and being placed in a nursing home, underreport or fail fully to disclose the true extent of their falls. People with dementia will not be able to provide accurate fall histories. In these cases, information should be obtained from family members, significant others, and health providers if available.

Once the fall history is obtained, past medical problems, current complaints, and medications should be reviewed. The latter is particularly important because recent prescription drug or dosage changes or the use of over-the-counter medications may provide a clue to the cause of falling.

Assessment of Gait and Balance

The next step is to examine the patient. In the absence of an identifiable medical cause of falling, an assessment should begin with an evaluation of the patient's mobility. The observation of gait and balance is a better predictor of altered mobility than the standard neuromuscular examination.[24] There are several instruments that can be used to assess an elderly person's mobility, including the Get Up and Go Test and the Performance-Oriented Assessment of Mobility (POMS).[25, 26] An example of a performance-oriented mobility instrument that one of the authors of this chapter (R.T.) designed from the aforementioned instruments is provided in Table 8.3. The POMS is a quick clinical screen that assesses a person's gait and balance and consists of observing the person perform a number of mobility tasks. Ask the individual to rise from a chair (not using the armrests or seat edge for assistive support), stand without assistive support, walk in a straight line (a distance of about 15 feet) and turn around (with assistive walking devices if used for ambulation), bend down and pick up an object from the ground, return to the chair and sit down. Lastly, ask the person to lie down on the floor and get up unassisted (to assess the risk of prolonged postfall lie times). A normal POMS is demonstrated if the person can accomplish each balance task (chair transfers, immediate standing, bending down) and floor-rising maneuver in a smooth and controlled manner, without difficulties or a loss of balance. Gait is normal when walking is continuous, without hesitation or excessive sway, and both feet clear the floor. Turning is normal when stepping is continuous, without staggering or balance loss.

At this point, a Romberg's test to assess proprioception and a sternal nudge or push test to assess postural competence should be performed. Romberg's test is performed with the person standing erect, the feet positioned together, arms placed by his or her sides, and both eyes closed. An abnormal response is demonstrated by increased sway and balance loss. The sternal nudge test is accomplished with the person in the standing position. The examiner, standing behind the person, nudges the person's sternum with enough pressure to elicit a displacement of balance backward. A normal response is demonstrated by a rapid step backward, often associated with a brisk forward movement of both arms (the righting reflex). An abnormal response consists of the person falling into the examiner's arms because of an ineffective stepping strategy (to preserve balance) or because of a complete absence of the righting reflex.

The POMS is useful in detecting mobility problems in elderly people with underlying neuromuscular diseases. Abnormalities discovered on the POMS may provide clues as to the cause of the person's falls (Table 8.4), localize the organ systems involved, and guide the clinician in performing the

Table 8.3 Performance-Oriented Mobility Screen

Instructions: Ask the patient to perform the following maneuvers. For each maneuver, indicate whether the patient's performance is normal or abnormal.

Ask Patient to	Observation	
	Normal	*Abnormal*
Sit down in chair (select a chair with armrests approximately 16–17 inches in seat height)	❏ Able to sit down in one smooth controlled movement without using armrests	❏ Sitting is not a smooth movement; falls into chair or needs armrests to guide
Rise up from chair	❏ Able to rise in one smooth movement without using armrests	❏ Uses armrests, moves forward in chair, or both to propel self up; requires several attempts to get up
Stand (for approximately 30 secs) after rising from chair	❏ Steady, able to stand without support	❏ Unsteady, loses balance
Stand with eyes closed (for approximately 15 secs)	❏ Steady, able to stand without support	❏ Unsteady, loses balance
Stand with eyes open; the examiner nudges the patient on the sternum with light pressure three times	❏ Steady, needs to move feet, but able to withstand pressure and maintain balance	❏ Unsteady, begins to fall
Walk in a straight line (approximately 15 feet) at "usual" pace, then back again	❏ Gait is continuous without hesitation; walks in a straight line and feet clear ❏ With aid ❏ Without aid	❏ Gait is noncontinuous, with deviation from straight path; feet scrape or shuffle on floor ❏ With aid ❏ Without aid
Walk a distance of 5 feet and turn around	❏ No staggering; steps are smooth and continuous ❏ With aid ❏ Without aid	❏ Staggering; steps are unsteady and discontinuous ❏ With aid ❏ Without aid

Note: If the patient uses a walk aid such as a cane or walker, the walking maneuvers are tested separately, with and without the aid. Indicate type of aid used:
❏ Cane ❏ Walker ❏ Other ❏ None

physical examination. The POMS provided useful information in the following case.

> *L.N. is an 86-year-old male with two recent falls. He stated that both falls occurred while transferring from a chair. The POMS confirmed a decreased ability to transfer independently from a chair and suggested proximal muscle weakness as a cause of L.N.'s falls. A directed physical and diagnostic examination revealed the presence of hypothyroidism. On receiving replacement treatment, the patient's falls subsided.*

Table 8.4 Differential diagnoses of abnormal Performance-Oriented Mobility Screen maneuvers

Impaired Maneuver	Intrinsic Factor	Extrinsic Factor
Chair transfer (possibly impaired bed, toilet, and bathtub transfers)	Parkinsonism Arthritis Deconditioning	Poor chair design (possibly faulty bed, toilet, and bathtub design)
Standing balance	Postural hypotension Vestibular dysfunction Adverse drug effects	
Romberg's test	Proprioceptive dysfunction Adverse drug effects	Poor illumination Overly absorptive footwear, carpeting, or both
Sternal nudge test	Parkinsonism Normal-pressure hydro- cephalus Adverse drug effects	
Bending down	Neuromuscular dysfunc- tion Adverse drug effects	
Walking or turning	Gait disorders (parkin- sonism, hemiparesis, or foot problem) Sensory dysfunction Adverse drug effects	Improper footwear Improper size or use of ambulation devices Hazardous ground surfaces (slippery, uneven)
Rising from floor	Neuromuscular dysfunc- tion	

Abnormalities on the POMS may also help in isolating environmental conditions contributing to dysmobility (see Table 8.4). In L.N.'s case, a decrease in chair transfers indicated that the patient might also have problems with other activities such as toilet and bathtub transfers. L.N. verified problems in performing these activities and was provided with appropriate assistive medical equipment.

Assessment of Fall Risk

As part of the medical evaluation, the elderly should always be assessed for fall risk by reviewing the medical history and identifying those conditions and medications that place them at risk (Table 8.5). The POMS is performed to assess the elderly person's mobility; any dysfunction of gait and balance detected is strongly correlated with fall risk. In the absence of identifiable risk factors and a normal POMS, the person is at low fall risk. The presence of one or more risk factors and any abnormalities discovered on the POMS, however, indicate fall risk and should trigger further investigation to search for modifiable factors.

Table 8.5 Fall risk factors

Postural hypotension
Lower-extremity weakness
Gait dysfunction
Balance dysfunction
Visual impairment
Cognitive impairment
Urinary dysfunction
Medications (e.g., psychotropics, sedatives)

Physical Assessment and Diagnostic Evaluation

The last steps in the evaluation process consist of a physical examination and obtaining diagnostic and laboratory studies. The extent of the physical examination is dictated by the information gathered from the fall history, risk factor assessment, and POMS. In the absence of historical information, the physical examination should focus on organ systems that affect gait and balance and consists of a comprehensive neuromuscular, cardiovascular, and cognitive analysis.

Diagnostic tests and laboratory studies used to investigate falls and fall risk should be selective, based on clinical suspicions derived from previous evaluations. Obtaining routine laboratory and diagnostic studies (chemistries, hematology, Holter monitoring, brain imaging, electromyogram) are rarely useful in the absence of symptoms or demonstrated physical findings.

Once the evaluation process is complete and a list of factors that contribute to either falls or fall risk is assembled, interventions aimed at ameliorating or eliminating the factors are addressed. Efforts at prevention must strike a balance between protecting the person from the risk of falls and maintaining mobility and personal autonomy.

REHABILITATIVE STRATEGIES

Those who fail to improve or respond to medical treatment may benefit from a trial of rehabilitative therapy. For those with chronic neuromuscular disorders, a program of exercises aimed at correcting gait and balance impairments may reduce fall risk.[27] For example, in those with degenerative joint disease, exercise directed toward improving joint flexibility and lower-extremity muscle strength may enhance ambulation and transfer mobility. For those with parkinsonism, a program of ambulation training, muscle strengthening, and postural exercise can improve mobility. For those with dementia, a daily program of walking can offset altered gait and balance that commonly result from immobility. Habitual exercise may improve cognitive functioning in demented patients and reduce falls that result from poor judgment (e.g., taking part in hazardous activities). In elderly women with osteoporosis, weight-bearing exercise such as walking and stair-climbing can minimize further bone loss, thereby reducing the risk of fracture. For those whose bone density is already well below the fracture threshold, exercise may be useful for its effect on proximal muscle strength and coordination of gait and balance, ultimately reducing the likelihood of falls. Also, exercise therapy helps restore confidence and reduce the fear of instability and falls. As any program of exercise will need to be designed in accordance with the patient's general health, it is prudent to refer patients to a physiatrist.

Elderly people at risk of falls who live alone and have difficulty getting up from the floor unassisted should be provided with a personal emergency alarm system. Alarm systems are designed to provide the elderly who fall with a means to summon help. Their basic elements include a portable help button worn as a necklace or bracelet, a console unit integrated with the telephone, and a response center that sends immediate help. Those unable to afford an alarm system or who refuse its use should be instructed on how to get up from the floor. Most can be taught to move themselves along the floor to a chair or sofa and, with its support, get themselves into a side-sitting position. From there, they assume a kneeling position with the support of the chair and, with the strongest knee, push themselves up onto the chair.

Attention to footwear can support safe patterns of gait. Shoes with rubber or crepe soles provide adequate slip resistance on most ground surfaces. Socks with nonskid treads are helpful for those who prefer to walk about bare-footed. For those with shuffling gait or poor steppage height, footwear with rubber soles may stick to ground surfaces and lead to tripping. Shoes with leather soles that glide along floor surfaces may be a better choice in these individuals. High-heeled footwear should be avoided, as it decreases the standing and walking BOS and promotes balance loss. Footwear with low heels (<3.5 cm in height) and broad surfaces (5.5 cm in width) are best suited to provide maximum balance support. For women who want to wear high heels, either for reasons of vanity or because a life-long use of high heeled footwear (resulting in short heel cords) necessitates their use, shoes with wedge heels should be recommended. The best way to ensure that footwear is adequate is to observe the person walking about in the home environment.

For those with gait and balance disorders, ambulation devices can be used to improve mobility. These devices function by increasing the person's standing and walking BOS and stability. Also, they provide a sense of confidence and a visual means of support that help reduce the fear of instability and falls. To ensure optimum function, canes and walkers need to be of the proper size, in good repair, and used properly.

ENVIRONMENTAL STRATEGIES

Environmental interventions consist of two approaches. First, identify and eliminate hazardous conditions in the home that interfere with mobility and increase fall risk. Table 8.6 lists some of the most common home environmental hazards and can be used as a checklist by elderly persons, family members, and clini-

Table 8.6 Environmental hazard checklist

Illumination
  Are lights bright enough to support vision and mobility?
  Are lights and lighting conditions glare-free?
  Are light switchplates and lamp pull cords/switches in all rooms and stairways both
    visually and physically accessible?
  Are light switchplates located by the entry way of all rooms and at the top and bot-
    tom of stairs (to avoid ambulation in the dark)?
  Are night-lights available in the bedroom and bathroom?
Floor surfaces
  Are floor surfaces slip-resistant?
  Are carpet edges tacked or taped down?
  Are throw rugs nonslip?
  Are pathways free of low-lying and difficult-to-visualize objects?
Stairways
  Are step surfaces in good repair and slip-resistant?
  Are handrails present to support mobility?
Furnishings
  Are beds low in height and stable to support transfers?
  Are chairs outfitted with armrests and stable to support transfers?
  Are bedside and dining room tables stable to support seating and walking mobility?
Bathroom
  Are toilet grab rails available to support transfers?
  Are bathtub grab rails available to support transfers?
  Are bathroom grab rails securely fastened to toilets and bathtub or mounted on
    walls?
  Are bathtub surfaces slip-resistant?

cians. Second, simplify or maximize mobility tasks through the modification of the environment and existing furnishings. This is best accomplished by observing patients function in their living environment and determining whether a particular area or furnishing is safe or hazardous. Ask the individual to walk through every room; over floor surfaces and door thresholds; transfer on and off the bed, chairs, and toilet; get in and out of the bathtub or shower; climb and descend stairs; reach up to obtain objects from kitchen and closet shelves; and bend down to retrieve objects from cabinets. Note which environmental features interfere with safe mobility so that adaptive modifications can be arranged.

The following discussion focuses on aspects of the environment most likely to contribute to unsafe mobility and suggests a number of modifications.

Lighting

Low lighting levels can be increased by using 100-watt light bulbs. Using light-colored wall coverings will increase the reflective quality of available light.

Rheostatic light switches or three-way light bulbs allow one to increase and decrease illumination levels as desired. Night-lights can be placed in high-risk fall locations, such as the top and bottom of stairways, bedrooms, and bathrooms. A "clapper light," a device that turns on lights automatically when it senses clapping the hands together, can be helpful. Glare from unshielded light bulbs can be eliminated by either using translucent shades or coverings or frosted light bulbs. Window glare can be controlled with sheer drapery or mylar-tinted shades that diffuse glare without reducing the amount of available light. Floor glare is reduced by using carpets or floor finishes that diffuse rather than reflect light.

Ground Surfaces

Carpets, rugs, and linoleum tiles that are patterned and those with checkered or floral designs should be avoided. These coverings tend to interfere with depth perception and balance stability. Floor coverings should be solid in color. Sliding throw rugs and carpets should be replaced. As an alternative, double-sided, slip-resistant, adhesive backing should be applied or nonslip matting placed underneath. Carpet edges that are prone to buckling or curling should be tacked or taped down. Linoleum and wooden floors are made slip-resistant by applying nonskid finishes. Bathroom tiles can be rendered slip-resistant by applying nonskid adhesive strips or decorative decals on the floor next to the toilet, sink, and bathtub. The use of indoor-outdoor carpeting on bathroom floors has similar benefits and also provides cushioning that may decrease the impact of a fall and reduce the risk of injury.

Beds

Elevated bed heights can be eliminated by replacing thick mattresses with those thinner in width. The mattress should be firm to support bed transfers. Within institutional settings, height-adjustable beds can be used to ensure proper bed height. For those who use the head- or footboard for assistance when transferring in and out of bed, their surfaces should be slip-resistant. The application of nonslip adhesive tape along the top length of foot- and headboards will help prevent hands from slipping. Half-side rails can be used as assistive devices to support safe transfers. Beds that slide away during transfers can be placed against a wall for support if feasible. If bed floor surfaces are slippery, have the patient wear traction-soled socks or slippers.

Chairs

To support seated transfers, all chairs used by elderly individuals should have armrests. Armrests provide leverage during rising, gradual deceleration when sitting, and can usually compensate for low seat heights. Armrests located approximately 7 inches above the seat and extending slightly beyond the front seat edge provide maximum support. A cushion can increase seating height, its thickness determined by the height needed to support independent transfers.

Bathrooms

The addition of a double armrest toilet grab bar compensates for low toilet heights. These devices are height- and width-adjustable and offer better support and leverage than conventional wall-mounted grab bars. Towel bars used for balance support should be replaced with wall-mounted grab bars. The grab bars should be slip-resistant, color-contrasted from the wall for visibility, and securely fixed to the studs of the wall for adequate support. Nonslip adhesive strips can be placed on the top of sink edges to guard against hand slippage if these surfaces are used for support. A rubber mat or nonslip adhesive strips applied to the bathtub floor surface provide stable footing. Wall-mounted grab bars in the bathtub provide support during tub transfers. Their location is determined by where the person customarily places his or her hands during transfers. The use of an adjustable grab bar that attaches onto the edge of bath rim can be used for further transfer support. In those with severe balance loss, the use of bathtub benches and extended shower hoses can serve as alternatives to ensure safe bathing.

Stairs

All stairways should be equipped with handrails for support. They should be round in shape, slip-resistant, and color-contrasted from the wall for visibility. The application of nonskid treads to all step edges reduces the likelihood of slipping.

Shelves

To remedy the problem of low or high shelf heights, frequently used items should be placed at a level that allows the person to avoid excessive bending or reaching. A hand-held reacher device can be employed as an alternative.

COMPLIANCE

The compliance of elderly individuals to environmental modifications and recommendations for durable medical equipment depends on a number of factors. Compliance is enhanced if the modification or equipment improves mobility, does not impose an excessive economic burden, is easily obtained, and is simple to implement.[28]

SUMMARY

Falls are a common problem for the elderly and are associated with significant mortality and morbidity. Falling is not an inevitable consequence of aging. Rather, most episodes are the result of identifiable acute and chronic disease processes, adverse medication effects, and environmental hazards in the home. Preventive interventions consist of medical strategies aimed at identifying the circumstances of falls and fall risk and attempting to modify the factors responsible. For those who remain at fall risk, rehabilitative and environmental strategies should be tried. In most cases, the approach to reducing fall risk includes components of each strategy.

REFERENCES

1. Tinetti ME, Speechley M, Ginter SF. Risk factors for falls among elderly persons living in the community. N Engl J Med 1988;319:1701.
2. Rubenstein LZ, Robbins AS, Schulman BL, et al. Falls and instability in the elderly. J Am Geriatr Soc 1988;36:266.
3. Blake AJ, Morgan K, Bendall MJ, et al. Falls by elderly people at home: prevalence and associated factors. Age Ageing 1988;17:365.
4. Campell AJ, Borrie MJ, Spears GF, et al. Circumstances and consequences of falls experienced by a community population 70 years and over during a prospective study. Age Ageing 1990;19:136.
5. Tinetti ME, Speechley M. Prevention of falls among the elderly. N Engl J Med 1989;320:1055.
6. Wild D, Nayak USL, Isaacs B. How dangerous are falls in old people at home? BMJ 1981;282:2132.
7. Melton LJ, Riggs BL. Risk factors for injury after a fall. Clin Geriatr Med 1985;1:525.
8. Evans JG, Prudham D, Wandless I. A prospective study of fractured proximal femur: incidence and outcome. Public Health 1979;93:235.
9. Nevitt MC, Cummings SR, Kidd D, Black D. Factors for recurrent nonsyncopal falls: a prospective study. JAMA 1989;261:2663.
10. Sheldon JH. On the natural history of falls in old age. BMJ 1960;2:1685.
11. Kolanowski AM. The clinical importance of environmental lighting to the elderly. J Gerontol Nurs 1992;18:10.
12. Kokeman E, Bossemyer RW, Barney J. Neurologic manifestations of aging. J Gerontol 1977;32:411.
13. Werner JS, Peterzell DH, Scheetz AJ. Light, vision, and ageing. Optom Vis Sci 1990;67:214.
14. Skinner HB, Barrack RL, Cook SD. Age-related decline in proprioception. Clin Orthop 1984;184:208.
15. Overstall PW, Exton-Smith AN, Imms FJ, Johnson AL. Falls in the elderly related to postural balance. BMJ 1977;1:261.
16. Sloan PD, Baloh RW, Honrubia A. The vestibular system in the elderly: clinical implications. Am J Otolaryngol 1986;10:422.
17. Larson L, Grimby G, Karlsson J. Muscle strength and speed of movement in relation to age and muscle morphology. J Appl Physiol 1979;46:451.
18. Whipple R, Wolfson LI, Amerman P. The relationship of knee and ankle weakness to falls in nursing home residents: an isokinetic study. J Am Geriatr Soc 1987;35:13.
19. Gabell A, Nayak USL. The effect of age on variability of gait. J Gerontol 1984;39:662.
20. Nelson DE, Sattin RW, Langlois JA, et al. Alcohol as a risk factor for fall injury events among elderly persons living in the community. J Am Geriatr Soc 1992;40:658.
21. Tideiksaar R. Falling in Old Age: Its Prevention and Treatment. New York: Springer, 1989;49.
22. Cummings SR, Nevitt MC. A hypothesis: the causes of hip fractures. J Gerontol 1989;44:107.

23. Nevitt MC, Cummings SR. Type of fall and risk of hip and wrist fractures: the study of osteoporotic fractures. J Am Geriatr Soc 1993;41:1226.

24. Tinetti ME, Ginter SF. Identifying mobility dysfunctions in elderly patients. JAMA 1988;259:1190.

25. Mathias S, Nayak US, Isaacs B. Balance in the elderly: the get-up and go test. Arch Phys Med Rehabil 1986;67:387.

26. Tinetti ME. Performance-oriented assessment of mobility problems in elderly patients. J Am Geriatr Soc 1986;34:119.

27. Elward K, Larson EB. Benefits of exercise for older adults. A review of existing evidence and current recommendations for the general population [review]. Clin Geriatr Med 1992;8:35.

28. Tideiksaar R. Environmental adaptations to preserve balance and prevent falls. Topics Geriatr Rehabil 1990;5:78.

9

Issues in the Management of Seizures in Elderly Patients

Tess L. Sierzant

Although aging can be thought of as beginning with conception, the term is most often associated with members of our society who are 65 years of age and older. Aging for this group is also associated with many developmental tasks. These include adjusting to changes in health status and physical strength, dealing with retirement and a reduced income, coping with changes in living arrangements, finding new meaning and satisfaction with life, adjusting to the reality of death, and accepting oneself as an aging person.[1]

Stereotypes haunt the elderly individual, and the management approach taken with elderly patients must take into account not only societal stereotypes but also health professionals' biases as well. These include perceptions that elderly people are dependent, asexual, pessimistic toward the future, meddlesome, insecure, and lonely; that they have memory loss; that they are undervalued by their families; that they have limited interests; and that they are in poor physical and mental health.[2]

A gerontologic nursing model described by McConnell[3] is based on several assumptions that challenge many of these stereotypes. In this model, the elderly individual is viewed as an open system capable of change. He or she is affected by a variety of factors in unique ways and is capable of making independent decisions. Thus, an elderly person is able to benefit from a variety of health services and from health promotion teaching.

Attitudes can influence the depth of assessments made, and areas of dysfunction may be incompletely dealt with when attributed exclusively to the aging process. A custodial focus can be changed by incorporating information about health promotion, teaching the individual to minimize the effects of chronic disease, and reinforcing positive coping measures.

As life expectancy increases, health professionals will encounter a greater number of patients older than age 65 years. With the incidence of epilepsy highest in the oldest segments of our population, the numbers of elderly individuals who develop seizures will increase. Management requires an integrated team approach to which nursing can make a strong contribution. In the hospital setting, nurses are able to make frequent observations of patients' behavior and may be the first to identify seizure activity in an elderly patient. Similarly, in nursing homes, home-care settings, and the community, nurses may play a key role in this process.

Assessment of the elderly individual is complex and challenging due to the multiple variables that influence the aging process, including lifestyle, genetic composition, family characteristics, personality patterns, the environment, and socioeconomic factors.[4] Marjory Gordon's Functional Health Patterns, first described in 1982,[5, 6] provide a framework for patient assessment and establishment of a database that can be used to identify areas of dysfunction and nursing diagnoses. Functional assessment aids in defining a patient's concerns. Patients may view illness as a degree of discomfort with restriction of activity rather than a medical diagnosis.[7] Patients may perceive themselves as healthy because they are still able to do the things they need and want to do. Functional assessment is useful in realistic goal-setting and in the selection of interventions, particularly in those patients with chronic, progressive, or irreversible conditions. The patterns are useful in a variety of settings, including hospitals, clinics, extended-care facilities, nursing homes, private homes, and the community. A single pattern cannot be understood without knowledge of the others. Each is influenced by biological, spiritual, developmental, social, and cultural factors and is an expression of biopsychosocial integration. The 11 functional health patterns provide a holistic and understandable framework for discussion of the management of the elderly individual with epilepsy.

HEALTH PERCEPTION AND HEALTH MANAGEMENT

In this pattern, the patient's perceptions of his or her health, well-being, and health management activities are assessed. These perceptions influence activities such as nutrition, exercise, use of alcohol and tobacco, safety practices, and adherence to health promotion activities. The patient's health perception provides insight into self-concept, need for education, and desire for change. Ability to articulate goals for health maintenance also provides insight.

In an elderly individual newly diagnosed with epilepsy, the relationship of the patient's concept of health to this diagnosis is explored. The elderly individual may have matured with negative stereotypes of epilepsy and may now perceive himself or herself as unhealthy or a different, less-valued person than previously. Determining the person's understanding of the cause of the seizures and factors in his or her lifestyle that contribute to their ongoing occurrence is important. Misconceptions may need clarification. The older adult may have difficulty gaining access to services important to health maintenance. Although the motivation and understanding may be present, decreased physical mobility, lack of transportation, or limited finances may contribute to the underutilization of services. Driving restrictions related to epilepsy may have an impact on health perception and health management. A fear of trying alternate means of transportation, lack of social support, or altered perceptions regarding the importance of follow-up care may alter health management. A thorough understanding of first aid for various seizure types improves the patient's confidence and ability to manage seizure occurrence, either alone or with the help of others.

Ongoing assessment of safety practices in the elderly individual should take place. As functional status is impaired only episodically, there is a tendency for staff to become lax with precautions. Judicious use of restraints, especially in elderly patients whose mobility is already impaired, is warranted. The potential for injury during seizures, as in any age group, must be balanced with maximum independence and participation in activities.

NUTRITIONAL AND METABOLIC STATUS

In this pattern, the relationship of food and fluid consumption to metabolic need is described. Type and quantity of food consumed, eating times, food preferences, and dietary supplements are described when assessing this pattern. Skin lesions; ability to heal; and the condition of the hair, nails, mucous membranes, and teeth are included along with body temperature, height, and weight. Difficulty with eating, swallowing impairment, and dietary restrictions are assessed. This pattern may be affected by ill-fitting dentures, inability to shop for groceries or prepare meals, appetite, and income status. A multitude of risk factors are associated with poor nutritional status in the elderly population, including inappropriate food intake with disproportionate intake of snack foods and sweets, social isolation, dependency and disability, and chronic medication use.[8]

Changes in nutritional needs occur throughout life. Although there is no single standard for establishing malnutrition, many signs of poor nutritional status in elderly individuals exist. These include weight loss, reduction in serum protein, change in functional status, sustained inappropriate intake, and presence of certain nutrition-related disorders including folate deficiency.[8]

Nutritional status may strongly relate to the effectiveness of antiepileptic medications (AEMs). Nutrition can influence an individual's tolerance of medications, the extent of side effects, absorption, distribution, and binding of medications. It is imperative to incorporate assessment of this pattern when evaluating efficacy of AEMs.

The importance of assessing and integrating data from all of the functional health patterns becomes more evident when epilepsy is present with other deficits or diseases. For instance, cerebrovascular disease is the most frequent cause of seizures after age 50, and mobility may be restricted in a stroke survivor with epilepsy, thus decreasing caloric need. With impaired swallowing that occurs after some cerebrovascular accidents, however, nutritional status may deteriorate. If protein becomes depleted, serum levels of AEMs may be affected. Some AEMs may alter appetite; thus, as medication regimens are altered, ongoing nutritional status assessment should take place.

ELIMINATION

This pattern describes the excretory function of the bowel and bladder. Use of laxatives, problems with control, frequency, character, and associated discomfort with bowel function are assessed. A decrease in the functional capacity of the gastrointestinal system is often linked to pathologic problems rather than specific age-related changes. A decrease in blood flow to the organs of the gastrointestinal tract, along with a decrease in the size of the organs, may occur with increasing age. Motility may also decrease.

Frequency, urgency, and problems in control are areas of assessment of the urinary elimination pattern. Loss of nephrons and a decrease in renal mass accompany increasing age. There is also a decrease in creatinine clearance, and endocrine functions associated with the kidney diminish. The bladder tissue is altered as smooth muscle and elastic tissue are replaced with fibrous connective tissue. Bladder capacity is decreased, and the likelihood of loss of bladder control increases.

Changes in continence of bowel or bladder may occur with seizures. Incontinence—one of the most common reasons older adults are institutionalized—and persistent seizures may compound the problem. Urinary incontinence is embarrassing and may result in feelings of guilt, isolation, and reluctance to report it to health professionals. Discussion of incontinence should emphasize the availability and success of treatment modalities in the majority of individuals.

Diarrhea in elderly individuals has implications for nutritional status and may have an impact on the absorption of AEMs. Impaired appetite may contribute to constipation; as a result, some individuals may independently alter their medications. Assessments of the nutritional-metabolic pattern and the elimination pattern are often closely related.

ACTIVITY AND EXERCISE PATTERN

In this pattern, exercise, leisure, recreation, and activities of daily living such as cooking, shopping, and home maintenance are assessed. Factors that interfere with these activities are noted, including neuromuscular changes, musculoskeletal deficits, and alterations in cardiopulmonary functioning. Normal aging results in a progressive decrease in stature, particularly in women. There are changes in body appearance and distribution of fat and lean body mass. Bone tissue changes with age, and bone metabolism slows. Likewise, muscle wasting occurs, and regeneration of muscle tissue slows. Prolongation of contraction time, latency period, and relaxation period of motor units are associated with the aging process. Joints become more prone to inflammation, stiffness, pain, and deformity.

With aging, changes in the heart, blood, and blood vessels include thickening and stiffening of the cardiac valves, decrease in pacemaker cells of the sinoatrial node, loss of elasticity of the aorta, decreasing sensitivity of the baroreceptors, and decrease in blood volume and hemopoietic activity. The activity-exercise pattern is also affected by changes in the respiratory system. Extrapulmonary changes such as musculoskeletal deformities, osteoporosis of the ribs and vertebrae, and weakening of the muscles of respiration will affect respiratory function. Intrapulmonary changes associated with aging include progressive loss of lung elastic recoil and reduction of alveolar surface area. Vital capacity and oxygen saturation are decreased, and there is a decline in exercise tolerance.

Several epilepsy-related factors may influence this pattern. The type, frequency, and severity of seizures may have a significant impact on activity and exercise. Activities of daily living such as shopping and cooking may be profoundly affected. In an individual with diminished reserves for recovery, a generalized tonic-clonic seizure increases the potential for injury. Frequent seizures lead to fear and social isolation, and activities such as eating, cooking, and home maintenance may be altered, resulting in compromised nutritional status. The elderly patient may refrain from involvement in previous activities that have played a role in stress management, relationships, and self-esteem. Medication side effects and the duration of the postictal period are important considerations. The postictal period may be prolonged, thus interfering with participation in activities. The elderly person is likely to be taking medications for other conditions, with many having prescriptions for five to 13 other medications.[9] The potential for adverse side effects is therefore increased.

SLEEP AND REST

Patterns of sleep, rest, and relaxation include a subjective assessment by the patient of the quality and quantity of sleep and rest, a report of energy level, daytime functioning, and alcohol and drug use. As age increases, the amount of sleep decreases. Older individuals may take longer to fall asleep and awaken more frequently at night. Alteration in the usual pattern may result in irritability, decreased ability to concentrate, and increased stress. In some patients with epilepsy, sleep deprivation increases seizure frequency. AEMs may alter the normal sleep-wake cycle, resulting in more or less daily sleep. Side effects and the postictal period contribute to the amount of time the patient spends in sleep. Sleep may become the primary coping mechanism for an individual unable to deal with a diagnosis of epilepsy. Other patterns, including the activity-exercise pattern and the health perception-health management pattern, are affected by alterations in the sleep cycle.

COGNITION AND PERCEPTION

In assessing the cognition and perception pattern, sensory-cognitive and perceptual functions are evaluated, including vision, hearing, taste, touch, and smell. The use of compensatory techniques and prosthetics is identified. Pain and pain management are explored, and language, memory, and decision-making ability are assessed.

Neuronal loss in the brain and spinal cord occurs with aging and is most evident after the age of 70 years. Reaction time, proprioception, and balance decline. In addition, sensory changes may have a significant impact on the quality of life. Changes in the eye include limitation of upward gaze due to loss of orbital fat, diminished tear secretion, decreased corneal sensitivity, increased difficulty with accommodation, and decreased pupillary size. Changes in vision include decreases in visual acuity, tolerance of glare, adaptability to the dark and light, and peripheral vision. Some degree of hearing loss is virtually inevitable. Conductive and sensorineural hearing losses result from a variety of causes and often result in diminished speech discrimination and comprehension. Changes in taste and smell may occur, although these may be related to environmental factors such as smoking. Likewise, changes in somesthetic sensitivity may be due to illnesses that affect these functions rather than the aging process.

Because seizures in the elderly are often due to cerebrovascular disease, brain tumor, trauma, or Alzheimer's disease, alterations in the senses are often present. Language, memory, and higher cognitive functions such as decision-making are likely to be affected. Cognitive deficits play a role in the patient's response to education provided about epilepsy and in his or her understanding of the disorder. Timing of education is important in this population, and if vision or hearing is impaired, stimulation of a variety of sensory modalities will improve the patient's understanding. For example, use of color to help in the identification of particular medications may need to be supplemented by information regarding shape or texture.

The manner in which medications are used in the treatment of epilepsy may be confusing for patients who are receiving numerous medications for other conditions. The concepts of steady state and half-life may be new to them, and the need to take AEMs regularly may not be clear. Assessing the patient's understanding of the effectiveness of the current AEMs is useful when carrying out an education program.

Many patients complain of memory problems as a side effect of AEMs. This perception of altered memory, especially in the context of underlying cognitive dysfunction, may be stressful, thus contributing to greater memory difficulties. Moreover, a seizure often results in memory lapses, which may be prolonged. All these factors must be assessed frequently in the elderly patient, and topics such as seizure first aid, management of medications, and the unique nature of epilepsy itself should be discussed.

SELF-PERCEPTION AND SELF-CONCEPT

The self-perception–self-concept pattern describes attitudes and perceptions of abilities, body image, and sense of self. Emotional patterns; sense of worth; and patterns of body movement, such as eye contact and voice, are assessed. The patient's sense of hope and perception of control are part of this pattern. Numerous aspects of a person's self-concept remain stable over time, including traits such as well-being, sociability, openness to experience, and degree of extroversion or introversion. Caution in pursuing in new endeavors or relationships may grow with age. Personality traits, learning ability, and attitudes generally remain stable in the absence of disease. Many factors contribute to a sense of self-worth, including the extent of physical change, emotional support systems, and the perceived degree of control and independence.

The elderly person may have beliefs and attitudes about epilepsy reflective of less enlightened times. Being diagnosed with epilepsy may significantly alter the self-perception–self-concept pattern of functioning. The loss of sense of control is present for many with epilepsy. For the elderly individual with limited income, diminished mobility, death of friends, and physical impairments, the thought of having a seizure can be overwhelming. The concept of being "an epileptic" may lead to feelings of worthlessness. The patient's sense of hope may be affected, especially if seizures are resistant to control, and activity, nutrition, and coping strategies may be affected. Alterations in self-concept may be reflected by changes in eye contact and degree of participation in care, and a feeling of loss of control.

ROLES AND RELATIONSHIPS

The patient's pattern of relationships and his or her roles of active engagement are explored. Responsibilities and degree of satisfaction with these roles are identified. The family structure, living situation, and the family's methods of coping are described, and the interdependence of patient and family are explored. The family's perception of epilepsy is part of this functional pattern. Identification of social groups, close friends, and neighborhood and community activities may be pertinent. Disturbances in family, work, and social relationships and responsibilities are assessed.

Identities are strongly influenced by the roles one plays. As the aging process proceeds, many roles are changed or lost. This may be due to age stratification, change in the role of a significant other, loss of social group members through death or relocation, and declining health status.[10] The range of role options available to a person may change with age. First-order roles, or those closest to the core of our beings, are changed through retirement or loss of a spouse. Replacement of first-order roles is more difficult than replacing second- or third-order roles such as "friend," "neighbor," or "volunteer." A person who is no longer "husband," "lawyer," "coach," "neighbor," "chauffeur," or "counselor" may become an "elderly person." Coping with the stereotypes related to being elderly and having epilepsy present added stress.

The diagnosis of epilepsy will affect the family members and their roles. In the case of an elderly person with epilepsy, role reversal may occur. The adult child may become overly protective of a parent and, in an attempt to prevent perceived harm from seizures, abridge the patient's independence.

The degree of participation in the social network may change. A decline in social participation may be reflective of the fear of having a seizure in front of friends. Activities that once were enjoyable may become less so. Transportation may be a contributing factor as well. The elderly individual is just as likely to be uncomfortable asking for a ride as anyone else. Loss of previous roles contributes to dissatisfaction with current roles, and grieving may occur. Incorporating new roles where others have been lost may be difficult.

SEXUALITY AND REPRODUCTIVE PATTERN

In this pattern, the satisfaction of sexual relationships is explored. Changes and problems in sexual functioning are identified. Of all of the functional health patterns in the elderly, this is the one most likely to be unaddressed.

Alterations in sexual functioning can have profound effects on self-concept and body image. Women experience atrophy of the external genitalia, vagina, and breasts due to loss of stimulation by estrogen and progesterone. The vagina becomes thinner and poorly lubricated, which may result in painful intercourse, vaginal infections, and pruritus.

In men, testicular volume and spermatogenesis decrease. Men may experience a decrease in blood flow to the penis, with a resulting decrease in erectile capacity. For both men and women, sexual response tends to be slower and less intense with increasing age.

Myths abound that older people have no interest in sex and are unable to enjoy it. When today's older person was maturing, discussion of sexual activity was less open. AEMs can contribute to alterations in libido and potency, but discussion of these difficulties may not be initiated by the elderly patient who values privacy over the risk of embarrassment. The differences in age between the elderly person and the health professional may play a role in the comfort surrounding such a discussion. Normalizing discussion about sexuality and reproductive aspects of the elderly individual's life can provide a greater degree of comfort with and trust in the health professional and lead to greater life satisfaction.

COPING AND STRESS-TOLERANCE

In this pattern, the patient's coping pattern and its effectiveness in relationship to stress tolerance are described. An understanding of the past patterns of coping will facilitate planning for care. Examination of approaches that have been effective in the past is useful in determining if they will continue to be effective. The patient's ability to meet challenges to self-integrity, the usual methods of coping with stress, and past and current support systems are identified. It is important to identify the elderly patient's perception of the major changes and crises that have taken place in life and how coping with them has been effective or ineffective. Use of medication, illicit drugs, and alcohol is also explored.

Coping, or active problem-solving, is influenced by a variety of factors, including the environmental demands for coping, personality traits, and social role modeling.[7] The patient may exhibit a variety of physical, cognitive, emotional, and behavioral signs when under stress. In some patients, an increased stress level may contribute to an increase in seizure frequency.

Snyder's Revised Epilepsy Stressor Inventory[11] is a useful tool in identifying the frequency and degree of certain stressors associated with epilepsy. Once stressors are identified, strategies for coping with them can be defined. Working within the patient's known pattern of coping with stress increases the likelihood of better stress management. Negative coping strategies, such as regular use of drugs and alcohol, may need to be addressed through specific treatment programs. A history of alcohol abuse is present in up to 25% of individuals with late-onset epilepsy.[12, 13]

VALUES AND BELIEFS

The pattern of values and beliefs deals with the goals, values, and beliefs that guide decision-making and choices. This pattern includes the individual's definition of quality of life, and perceived conflicts in values, beliefs, and expectations related to health. Knowledge of an elderly patient's values and beliefs is essential in aiding health professionals in contributing ethically to the promotion of health and coping with illness.

There may be conflict between the values of health professionals and elderly patients. Total seizure control, for example, may not be the patient's goal if transportation to and from the clinic is a problem, the expense of the AEM is too great, or there is confusion with respect to medications. Nonjudgmental interaction is key to gaining an understanding of the patient's values and beliefs and how they are in concert with the management of his or her epilepsy.

NURSING DIAGNOSES

An in-depth assessment of the elderly individual with epilepsy using Gordon's Functional Health Patterns provides a sound basis for nursing diagnoses and development of an individualized management plan. Some of the most frequent nursing diagnoses related to alterations in functional health patterns in the elderly population include the following:

- *Health perception-health management pattern:* ineffective management of therapeutic regimen, high risk for infection, altered health maintenance, high risk for injury
- *Nutritional-metabolic pattern:* altered nutrition: more than body requirements, altered nutrition, less than body requirements, impaired swallowing, high risk for impaired skin integrity
- *Elimination pattern:* constipation, diarrhea, altered urinary elimination pattern
- *Activity-exercise pattern:* high risk for activity intolerance, impaired physical mobility, total self-care deficit, impaired home maintenance management, impaired gas exchange, decreased cardiac output, altered tissue perfusion
- *Sleep-rest pattern:* sleep pattern disturbance
- *Cognitive-perceptual pattern:* pain, sensory-perceptual alterations: input deficit or sensory deprivation, sensory-perceptual alterations: input excess or sensory overload, knowledge deficit
- *Self-perception–self-concept pattern:* fear, anxiety, hopelessness, self-esteem disturbance, chronic low self-esteem, situational low self-esteem, body image self-disturbance
- *Role-relationship pattern:* anticipatory grieving, dysfunctional grieving, disturbance in role performance, social isolation, impaired social interaction, altered family processes
- *Sexuality-reproductive pattern:* sexual dysfunction, altered sexuality patterns
- *Coping–stress-tolerance pattern:* ineffective coping, impaired adjustment, ineffective family coping
- *Value-belief pattern:* spiritual distress (distress of the human spirit)

Epilepsy plays a role in each of the elderly patient's functional health patterns. Desired outcomes must be identified and individualized, interventions implemented, and ongoing evaluation of success carried out. The interconnections among the patterns emphasizes the holistic nature of patients. A greater understanding of one pattern enhances our understanding of all of the patterns and ultimately contributes to our understanding of body, mind, and spirit of the elderly individual with epilepsy.

REFERENCES

1. Havighurst RJ. Social Roles, Work, Leisure and Education. In C Eisdorfer, MP Lawton (eds), The Psychology of Adult Development and Aging. Washington DC: American Psychiatric Association, 1973.
2. Solomon K. Social antecedents of learned helplessness in the health care setting. Gerontologist 1982;22:282.
3. McConnell ES. A Conceptual Framework for Gerontological Nursing Practice. In MA Matteson, ES McConnell (eds), Gerontological Nursing Concepts and Practice. Philadelphia: Saunders, 1988;5.
4. Lekan-Rutledge D. Functional Assessment. In MA Matteson, ES McConnell (eds), Gerontological Nursing Concepts and Practice. Philadelphia: Saunders, 1988;57.
5. Gordon M. Nursing Diagnosis: Process and Application. St. Louis: Mosby, 1982.
6. Gordon M. Manual of Nursing Diagnosis. St. Louis: Mosby, 1993.
7. Sehy YA, Williams MP. Functional Assessment. In WC Chenitz, JT Stone, SA Salisbury (eds), Clinical Gerontological Nursing: A Guide to Advanced Practice. Philadelphia: Saunders, 1991;119.
8. Nelson RC, Franzi LR. Nutrition. In RJ Ham, PD Sloane (eds), Geriatrics: A Case-Based Approach. St. Louis: Mosby, 1992;162.
9. Kurfees JF, Dotson RL. Drug interactions in the elderly. J Fam Pract 1987;25:477.
10. McConnell ES, Matteson MA. Psychosocial Aging Changes. In MA Matteson, ES McConnell (eds), Gerontological Nursing Concepts and Practice. Philadelphia: Saunders, 1988;431.
11. Snyder M. Revised epilepsy stressor inventory. J Neurosci Nurs 1993;25:9.
12. Dam AM, Fuglsang-Frederiksen A, Svarre-Olsen U, Dam M. Late-onset epilepsy: etiologies, type of seizure and value of clinical investigation, EEG and computerized tomography scan. Epilepsia 1985;26:227.
13. Lopez JLP, Lonzo J, Qiuntana F, et al. Late onset epileptic seizures. Acta Neurol Scand 1985;72:380.

SUGGESTED READINGS

Beyea S, Matzo M. Assessing elders using the functional health pattern assessment model. Nurse Educator 1989;14:32.
Birchenall JM, Streight ME. Care of the Older Adult (3rd ed). Philadelphia: Lippincott, 1992.
Lannon SL. Epilepsy in the elderly. J Neurosci Nurs 1993;25:273.
Luhdorf K, Jensen LK, Plesner AM. Epilepsy in the elderly: incidence, social function, and disability. Epilepsia 1986;27:135.
McDowell FH. Antiepileptic Drugs in the Elderly. In SR Resor Jr, H Kutt (eds), The Medical Treatment of Epilepsy. New York: Marcel Dekker, 1992;65.
Wold G. Basic Geriatric Nursing. St. Louis: Mosby, 1993.

III

Diagnosis of Seizures in the Elderly

10

The Altered Presentation of Seizures in the Elderly

Paolo Tinuper

Epileptic seizures result from a paroxysmal disturbance of the brain, whereas the epilepsies are diseases characterized by spontaneous recurrent epileptic seizures due to functional or structural damage affecting the brain locally or diffusely. Both epilepsy and seizures have many causes and vary in their incidence according to the age group in question. For example, febrile seizures, birth trauma, encephalitis, and cerebral malformations underlie the majority of infantile epilepsies, whereas tumors, traumatic head injury, and cerebrovascular disease are the most common causes of epilepsy in adults and the elderly population.

It has long been thought that epilepsy is rare in the aged.[1–3] Indeed, previous work suggested that 75% of all epilepsies begin before age 20 years,[4, 5] whereas the incidence of epilepsy was thought to decline over subsequent decades.[6–9] More recently, epidemiologic studies have demonstrated that the highest incidence of seizures and epilepsy occurs at the extremes of life. In fact, the incidence of epilepsy in those older than the age 75 years appears to be higher than in the first decade of life.[10–21]

In older life, the differential diagnosis between epileptic seizures and other paroxysmal cerebral events is often difficult.[22–29] It therefore is important to establish a semiology of epileptic seizures in elderly patients and to determine whether clinical seizure expression is altered over time.

LATE-ONSET EPILEPSY: PARTIAL OR GENERALIZED SEIZURES?

Seizure semiology has been carefully studied and well described in the pediatric and younger adult populations. This advance was made possible with the development of electroencephalographic (EEG)-video monitoring, particularly during evaluation for epilepsy surgery. Elderly patients are rarely considered for epilepsy surgery; thus, we have limited information concerning the details of seizure phenomenology in this population.

In infancy, epilepsy presents most frequently with seizures of generalized onset. In older children and adults, the incidence of epilepsies of partial onset and generalized seizures is approximately equal. In elderly patients, however, there is a marked increase in the incidence of partial onset attacks. This may be

123

explained only in part by the higher frequency of identifiable focal lesions in this age group. Vascular accidents, for example, account for only approximately one-third of all elderly patients with epilepsy.

Generalized tonic-clonic seizures are the expression of diffuse brain pathology and therefore are supposed to be relatively frequent in the elderly. Most authors, however, believe that generalized seizures in older patients have a partial onset that is difficult to appreciate. Generalized clonic or tonic-clonic seizures have been described in patients with Alzheimer's disease and other forms of dementia,[30, 31] but it is not clear whether or not these seizures differ in their characteristics from the tonic-clonic attacks associated with the idiopathic generalized epilepsies.

Many studies describe partial (focal onset) seizures in the elderly, but few of them focus on the semiologic aspects of the events. Such seizures are usually described as complex partial in type without further elaboration. Thus, there is little information regarding the characteristics of these events in the elderly and how they may differ from those occurring in a younger age group. Some ictal events, however, have been described in detail, in particular, nonconvulsive status epilepticus (see Chapter 16). Furthermore, there are reports of attacks in the elderly that present as transient memory disturbances.[32, 33]

EPILEPTIC AMNESTIC SEIZURES

This condition is characterized by the appearance of frequent, severe amnesic attacks in elderly, previously healthy individuals. Interictal EEG tracings show epileptiform abnormalities, mainly in the temporal regions. Ictal recordings disclose that the amnesic spells are preceded by a temporal lobe seizure that was not appreciated by relatives and therefore not reported in the history. The memory disturbance is therefore a postictal state that occurs after a complex partial seizure, a kind of Todd's paresis of the memory circuitry. In one patient described by Tassinari et al.,[34] seizures recurred in clusters, intermingled with amnesic states. Antiepileptic drug therapy may lead to marked improvement. Why this condition affects only elderly patients is an open question, but it is important to consider this diagnosis in patients with late-onset isolated memory disturbances or frequent episodes of transient amnesia. These events are to be differentiated from transient global amnesia. In the latter condition, episodes are infrequent and more prolonged than in the case of complex partial seizures. Furthermore, the EEG findings during the amnestic episode are normal, and interictal EEG findings do not contain epileptiform activity. A careful history will usually suggest the correct diagnosis.

DO THE CHARACTERISTICS OF SEIZURES CHANGE OVER TIME?

Some epileptic syndromes demonstrate changes in seizure manifestations over time. For example, the infantile spasms of West's syndrome may evolve into the tonic or atonic seizures of the Lennox-Gastaut syndrome. Thereafter, the patient may develop typical partial seizures. The primary generalized epilepsies also demonstrate age-related changes—in most cases absence attacks tend to diminish and disappear during adolescence. At the same time, there are studies[35] describing patients with long histories of absence attacks with minor changes in seizure characteristics and EEG patterns over time.

Generalized tonic-clonic seizures may occur at any age. Primarily generalized seizures are, however, rare in older people, and most generalized seizures have a partial onset. The incidence of primarily generalized tonic-clonic seizures in the elderly is unknown.

There are no studies dealing with the possible changes in semiology in the chronic partial epilepsies. In particular, there are no investigations of the possible evolution of clinical characteristics of complex partial seizures that extend to the elderly.

At the Epilepsy Center of the Neurological Institute of Bologna, Italy, a series of outpatients older than age 60 years were followed for more than 20 years. The mean duration of epilepsy was 45 years. In this group, secondarily generalized seizures disappeared over time in 80% of cases. Complex partial seizures may remain identical for many years, but in 38% of patients the motor components of the seizures subsided over time. In particular, gestural automatisms are reported less frequently. Serial EEG tracings showed a comcomitant decrease in interictal epileptiform activity. Despite the resistance of seizures in this group to pharmacotherapy, these elderly patients do not suffer from severe epilepsy. They indeed appear to lead well integrated family and social lives.

ILLUSTRATIVE CASE HISTORIES

An 87-year-old woman developed seizures at the age of 2 after a prolonged febrile convulsion. Since the age of 50, she has been followed at the Neurological Institute of Bologna. In her youth, her husband recalled that her seizures consisted of a rising epigastric sensation, oral and gestural semipurposeful automatisms, and confusion. From time to time she experienced a secondarily generalized tonic-clonic convulsion. EEG studies at an early stage demonstrated a right frontotemporal spike focus. At age 60 years, her generalized seizures disappeared, and her partial seizures were less elaborate, consisting mainly of the usual rising epigastric sensation. A recent EEG (Figure 10.1A) demonstrated slight bitemporal abnormalities without epileptiform activity. The computed tomography (CT) scan (Figure 10.1B) showed only diffuse atrophy. Despite her 85-year history of epilepsy, this patient had a normal family and social life.

In our series of 56 patients, only four (7.5%) experienced marked change in their seizure patterns with the appearance of secondarily generalized tonic-clonic seizures. These were individuals who acquired a cerebrovascular lesion in older age. It was also noted that these patients experienced progressive mental deterioration along with increased seizure frequency and more severe EEG abnormalities.

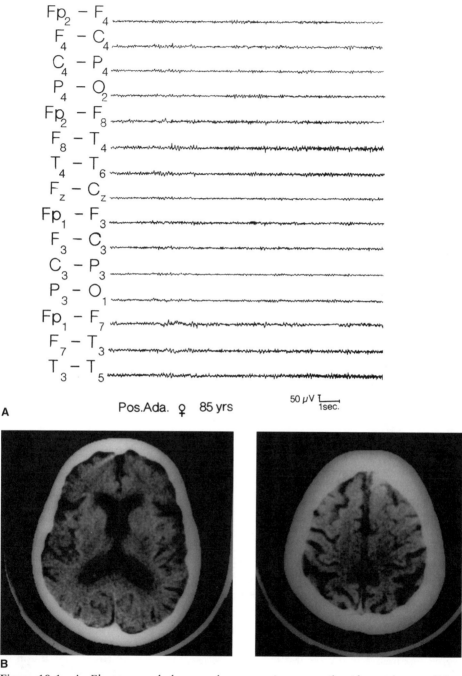

Figure 10.1 A. Electroencephalogram demonstrating nonepileptiform abnormalities, more evident over the left temporal region. B. Computed tomography scan showing mild diffuse atrophy without focal lesions.

A 63-year-old woman developed complex partial seizures at the age of 30 years without apparent etiologic factors. Early EEGs showed nonepileptiform temporal abnormalities. A CT scan of the head was normal. During her later years, the seizures worsened, with the appearance of tonic-clonic convulsions. Her complex partial seizures became prolonged, with associated screaming, spitting, and lip-smacking. There were violent automatisms and frequent sudden falls. A recent EEG showed multiple, independent spike foci over the temporal lobes (Figure 10.2A). Magnetic resonance imaging of the brain showed multiple areas of infarction (Figure 10.2B). Her seizures have been refractory to multiple drug regimens. In addition, she has experienced severe cognitive deterioration with memory disturbances and a limited social life.

SUMMARY

Epileptic seizures may occur at any age, and epidemiologic studies have demonstrated a high incidence in the elderly population. Epilepsy and epileptic syndromes may last a lifetime, and with aging the clinical expression of seizures may change. Evolution of seizure characteristics is well known in infantile epileptic encephalopathies, but modification of seizure patterns may also occur during old age.

The detailed characteristics of epileptic seizures in the elderly have not been studied systematically. Moreover, the possible alteration of seizure patterns over time, particularly with respect to epilepsies extending into late life, is not known. Seizures starting in the elderly usually are of focal onset; however, the well known characteristics of partial seizures in the younger population are not recognizable in the elderly. In our preliminary study in a selected group of outpatients referred to the Epilepsy Center in Bologna, partial seizures appear to become less elaborate in the elderly, and the epilepsy itself seems to be more tolerable. Detailed physiologic studies, including EEG-video monitoring, will be required to improve our understanding of seizure characteristics and their relationship to cerebral pathology in the elderly. In addition, long-term prospective studies are also required to document the natural history, clinical changes, and outcome in elderly patients with epilepsy.

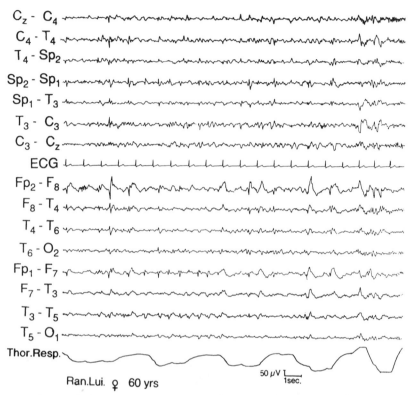

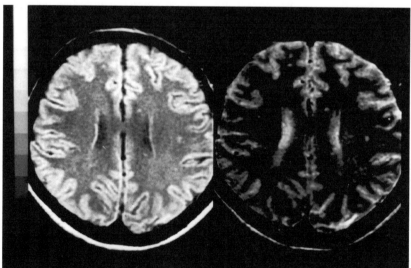

Figure 10.2 A. Electroencephalogram showing multiple independent spike foci over both temporal regions. B. Magnetic resonance imaging showing disseminated vascular lesions.

REFERENCES

1. Baldwin R, Davens E, Harris VG. The epilepsy program in public health. Am J Public Health 1953;43:452.
2. Otomo E. Convulsions in the aged. Folia Psychiatr Neurol (Jpn) 1981;35:295.
3. Gastaut H. "Benign" or "functional" (versus "organic") epilepsies in different stages of life: an analysis of corresponding age-related variations in the predisposition to epilepsy. Electroencephalography 1982;35(Suppl 1):17.
4. Gowers WR. Epilepsy and Other Chronic Convulsive Disorders. London: Churchill, 1981.
5. Lennox WG, Lennox MA. Epilepsy and related disorders (Vol. 1). Boston: Little, Brown, 1960;66.
6. Crombie DL, Cross KW, Try J, et al. A survey of the epilepsies in general practice. BMJ 1960;2:416.
7. Brewis M, Poskanzer DC, Rolland R, Miller M. Neurological disease in an English city. Acta Neurol Scand 1966;42(Suppl 24):1.
8. Gudmundsson G. Epilepsy in Iceland. A clinical and epidemiological investigation. Acta Neurol Scand 1966;(Suppl 25):1.
9. de Graaf AS. Epidemiological aspects of epilepsy in northern Norway. Epilepsia 1974;15:291.
10. Hauser WA, Kurland LT. The epidemiology of epilepsy in Rochester, Minnesota, 1935–1968. Epilepsia 1975;16:1.
11. Hauser WA, Annegers JF, Kurland LT. Prevalence of epilepsy in Rochester, Minnesota, 1940–1980. Epilepsia 1991;32: 429.
12. Lüdhorf K, Jensen LK, Plesner AM. Etiology of seizures in the elderly. Epilepsia 1986;27:458.
13. Lüdhorf K, Jensen LK, Plesner AM. Epilepsy in the elderly: incidence, social function and disability. Epilepsia 1986;27:135.
14. Keränen T, Riekkinen PJ, Sillanpää M. Incidence and prevalence of epilepsy in adults in eastern Finland. Epilepsia 1989;30:413.
15. Hauser WA. Seizure disorders: the change with age. Epilepsia 1992;33(Suppl 4):S6.
16. Forsgren L. Prospective incidence study and clinical characterisation of seizures in newly referred adults. Epilepsia 1990;31:292.
17. Forsgren L. Prevalence of epilepsy in adults in northern Sweden. Epilepsia 1992;33:450.
18. Loiseau J, Loiseau P, Duche B, et al. A survey of epileptic disorders in southwest France: seizures in the elderly patients. Ann Neurol 1990;27:232.
19. Loiseau J Loiseau P, Guyot M, et al. Survey of seizure disorders in the French southwest. Incidence of epileptic syndromes. Epilepsia 1990;31:391.
20. Tallis R. Epilepsy in old age. Lancet 1990;336:295.
21. Tallis R, Hall G, Craig I, Dean A. How common are epileptic seizures in old age? Age Ageing 1991;20:442.
22. Godfrey JW, Roberts MA, Caird FI. Epileptic seizures in the elderly: II. Diagnostic problems. Age Ageing 1982;11:29.
23. Godfrey JBW. Misleading presentation of epilepsy in elderly people. Age Ageing 1989;18:17.
24. Roberts MA, Godfrey JW, Caird FI. Epileptic seizures in the elderly: I. Etiology and type of seizures. Age Ageing 1982;11:24.
25. Dam AM, Fuglsang-Frederiksen A, Svarre-Olsen U, Dam M. Late onset epilepsy: etiology, types of seizures and value of clinical investigation, EEG and computerized tomography scan. Epilepsia 1985;26:227.
26. Lesser RP, Luders H, Dinner DS, Morris HH. Epileptic seizures due to thrombotic and embolic cerebrovascular disease in older patients. Epilepsia 1985;26:622.

27. Mahaler ME. Seizures: common causes and treatment in the elderly. Geriatrics 1987;42:73.
28. Roberts RC, Shorvon SD, Cox TC, Gilliatt RV. Clinically unsuspected cerebral infarction revealed by computer tomography scanning in late onset epilepsy. Epilepsia 1988;29:190.
29. Sung CY, Chu NS. Epileptic seizures in elderly people: aetiology and seizure type. Age Ageing 1990;19:25.
30. Hauser WA, Morris ML, Heston LL, Anderson VE. Seizures and myoclonus in patients with Alzheimer's disease. Neurology 1986;36:1226.
31. McAreavey MJ, Ballinger BR, Fenton GW. Epileptic seizures in elderly patients with dementia. Epilepsia 1992;33:657.
32. Gallassi R, Morreale A, Lorusso S, et al. Epilepsy presenting as memory disturbances. Epilepsia 1988;29:624.
33. Gallassi R, Morreale A, Di Sarro R, Lugaresi E. Epileptic amnesic syndrome. Epilepsia 1992;33(Suppl 6):S21.
34. Tassinari CA, Ciarmadori C, Alesi C, et al. Transient global amnesia as a postictal state from recurrent partial seizures. Epilepsia 1991;32:882.
35. Gastaut H, Zifkin BJ, Mariani E, Salas Puig J. The long term course of primary generalized epilepsy with persisting absences. Neurology 1986;36:1021.

11

Differential Diagnosis of Seizures in the Elderly

Frederick Andermann

One of the main clinical problems encountered in the elderly is the distinction of intermittent ischemic attacks from epileptic seizures.[1, 2] The duration of seizures is often shorter, and the associated clonic movement may present an important clue. In somatosensory or visual attacks, however, the differential diagnosis may be particularly difficult. When there is some doubt about the nature of the events, electroencephalographic (EEG)-video monitoring to clarify the nature of the behavioral manifestations and their electrical correlates, if any, may be indicated. This certainly would be preferable to a trial of antiepileptic medication, which is undesirable in individuals who may be quite sensitive to additional drugs.

The visual hallucinations of the blind and the auditory hallucinations of the deaf may bring about some difficulty in diagnosis.[3] This is particularly the case if the physician is not aware of the presence of hallucinations related to these forms of sensory deprivation. The details of the history and, above all, awareness of these conditions are crucial in making an accurate diagnosis.

Syncopal attacks are relatively frequent in the elderly. The lack of elasticity of the vasculature has often been invoked to explain the increased number of such episodes. The circumstances, the associated posture, and the pallor are characteristic, just as in younger individuals. Some confusion after syncope is not unusual in older patients, and even a mild degree of automatism may be encountered.[4–18] If the diagnosis is not clear, monitoring of both the EEG and the electrocardiogram for prolonged periods may be essential. Inasmuch as these events are episodic and at times separated by long intervals, clarification may not be easy.

Cardiac arrhythmia is common in this population. The occurrence of missed beats or a sensation of choking before loss of consciousness orient one toward the presence of cardiac arrhythmia as opposed to an epileptic etiology. Intensive EEG-video monitoring may resolve the question but again may not be conclusive, as the events may be clustered during certain periods and may be absent for long stretches.[19]

The differential diagnosis of falling attacks in the elderly is at times difficult. The advent of de novo atonic or tonic epileptic attacks in this age group would be unusual. Most such attacks are syncopal or perhaps cardiogenic.[20, 21]

Their significance lies primarily in the injuries they bring about, particularly fracture of the hip.[22] Here, too, their periodic or occasional appearance makes accurate diagnosis difficult, and supporting evidence from EEG, and more importantly from electrocardiogram, is valuable.

The effect of various medications, particularly the hypotension associated with some, must be taken into account. Vasodilator and antihypertensive agents may lead to hypotensive episodes and syncopal attacks.[11, 16, 23–26] Occasionally, some drugs can lead to paroxysmal movement disorders, for example, paroxysmal choreoathetosis induced by taking methyldopa.

Migraine with aura may occur in elderly people, and indeed acephalgic migraine attacks are more common in this age range compared with younger individuals. The classic march often present in people with acephalalgic migraine enables one to make the diagnosis. A major problem is the differential diagnosis between migraine with aura and intermittent cerebral ischemia in the posterior circulation.[27–30]

GENERALIZED EPILEPSIES IN THE ELDERLY

Petit mal status developing de novo in this age group has been well recognized.[31] The causes are unclear, and it is likely that some systemic disorder may activate a previously dormant genetic predisposition. In some of the patients, maturity-onset diabetes is found, but this is by no means the rule. Benzodiazepine withdrawal has been found to be a major causal factor.[32, 33] The confusional states and amnesia associated with petit mal status have led to an extraordinary number of publications over the years that attempt to alert physicians in emergency departments to the possibility of this somewhat unusual seizure pattern. Quivering of the chin, myoclonus of the eyelids, and low-amplitude myoclonus of the hands are some of the features that are helpful in suggesting this diagnosis. It is important to remember that the severity of the absence status varies greatly, from self-perceived lack of clarity of thought all the way to deep stupor.[31]

Patients with a previous history of having primary generalized epilepsy and spontaneous remission for many years may develop absence status as they age. In such individuals, awareness of the previous history is crucial for making the diagnosis.[32, 33]

The antiepileptic treatment of petit mal status in this age group presents certain problems. Patients are more prone to the appearance of familial or essential tremor activated by their valproic acid. When this is pronounced, parkinsonian features may appear as well and may add to gait difficulty and consequent risk of falling in already frail individuals.

The progressive myoclonus epilepsies characteristically are disorders of the second decade.[34, 35] They do, however, occasionally develop de novo in elderly individuals, particularly myoclonus epilepsy with ragged-red fibers (MERRF). In one such sporadic patient, the onset of the myoclonus was in the early 70s. The absence of a family history does not exclude this diagnosis, and it must be kept in mind when myoclonus appears in the elderly.

Occasionally in families with a well-documented MERRF mutation, some members may develop myoclonus and other manifestations of the illness when they are in their late 50s or 60s.[36] Mitochondrial encephalomyopathy with lactic acidosis and stroke-like episodes (MELAS) may also present with seizures and at times with myoclonus in the elderly age range. In one family with a proven MELAS mutation, the only manifestation in early adult life was hearing loss. Seizures, stroke, and myoclonus developed in the 50s and 60s.[37]

Myoclonus that occurs in the elderly may be a manifestation of Alzheimer's disease. It is often combined with generalized tonic-clonic seizures, and its appearance may precede other features of the illness. Myoclonus and generalized seizures accompanied by the characteristic periodic discharges in the EEG are features of Creutzfeldt-Jakob disease.[38–41]

Some features of idiopathic generalized epilepsy that are present in the young and in early adult life are conspicuous by their absence in the older population. Myoclonus, a typical feature of juvenile myoclonic epilepsy, is uncommon in older individuals. The prognosis of juvenile myoclonic epilepsy is considered to be poor, with a lifetime risk of recurrence of 80%. This is probably an overestimate, as in older individuals the myoclonus is certainly not apparent, and even the recurrence of seizures may be considerably lower. Conclusive studies of this issue are, however, not available.

Complications of antiepileptic medications may appear in the elderly after many years of trouble-free seizure control. The appearance of progressive ataxia in patients who have taken phenytoin at levels that were not obviously toxic may not be recognized as a complication of phenytoin therapy. The ataxia may be such as to make one suspect the presence of malignancy or of spinocerebellar degeneration. Stabilization of the ataxia after replacement of that medication confirms the diagnosis.

PARTIAL EPILEPSIES

Epileptic confusional episodes may be manifestations of partial epilepsy as well as the generalized form of the disease. Confusional status epilepticus of frontal lobe origin is not common but is particularly well recognized. It tends to occur de novo in elderly individuals and may be due to a vascular lesion. The EEG changes may be similar to those of petit mal status or may be more clearly localized. Correlation with imaging findings should lead to the diagnosis.[42–44]

Partial complex status of temporal lobe origin may develop in patients with a well established diagnosis of temporal lobe epilepsy, or it may arise without an antecedent history of epilepsy. The nature of the associated, sometimes subtle, automatisms and the electroclinical correlation enable the diagnosis. Distinction between petit mal and partial complex status may at times be difficult and, on the basis of the EEG findings alone, impossible.[45]

Seizures may occur in patients with chronic subdural hematoma. It was thought earlier that subdural hematomata are not associated with seizures, but exceptions to this rule have now been well recognized. The diagnosis of subdural hematoma, of course, is much easier since the advent of modern imaging procedures, and in elderly patients with slow or rapid deterioration, the diagnosis must be kept in mind.[46–49]

Late onset of temporal lobe epilepsy is not uncommon. In these patients, the question always remains as to whether there is activation of a long-standing underlying process or whether a new disorder is developing. In some of the patients, there is evidence of enlargement of the temporal horn, and other features of atrophy may be present. The possibility of an otherwise asymptomatic vascular event in anterior and inferomesial temporal areas is often suspected, but pathologic evidence for such vascular lesions is not available. Tumors and other lesions in this age group may lead to seizures as well.

Patients with a well documented history of temporal lobe epilepsy over many years may develop atonic seizures or falling attacks. These seizures, previously referred to as temporal lobe syncope, may be due to rapid spread of epileptic discharge contralaterally and to frontal areas, also involving reticular mechanisms. Falling seizures in addition to minor complex partial attacks represent a considerable addition to the patients' disability and may motivate some of them to consider surgical treatment in later adult life. It is the previous presence of well documented partial complex seizures that enables this diagnosis to be established.[50]

Patients with maturity-onset diabetes have at times been reported to develop reflex epilepsia partialis continua with seizures induced by movement, related to the presence of nonketotic hyperglycemia. The recognition of this syndrome and correction with the metabolic disorder are essential for successful treatment.[51–54]

Patients with long-standing hemiparesis may occasionally develop status epilepticus de novo in middle age (personal observations). The reasons of such activation of epileptogenic activity in the presence of a long-standing fixed lesion are not clear, but hypoxia or as yet unidentified metabolic factors may play a role. The major problem in such patients is to decide whether antiepileptic medication should be continued indefinitely, mainly because of the serious risk of status epilepticus in this age group.

Alcoholism in elderly individuals is not uncommon, and the possibility of withdrawal seizures much be kept in mind.[55–65] Cessation of various medications such as barbiturates and benzodiazepines may lead to the appearance of withdrawal attacks.[58, 59, 64] Continued treatment with antiepileptic medication in such individuals is not advisable. The difficulty in diagnosis, however, is illustrated by a patient in whom a diagnosis of withdrawal seizures was made initially but who was later proved to have not one but two distinct cerebral tumors.

Patients who have received maintenance electroconvulsive therapy for long periods may occasionally develop recurrent spontaneous seizures.[66–69] These are probably related to temporal lobe abnormalities and would represent examples of kindling in the human.

A particular reason for the urgency to establish an accurate diagnosis in this age group is related to the side effects of the antiepileptic medications. In the elderly, numerous other drugs are at times prescribed, leading to drug interactions and above all to poorly tolerated side effects. The need for continued antiepileptic medication must be continuously reassessed and the benefits weighed against the risks of seizure recurrence.

REFERENCES

1. Fiorini E, Regli F, Bogousslavsky J. Transitory carotid ischemic attacks: clinical and pathogenic aspects. Schweiz Arch Neurol Psychiatr 1991;142:485.
2. Barolin GS. Seizures in old age. Wien Med Wochenschr 1991;141:156.
3. Klostermann W, Vierregge P, Kompf D. Musical psuedo-hallucination in acquired hearing loss. Fortschr Neurol Psychiatr 1991;60:262.
4. Rutan GH, Hermanson B, Bild DE, et al. Orthostatic hypotension in adults. Hypertension 1992;19:508.
5. Schoenberger JA. Drug induced orthostatic hypotension. Drug Saf 1991;6:402.
6. Kenny RA, Traynor G. Carotid sinus syndrome—clinical characteristics in elderly patients. Age Ageing 1991;20:449.
7. Dougnac A, Gonzalez R, Kychenthal A, et al. Syncope: etiology, prognosis, and relationship to age. Aging (Milano) 1991;3:63.
8. Hackel A, Linzer A, Anderson N, Williams R. Cardiovascular and catecholamine responses to head-up tilt in the diagnosis of recurrent unexplained syncope in elderly patients. J Am Geriatr Soc 1991;39:663.
9. Davidson E, Rotenbeg Z, Fuchs J, et al. Transient ischemic attack-related syncope. Clin Cardiol 1991;14:141.
10. Nozzoli C, Buomono C, Simone F. Syncopes with reference to sex and age. Funct Neurol 1990;5:215.
11. Hanlon JT, Linzer M, MacMillan JP, et al. Syncope and presyncope associated with probable adverse drug reaction. Arch Intern Med 1990;150:2309.
12. Olsky M, Murray J. Dizziness and fainting in the elderly. Emerg Med Clin North Am 1990;8:449.
13. Hoefnagels WA, Padberg GW, Overweg J, et al. Syncope or seizure? The diagnostic value of the EEG and hyperventilation test in transient loss of consciousness. J Neurol Neurosurg Psychiatry 1991;54:953.
14. Bonema JD, Maddens ME. Syncope in elderly patients. Why their risk is higher. Postgrad Med 1992;91:129.
15. Maloney JD, Jaeger FJ, Rizo-Patron C, Zhu DW. The role of pacing for the management of neurally mediated syncope: carotid sinus syndrome and vasovagal syncope. Am Heart J 1994;127:1030.
16. Hopson JR, Rea RF, Kienzle MG. Alterations in reflex function contributing to syncope: orthostatic hypotension, carotid sinus hypersensitivity and drug-induced dysfunction. Herz 1993;18:164.
17. Frazier HS. The diagnosis of syncope in the elderly. Int J Tech Assessment Health Care 1993;9:102.
18. Grubb BP, Wolfe D, Samoil D, et al. Recurrent unexplained syncope in the elderly: the use of head-upright tilt table testing in evaluation and management. J Am Geriatr Soc 1993;40:1123.
19. McIntosh S, Da Costa D, Kenny RA. Outcome of an integrated approach to the investigation of dizziness, falls and syncope in elderly patients referred to a 'syncope' clinic. Age Ageing 1993;22:53.
20. McLaren AJ, Lear J, Daniels RG. Collapse in an accident and emergency department. J R Soc Med 1994;87:601.
21. Partridge R, Hashemi K. What is collapse? A differential diagnosis in the elderly. Br J Clin Pract 1990;44:60.

22. Lindberg EJ, Macias D, Gipe BT. Clinically occult presentation of comminuted intertrochanteric hip fractures. Ann Emerg Med 1992;21:1511.
23. Berigaud S, Saint Jean O, Praet JP. Properties of drug complications in elderly patients. Revue de Praticien 1990;40:1366.
24. Mets T, De Bock V, Praet JP. First-dose hypotension, ACE inhibitors, and heart failure in the elderly. Lancet 1992;339:1487.
25. Heseltine D, Dakkak M, Woodhouse K, et al. The effect of caffeine on postprandial hypotension in the elderly. J Am Geriatr Soc 1991;39:160.
26. Hug CC Jr, McLeskey CH, Nahrwold ML, et al. Hemodynamic effects of propofol: data from over 25,000 patients. Anesth Analg 1993;77(Suppl 4):521.
27. Stewart WF, Lipton RB, Celentano DD, Reed ML. Prevalence of migraine headache in the United States. Relation to age, income, race, and other sociodemographic factors. JAMA 1992;261:64.
28. Diamond S. Management of headaches. Focus on new strategies. Postgrad Med 1990;87:189.
29. Silberstein SD, Lipton RB. Epidemiology of migraine. Neuroepidemiology 1993;12:179.
30. Blau JN. Classical migraine: symptoms between visual aura and headache onset. Lancet 1992;340:355.
31. Andermann F, Robb JP. Absence status. A reappraisal following review of thirty-eight patients. Epilepsia 1972;13:177.
32. Thomas P, Beaumanoir A, Genton P, et al. De novo absence status. Report of 11 cases. Neurology 1992;42:104.
33. Thomas P, Andermann F. Late Onset Absence Status Epilepticus Is Most Often Situation-Related. In A Malafosse, P Genton, E Hirsch, et al. (eds), Idiopathic Generalized Epilepsies. Harlow/Essex, England: John Libbey 1994;94.
34. Berkovic SF, Anderman F, Carpenters S, Wolfe LS. Progressive myoclonus epilepsies: specific causes and diagnosis. N Engl J Med 1986;315:396.
35. Berkovic SF, Cochius J, Andermann E, Andermann F. Progressive myoclonus epilepsies: clinical and genetic aspects. Epilepsia 1993;34(Suppl 3):19.
36. Berkovic SF, Carpenter S, Evans A, et al. Myoclonus epilepsy and ragged red fibers (MERRF). 1. A clinical, pathological, biochemical, magnetic resonance spectroscopy and positron emission tomographic study. Brain 1989;112:1231.
37. Desbiens R, Andermann E, Shoubridge E, et al. An unexpected phenotype of MELAS syndrome: maturity-onset dementia and strokes. Neurology 1992;42(Suppl 3):281.
38. Kennedy AM, Newman S, McCaddon A, et al. Familial Alzheimer's disease. A pedigree with a mis-sense mutation in the amyloid precursor protein gene (amyloid precursor protein 717 valine—glycine). Brain 1993;117(Pt 2):309.
39. Barcikowska M, Mirecka B, Papierz W, et al. A case of Alzheimer's disease simulating Creutzfeldt-Jakob disease. Neurol Neurochir Pol 1992;26:703.
40. Bergamini L, Pinesse L, Rainer I, et al. Familial Alzheimer's disease. Evidence of clinical and genetic heterogeneity. Acta Neurol Scand 1991;13:534.
41. James AJ. Down's syndrome, dementia and myoclonic jerks. Br J Psychiatry 1990;157:938.
42. Nierdermeyer E, Fineyre F, Riley T, Uematsu S. Absence status (petit mal status) with focal characteristics. Arch Neurol 1979;36: 417.
43. Aguglia U, Tinuper P, Farnarier G. Etat confusionnel critique a point de depart frontal chez le sujet age. Rev Electroencephal Neurophysiol Clin 1983;13:174.
44. Rey M, Papy JJ. Etats d'obnubilation critique d'origine frontale: un diagnostic clinique difficle. Rev Electroencephal Neurophysiol Clin 1987;17:377.
45. Thomson P, Lebrun C, Chatel M. True and false nonconvulsive confusional status epilepticus. J Neurol 1992;239(Suppl 2):72.
46. Rubin G, Rappaport ZH. Epilepsy in chronic subdural hematoma. Acta Neurochir (Wien) 993;123:39.

47. Nicoli F, Milandre L, Lemarquis P, et al. Chronic subdural hematoma and transient neurologic deficits. Rev Neurol (Paris) 1990;146:256.
48. Koywica Z, Brzeinski J. Epilepsy in chronic subdural hematoma. Acta Neurochir (Wien) 1991;113:118.
49. Jamjoom AN, Kane N, Sandeman D, Cummins B. Epilepsy related to traumatic extradural hematomas. BMJ 1991;302:448.
50. Gambardella A, Reutens DC, Andermann F, et al. Late onset drop attacks in temporal lobe epilepsy: a reevaluation of the concept of temporal lobe syncopy. Neurology 1994;44:1074.
51. Hennis A, Corbin D, Fraser H. Focal seizures and non-ketotic hyperglycemia. J Neurol Neurosurg Psychiatry 1992;55:195.
52. Linazasoro G, Urtasun M, Poza JJ, et al. Generalized chorea induced by nonketotic hyperglycemia. Mov Disord 1993;8:119.
53. Carril JM, Guijarro C, Portocarrero JS, et al. Speech arrest as manifestation of seizures in non-ketotic hyperglycemia. Lancet 1992;340:1227.
54. Tedrus GM, Albertin MC, Odashima NS, Fonseca LC. Partial motor seizures induced by movement in diabetic patients. Arq Neuropsiquiatr 1991;49:442.
55. Kashner TM, Rodell DE, Ogden SR, et al. Outcomes and costs of two VA inpatient treatment programs for older alcoholic patients. Hosp Community Psychiatry 1992;43:985.
56. Dunne FJ. Misuse of alcohol or drugs by elderly people. BMJ 1994;308:608.
57. McInnes E, Powell J. Drug and alcohol referrals: are elderly substance abuse diagnoses and referrals being missed? BMJ 1994;308:444.
58. Jones TV, Lindesy BA, Yount P, et al. Alcoholism screening questionnnaires: are they valid in elderly medical outpatients? J Gen Intern Med 1993;8:674.
59. Bercsi SJ, Brickner PW, Saha DC. Alcohol use and abuse in the frail, homebound elderly: a clinical analysis of 103 persons. Drug Alcohol Depend 1993;33:139.
60. Adams WL, Yuan Z, Barboriak JJ, Rimm AA. Alcohol-related hospitalizations of elderly people. Prevalence and geographic variation in the United States. JAMA 1993;270:1222.
61. Fulop G, Reinhardt J, Strain JJ, et al. Identification of alcoholism and depression in a geriatric medicine outpatient clinic. J Am Geriatr Soc 1993;41:737.
62. Thibaut JM, Maly RC. Recognition and treatment of substance abuse in the elderly. Prim Care 1993;20:155.
63. Gupta KL. Alcoholism in the elderly. Uncovering a hidden problem. Postgrad Med 1993;93:203.
64. Laforge RG, Mignon SI. Alcohol use and alcohol problems among the elderly. R I Med J 1993;76:21.
65. Miller NS, Belkin BM, Gold MS. Alcohol and drug dependence among the elderly: epidemiology, diagnosis and treatment. Compr Psychiatry 1991;32:153.
66. Dubin WR, Jaffe R, Roemer R, et al. The efficacy and safety and maintenance ECT in geriatric patients. J Am Geriatr Soc 1992;40:706.
67. Monroe RR Jr. Maintenance electroconvulsive therapy. Psychiatr Clin North Am 1991;14:947.
68. Loo H, Galinoski A, De Carvalho W, et al. Use of maintenance ECT for elderly depressed patients. Am J Psychiatry 1991;148:810.
69. Thienhaus OJ, Margletta S, Bennett JA. A study of the clinical efficacy of maintenance ECT. J Clin Psychiatry 1990;51:141.

12

Electroencephalography and Seizures in the Elderly

Kyusang S. Lee and Timothy A. Pedley

INTRODUCTION

A number of changes occur in the electroencephalogram (EEG) as part of normal aging. In his Fifth Report in 1932, Berger described slowing of the alpha rhythm in elderly patients with intellectual deterioration.[1] Because he did not observe this in healthy elderly people, Berger concluded that slowing of EEG frequency was due to pathologic processes rather than age alone. Since Berger's report, there have been many studies of the EEG changes seen in elderly people, and a corresponding amount of controversy has developed regarding which findings can be attributed to the aging process and which reflect cerebral pathology. Unfortunately, few studies have rigorously selected subjects free of disease as controls. Nonetheless, several EEG findings appear consistently across reports of elderly people, including slowing of the alpha rhythm, alteration in fast activity, increased diffuse slow-frequency activity, and the emergence of focal slow-wave activity.

EEG is an essential and probably the single most useful laboratory test in evaluating patients with seizures or epilepsy.[2–4] The incidence and prevalence of seizures and epilepsy rise substantially in people older than age 65 years,[5–7] but a comparable increase in the incidence of interictal EEG epileptiform activity has not been described.[5–10] Elderly individuals are also at increased risk for certain diseases of the aging brain that may result in epileptiform discharges. In addition, there are a few "benign" EEG patterns that occur with increasing frequency in the older population that may be falsely interpreted as epileptogenic.

Use of the EEG in evaluating elderly patients with seizures or epilepsy does not differ substantially from its application in younger patients. The main difference relates to recognizing EEG changes that occur normally with aging or are seen commonly in patients with either occult or symptomatic disease of the aging brain.

139

WAKING ELECTROENCEPHALOGRAPHIC ACTIVITY IN THE ELDERLY

Alpha Rhythm

The alpha rhythm has been the most consistently studied EEG variable as a function of aging, and slowing of alpha rhythm frequency is the most commonly reported finding with advancing years.[11–13] In large, unselected populations of young adults, the mean frequency of the alpha rhythm averages 10.0–10.5 Hz.[14, 15] The frequency of the alpha rhythm in mentally normal elderly subjects is significantly lower, averaging 9.0–9.5 Hz at age 70, and 8.5–9.0 Hz after 80 years of age.[11–13, 16–18] Mundy-Castle et al.[19] reported that the mean alpha frequency was 9.4 Hz in normal subjects who had a mean age of 75 years. In nursing home residents, Obrist[20] found that the mean alpha frequency was 9.1 Hz in those in their seventh and eighth decades of life, and 8.6 Hz in those beyond 80 years of age.[20] Hubbard and associates[21] studied 10 centenarians and found that the mean alpha rhythm frequency was 8.6 Hz in the seven individuals judged to be mentally normal. In a longitudinal study of healthy volunteers ranging in age from 59 to 85 years, Wang and Busse[22] found that the alpha rhythm frequency was 10.5 Hz at age 60, 9.5 Hz at age 70, and 8.5 Hz at age 85 years. This was interpreted as showing that increasing age is normally associated with predictable and progressive slowing of the mean alpha rhythm frequency at a rate that approximates 0.08 Hz per year after age 60 years. Katz and Horowitz[23] reported that the mean alpha rhythm frequency was 9.8 Hz in a cohort of 52 septuagenarians determined to be mentally normal by a battery of neurologic and psychometric tests.

Several investigators have used computer-assisted EEG analysis to evaluate changes in the alpha rhythm in the elderly. These studies have also found that the frequency of the alpha rhythm slows normally with age.[24, 25] Roubicek[26] used spectral analysis to study the EEG of 106 normal subjects. He reported that the mean alpha rhythm frequency was 9.0 Hz at age 60 years but only 7.0 Hz between the ages of 80 and 90 years. Using computerized EEG frequency analysis, Oken and Kaye[27] compared the peak frequency of the dominant posterior rhythm in subjects older than age 84 years with those who were younger. They found that those younger than age 84 years maintained an alpha frequency of more than 8.0 Hz, but that normal people older than age 84 years had a mean frequency between 7.0 Hz and 8.0 Hz.

Some investigators have denied that the frequency of the alpha rhythm declines in older individuals who are neurologically normal and healthy. Giaquinto and Nolfe[28] studied EEG recordings from normal middle-aged and normal elderly subjects and from demented patients using computer-assisted analysis and a fast Fourier transform algorithm. They found that the frequency of the alpha rhythm decreased by only 0.5 Hz over the entire life span, and that there was no significant difference between the normal middle-aged and normal elderly groups. Duffy et al.[29] also found no correlation between age and dominant background frequency in subjects participating in the Normative Aging Study. These individuals were monitored by EEGs while they performed specific tasks to help control for state.

Many factors can influence the frequency of the alpha rhythm, including neurologic and cardiovascular status, drug history, and metabolic factors. Andermann and Stoller[30] compared EEG findings of elderly patients from a psychiatric hospital, a convalescent home, and the community. The average age of study subjects was 70 years. The mean alpha frequency was 7.0–9.0 Hz in the psychiatric group, 9.0–9.5 Hz in convalescent home patients, and 11.0 Hz in community volunteers. Otomo[16] reported similar findings: Alpha rhythm frequency averaged 9.5 Hz in healthy individuals older than age 60 years, 9.0 Hz in neurologically intact patients with medical illnesses, and 8.6 Hz in patients with neurologic disease. Obrist and Bissell[31] reported a significant correlation between electrocardiographic changes suggestive of atherosclerosis and EEG slowing.

How or whether age affects the voltage of the alpha rhythm is less clear. Some authors have reported that the amplitude of the alpha rhythm decreases with age.[19, 32] Duffy et al.,[29] however, found only a weak correlation between amplitude of the alpha rhythm and age, and Pollock et al.[33] could find no statistically significant relation between log-transformed EEG voltages and age in subjects 56–76 years old.

Some authors have described a diminished alpha blocking response, less reactivity, and reduced photic driving in older people,[3, 29, 34, 35] but these findings have not been confirmed by others.[36]

EEGs obtained in people older than age 50 years often reveal activity over one or both temporal areas that is similar to the occipital alpha rhythm in morphology, regulation, and manner of occurrence (Figure 12.1).[37] When bilateral, this so-called temporal alpha is characteristically asynchronous on the two sides and, in the majority of cases, predominates on the left. The voltage of temporal alpha is commonly greater than that of the occipital alpha rhythm. Occasionally, a 4.0- to 5.0-Hz subharmonic may be intermixed. Fragments of this temporal alpha activity, especially when sharply contoured, may appear as "wicket spikes" or be misinterpreted as "epileptiform."

Beta Frequencies

There is somewhat less consensus about the effect of aging on beta frequencies. Gibbs et al.[38] reported that the amount of EEG activity in the 14.0–30.0 Hz range increased with aging. Other investigators have agreed with this conclusion and, additionally, noted that the effect was most marked over the central areas.[26, 39, 40] Some authors have found that age-related increases in fast activity are more common in women.[28] McAdam et al.[41] suggested that hormonal changes may play a role, because in their study significantly greater amounts of beta activity were observed in postmenopausal women than in premenopausal women. Mundy-Castle[42] found that the mean amplitude of beta activity was significantly greater in elderly than in younger individuals. Using computerized-frequency analysis, Roubicek[26] separated beta activity into two subtypes: *fast* beta

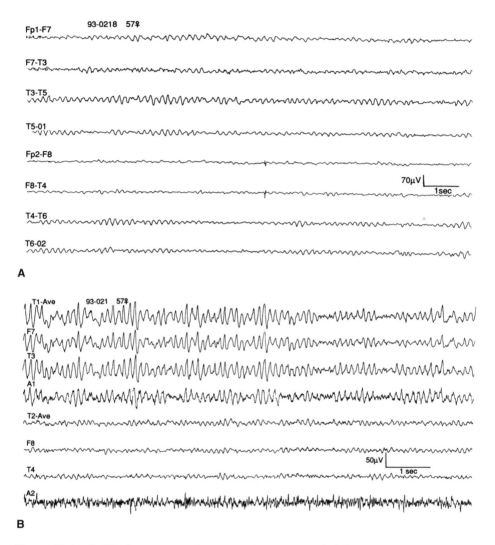

Figure 12.1 A. Bipolar montage demonstrating "temporal alpha" activity that is maximal in the left anterior to the midtemporal area. B. Referential (average) montage from another patient showing the wide distribution of the temporal alpha activity.

(>30.0 Hz), which reportedly increases with age, and *slow* beta (25.0–30.0 Hz), which reportedly decreases.

Not all investigators have found a consistent change in beta activity with aging.[39] Differences among studies are often difficult to account for because the varying methods of analysis, failure to account for medication history, and different circumstances of recording make comparisons difficult.

The significance of age-related changes in beta activity is unknown. Some authors have noted a positive correlation between fast activity and well preserved mental abilities.[11, 18] Thompson and Wilson[43] even reported that subjects with abundant fast activity had superior learning abilities. The other side of this coin is that decreased beta activity has been interpreted as an early sign of intellectual loss and mental impairment.[39]

Theta and Delta Frequencies

It is widely accepted that the amount of slow frequency activity increases with age and that this increase can occur both diffusely and either simultaneously or independently in a more localized fashion. In general, 4.0- to 7.0-Hz slow activity (theta) is likely to be less significant than comparable amounts of slow activity of less than 4.0 Hz (delta). The amount and severity of slow frequency activity correlate with diminished mental function and decreased longevity.[44, 45] The correlation is best for moderate to severe changes, because mild slowing of EEG background activity does not preclude normal intellectual function.[11–13]

Diffuse Slowing

Diffuse slow activity consists of theta activity, delta activity, or both that is randomly distributed bilaterally and shows no persistent focality (Figure 12.2). Compared with other age-related EEG characteristics, diffuse slow activity is less common among community volunteers during early senescence than in patients with medical or neurologic disorders.[11, 45, 46] Obrist and Busse[12] found diffuse slowing in 7% of subjects younger than 75 years old. At more advanced ages, however, there was a significant increase in the number of people showing diffuse slow activity, for example, in up to 20% of community volunteers.[11, 12, 45, 47]

Diffuse slow activity, more than any other EEG variable, correlates with impaired intellectual function.[11] Using various measures, numerous studies have found a strong correlation between abnormalities of mental function and diffuse EEG slowing: The more severe the slowing, the worse the intellectual impairment.[39] In studies of elderly community volunteers and other healthy elderly subjects who exhibit only mild EEG slowing, there is often a poor correlation with intellectual changes.[46, 48] On the other hand, in institutionalized subjects who display more pronounced EEG changes, there is a significant relationship between the degree of EEG slowing and the extent of cognitive impairment.[49, 50] This is consistent with the finding of significantly lower intelligence scores in clinic and hospital patients with diffusely slow, in contrast to normal, EEG findings.[51–53] Because of this relationship, the presence of marked diffuse slowing on EEG has been one criterion used in differentiating organic brain syndromes from senile depression or psychosis.[11, 54]

Diffuse slow activity may also be related to prognosis and life expectancy. Obrist and Henry[54] found that a majority of elderly patients with diffuse slow activity either remained hospitalized or died within a year after the EEG. Patients with normal EEG tracings, on the other hand, tended to be discharged or trans-

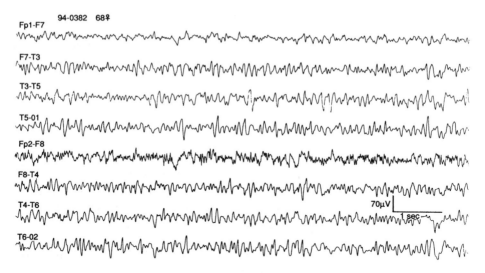

Figure 12.2 Neurologically and mentally normal 68-year-old woman whose electroencephalogram shows a moderate amount of admixed arrhythmic theta and delta activity diffusely.

ferred to nursing homes. Cahan and Yeager[55] claimed that normal EEG findings in elderly psychiatric patients carried twice the prognostic advantage for survival.

The cause of diffuse EEG slowing remains speculative, but changes in cerebral blood flow and metabolism may play a role. It is well established that cerebral ischemia and anoxia produce EEG slow activity.[56] In elderly patients with organic brain disease and diffuse EEG slow activity, Obrist et al.[57] found a significant negative correlation between cerebral oxygen uptake, cerebral blood flow, and the amount of slow activity. These findings have been confirmed in patients with cerebrovascular disease and organic dementia.[58, 59] Several investigators have found a relationship between blood pressure and EEG abnormalities.[60–62] Elderly subjects with hypertension tended to have relatively less diffuse slowing than those with low blood pressure. In addition, Obrist[63] found that when low blood pressure occurred in combination with detectable vascular disease, at least 70% of patients had EEGs showing diffuse slow activity. From associations such as these, it has been hypothesized that EEG slowing in the elderly most often results from diminished cerebral blood flow and reduced metabolism, although which is the primary disturbance is unclear. Chronic cerebral ischemia from cerebrovascular insufficiency may also play a role.

Focal Slowing

Elderly individuals have a high incidence of focal theta and delta activity that is characteristically most prominent over the temporal regions, especially the left.

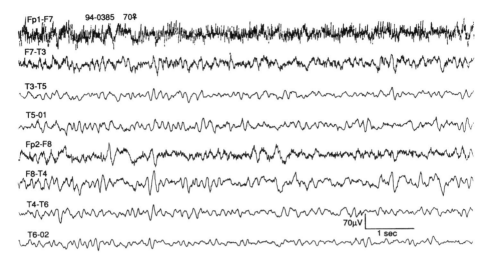

Figure 12.3 Moderate bitemporal arrhythmic theta and delta activity with poorly formed alpha rhythm in a 70-year-old woman with Alzheimer's disease.

Focal slowing of the elderly is enhanced by drowsiness (Figure 12.3). Such slowing is typically intermittent and polymorphic, although it can be more rhythmic, especially during drowsiness.[34, 45, 64] The amount or severity of the focal slowing usually continues to increase with advancing age.

Busse et al.[65] and Obrist[20] first reported the association of focal slowing and increasing age. They found that 30–40% of their community volunteers older than age 60 years had focal slow activity in their EEGs, predominantly over the left temporal area. Silverman et al.[45] observed that 75% of all focal abnormalities in elderly individuals were lateralized to the left hemisphere, and 80% of these were maximal over the anterior temporal region. They also reported that voltage asymmetries were common. Mundy-Castle[66] reported that 50% of residents in a nursing home had focal slowing, predominantly over the left temporal lobe. Kooi et al.[64] studied temporal abnormalities in 218 neurologically intact adults, of whom 37 were older than age 60 years. Two-thirds of these had focal temporal theta activity, and one-third had temporal delta activity. In a study of 3,476 normal control subjects, Gibbs and Gibbs[67] found minimal temporal slow-wave activity in 3.2% of their subjects older than age 60 years.

A high incidence of temporal EEG changes has also been reported in studies of hospitalized elderly patients. In contrast to community volunteers, however, the focal slowing in this group was more prominent and had a wider distribution. In patients with organic brain syndromes, temporal slowing and sometimes frontal slowing were often superimposed on diffuse background slow activity.[11] Therefore, although some degree of focal temporal slowing is common in healthy, asymptomatic elderly individuals, diffuse organic brain dysfunction is suggested when temporal slowing is combined with more widespread slow-wave activity.

As previously noted, "normal" focal temporal slowing of the elderly is intermittent and usually relatively infrequent. Its appearance is enhanced by drowsiness and arousal,[11, 12, 64] but it usually disappears or becomes much less evident as sleep deepens.

Not all investigators agree that temporal slow-wave activity is a normal consequence of aging.[68] In a highly selected group of neurologically and psychologically normal septuagenarians, Katz and Horowitz[23] found focal slowing (mainly theta activity) in only 17% of EEGs. Furthermore, when present in this group, it occupied less than 1% of the tracing.

Whether considered completely normal or not, focal temporal slowing of the elderly is a common, asymptomatic finding in those older than age 60 years. Drachman and Hughes[69] found no differences in memory ability between normal elderly subjects with and without temporal foci. Similarly, routine psychological testing has not revealed any consistent correlations between specific cognitive abnormalities and EEG temporal slow-wave activity.[11] Selecting from a large sample of community volunteers, Obrist[11] compared 20 subjects with prominent focal EEG slowing with 20 subjects with normal EEG findings matched for age and education. He was unable to find any significant differences between the two groups on measures of verbal learning, immediate or delayed recall, or intelligence.

The pathophysiology of focal temporal slowing is unknown. Decreased cerebral blood flow has been implicated as a causative factor, although this does not explain the striking left-sided predominance.[11, 13] In a group of elderly clinic patients, all of whom had moderately prominent EEG temporal slow-wave foci, Bruens et al. found that 89% had neurologic findings suggesting vascular disease. They also noted that hyperventilation, compression of the carotid artery, or inhalation of low oxygen mixtures increased the slowing, whereas breathing carbon dioxide tended to reduce it.[70] Niedermeyer[71] found that patients with chronic vertebrobasilar artery insufficiency commonly had minor temporal slow-wave abnormalities. Furthermore, rhythmic temporal theta may be associated with cerebrovascular disease in the absence of a major neurologic disease.[72] Some investigators believe that this pattern of slowing is caused by cerebrovascular disease and not simply by aging.

Although cerebrovascular insufficiency can give rise to focal EEG changes, other causes must be considered. For instance, relatively localized degenerative changes in the temporal lobes may occur as a part of the normal aging process but then be further accelerated by superimposed pathologic events.[11] Brody[73, 74] performed quantitative histologic studies on the brains of normal aged subjects and found a high degree of neuronal depopulation in the temporal and frontal areas relative to other cortical regions.

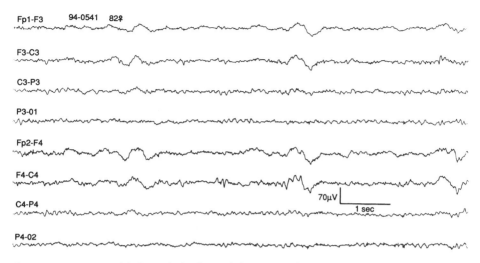

Figure 12.4 Normal bifrontal rhythmic delta waves during drowsiness in a neurologic-ally normal 82-year-old woman with depression.

SLEEP ELECTROENCEPHALOGRAPHIC ACTIVITY IN THE ELDERLY

Slow-Wave Sleep

EEG patterns during slow-wave (non–rapid eye movement [NREM]) sleep show many changes with aging. During stage 1 sleep (drowsiness), frontal rhythmic delta activity is a common finding (Figure 12.4).[75] Gibbs and Gibbs[67] referred to this as "anterior bradyrhythmia," and Katz and Horowitz[75] described it as "sleep-onset FIRDA" (frontal intermittent rhythmic delta activity). Frontal rhythmic delta activity of drowsiness is usually low-voltage, does not extend far posteriorly, and tends to occur in 1- to 3-second bursts. It is a normal, age-related finding but must be distinguished from "true" FIRDA, which can be seen in a variety of diffuse encephalopathies. Elderly people spend correspondingly more time in stage 1 sleep because of frequent transient arousals.

The amount of delta activity is both of lower voltage[76] and reduced quantity[77–82] in healthy older individuals. Some investigators have reported that there is a shift in the NREM sleep frequency spectrum toward the theta range[79] and that the remaining delta activity is more fragmented than in younger individuals. As a consequence, the amount of stage 3 and especially stage 4 sleep is decreased in older people. For unknown reasons, this reduction in slow-wave sleep is most pronounced in men.[83]

In older age, there is a significant reduction in the number, duration, and voltage of sleep spindles, as well as reduced numbers of vertex waves and K complexes during stage 2 sleep. Vertex waves also tend to be less complex, of longer duration, and lower voltage.[84–86] Finally, there is a decline in the number of positive occipital sharp transients after 70 years of age.[87] The physiologic basis of these changes is unknown.

Rapid Eye Movement Sleep

Both rapid eye movement (REM) density and associated motor twitches decrease with age, and REM latency usually shortens. The duration of REM episodes decreases slightly, but the percentage of REM in relation to total sleep time remains relatively constant. Saw-toothed waves are more prominent. Although not known with certainty, it is likely that these changes reflect the effects of normal aging on the pontine centers that regulate REM sleep.[88]

ELECTROENCEPHALOGRAPHIC PATTERNS OF NO OR UNCERTAIN SIGNIFICANCE

Subclinical Rhythmic Electrographic Discharge of Adults

Subclinical rhythmic electrographic discharge of adults (SREDA) is an uncommon but very striking EEG pattern seen mainly in older adults, especially those older than age 50 years. It was described first by Naquet and his colleagues,[89] who termed it "décharges paroxystiques" and attributed it to cerebrovascular insufficiency within middle cerebral artery and posterior cerebral artery watershed areas. The term *SREDA* was coined by Westmoreland and Klass.[90] At first glance, the pattern resembles an ictal discharge, but patients exhibit no behavioral or cognitive alterations during the EEG event, and it occurs with equal frequency in epileptic and nonepileptic patients.[90, 91]

SREDA is a stereotyped event that begins and ends abruptly (Figure 12.5). It consists predominantly of sharply contoured theta activity that is maximal over the parietal–posterior temporal areas. It is usually bilateral but is often asymmetric and may be unilateral. Onset is often with a series of monophasic delta waves followed by a sustained 5.0- to 7.0-Hz discharge that may gradually increase in frequency and diminish in amplitude, the reverse of the voltage/frequency sequence exhibited by most epileptic events. SREDA does not show continued evolution once established, a feature that is also atypical for ictal activity. It is often triggered by hyperventilation, and, once present, SREDA is usually seen in all subsequent EEG recordings.[90–92] The discharge lasts 40–80 seconds.

Small Sharp Spikes

Small sharp spikes (SSSs), also termed *benign epileptiform transients of sleep* or *benign sporadic sleep spikes* also occur with increasing frequency in older individuals, although they can be seen at any age.[92, 93] SSSs are maximal over the temporal region and commonly show a horizontal dipole from anterior to poste-

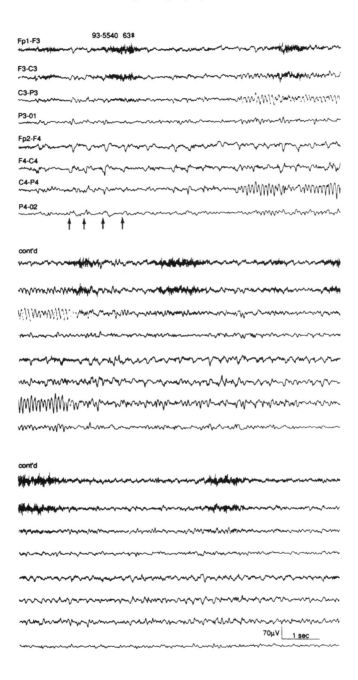

Figure 12.5 Subclinical rhythmic electrographic discharge in adults in a 63-year-old woman with vertigo. There was no history of seizures or stroke, and the patient was otherwise neurologically normal. Onset of the subclinical rhythmic electrographic electroencephalographic discharge of adults pattern begins with repetitive sharp waves (arrows).

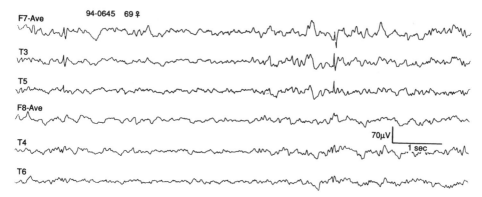

Figure 12.6 Small sharp spikes (benign epileptiform transients of sleep) in a 69-year-old woman with syncope. In this sample, the small sharp spikes are seen only on the left; in other portions of the electroencephalogram, they occurred independently on the right as well.

rior temporal areas. They are most evident using montages that employ long interelectrode distances (e.g., referential or nasopharyngeal linkages). The morphology is distinctive (Figure 12.6) and the best clue to recognition: a fast diphasic spike lasting less than 50 msec with positive and negative phases of equal amplitude. SSSs occur sporadically but are most common during waking–sleep transitions and during light sleep. Other identifying features include their sporadic occurrence, shifting laterality, and lack of associated focal slowing. Even when predominant on one side, SSSs almost never show persistent repetition or give the impression of a "focus."

EPILEPTIFORM ACTIVITY

Although the incidence of epilepsy increases in the elderly, general criteria for defining and classifying epileptiform activity are the same in elderly subjects as in younger individuals. Epileptiform discharges are recognized by several discriminators, including morphology, separateness from ongoing background activity, topographic distribution, repetition rate, associated abnormalities of background activity, and response to stimulation or state change.

EEG has been used to identify stroke patients at risk for later seizures, but there have been few systematic studies; available data are inconclusive or contradictory. EEG tracings collected after cerebral infarction has occurred may show either focal or generalized slowing with sharp-wave or spike-wave foci. Chartian et al.[94] described a number of patients in whom periodic, lateralized epileptiform discharges (PLEDs) appeared shortly after the infarct and were frequently associated with seizures (Figure 12.7). Holmes[95] also found that patients with postinfarction seizures had a higher incidence of PLEDs and other epileptiform patterns than poststroke patients without seizures. He noted, however, that

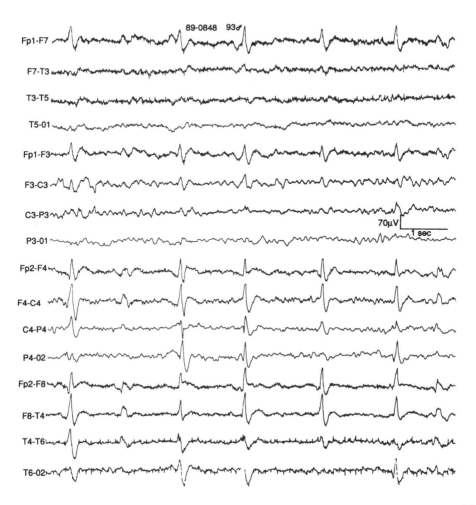

Figure 12.7 Right-sided periodic lateralized epileptiform discharges in a 93-year-old man with an acute stem occlusion of the right middle cerebral artery.

at least 70% of the patients who developed seizures did not have epileptiform abnormalities on their interictal EEG. Furthermore, there were no differences in the EEGs of patients with early (occurring within 2 weeks of infarction) versus late seizures. Epileptiform discharges were most frequent in patients with embolic strokes, and these patients had a very high risk of developing seizures. In the Seizures after Stroke study, however, there was no association between risk of seizures and cardioembolic stroke.[96] Furthermore, EEG findings were unhelpful in predicting onset or recurrence of seizures.

PLEDs can be seen in a variety of other acute or subacute conditions, including Binswanger's encephalopathy, Creutzfeldt-Jakob disease, herpes sim-

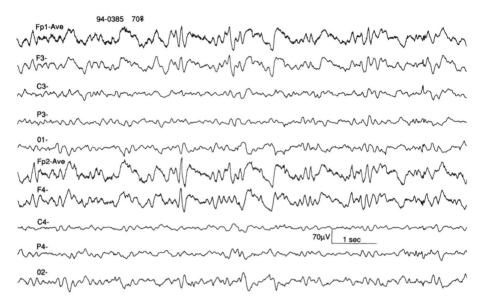

Figure 12.8 Bifrontal sharp waves mixed with high-voltage delta waves in a 70-year-old woman with Alzheimer's disease.

plex encephalitis, cerebral hemorrhage, and metastatic brain disease. Although a majority of patients with PLEDs have seizures, retrospective studies indicate that at least 20% do not. Antiepileptic drugs do not definitely affect PLEDs, nor is there evidence to suggest that their prophylactic use influences the development of later seizures.[3]

Epileptiform discharges (not PLEDs) may be seen in Alzheimer's disease (Figure 12.8).[97, 98] These are usually of low voltage and most often seen over the temporal areas; rarely, they are generalized. Occasionally, the epileptiform activity in Alzheimer's disease is more dramatic and may simulate a periodic pattern that superficially resembles that of Creutzfeldt-Jakob disease. Although both seizures and myoclonus occur in Alzheimer's disease, there have been no studies that have correlated either clinical manifestation with EEG findings, especially epileptiform activity.

There have been no prospective studies that have specifically addressed the role of EEG as a risk factor for recurrence in elderly patients with single unprovoked seizure or, similarly, as a risk factor for relapse after antiepileptic drug withdrawal.

Admixed slow-wave activity may produce combination wave forms that resemble epileptiform discharges. A common occurrence is the formation of an apparent temporal sharp slow-wave complex because of the coincidence of a sharp temporal alpha component with an isolated theta or delta slow-wave transient. The interpretive problem caused by combination waveforms and commingling of frequencies to produce pseudoepileptiform transients is even greater in EEGs showing prominent rhythmic beta activity (e.g., from benzodiazepines or other sedative drugs) and in patients with a breach rhythm resulting from a burr hole or craniotomy defect. Recognizing a sharp or "spiky" waveform as having a sinusoidal morphology and being part of a sequence of waves rather than a distinctly separate event is helpful in not overinterpreting transients as epileptiform.

ROLE OF LONG-TERM ELECTROENCEPHALOGRAPHIC MONITORING IN THE ELDERLY

Nonepileptic conditions may produce transient or paroxysmal symptoms that can be confused with epileptic seizures.[99] These symptoms may be secondary to neurologic, systemic, or psychogenic disorders. The approach to differential diagnosis of seizures in the elderly is similar to that in other age groups, although the diseases and conditions that may mimic epileptic seizures are, of course, different. Syncope presents the most common diagnostic problem. Transient ischemic attacks, transient global amnesia, drop attacks, movement disorders, and other kinds of spells may all, at times, prove perplexing to the physician and, depending on the circumstances, raise the question of seizures. Psychogenic seizures occur in a minority of elderly patients with depression. Finally, new-onset seizures may require diagnostic confirmation or present a dilemma in classification. As in other age groups, long-term EEG-video monitoring may be the most efficient way to establish a diagnosis of epilepsy and to distinguish nonepileptic from epileptic events.

CONCLUSIONS

The distinction between the normal and abnormal EEG is increasingly blurred with age. In the absence of quantitative measurements made in large samples of the normal population, EEG interpretation remains qualitative and subjective. Most age-related changes in EEG activity are probably due to various pathologic processes that affect the aging brain, but much of the time these are otherwise asymptomatic and of little or no clinical significance. Thus, in elderly patients with seizures, changes in EEG background activity may be related to concurrent disorders affecting the brain and not directly to the seizures themselves, which may arise from other conditions. Although the incidence and prevalence of epilepsy increase in older people, there are no changes in the EEG specifically associated with this increase. It is important to recognize that some age-related patterns mimic epileptic EEG activities but have no significance for the diagnosis of epilepsy. At the same time, interictal epileptiform discharges can occur with many diseases of old age that may or may not manifest with seizures.

There are a number of unanswered questions that pertain to the use of EEG in elderly patients with seizures:

1. What is the sensitivity and specificity of epileptiform discharges for epilepsy in the elderly?

2. Are EEG findings a risk factor for seizure recurrence as they are in younger age groups?
3. Are EEG findings related to risk of relapse following antiepileptic drug withdrawal?
4. Do EEG findings predict mortality as has been suggested for PLEDs in stroke?
5. Do antiepileptic drugs affect EEG findings in elderly patients?
6. Are there definable epilepsy syndromes of the elderly?

REFERENCES

1. Berger H. Über das Elektrenkephalogramm des Menschen V. Arch Psychiatr Nervenkr 1932;97:6. (English translation by Gloor P. "Hans Berger on the electroencephalogram of man.") Electroencephalogr Clin Neurophysiol 1969;28(Suppl):75.
2. Cooper R, Osselton JW, Shaw JC. EEG Technology (3rd ed). London: Butterworths, 1986;124.
3. Daly DD. Epilepsy and Syncope. In DD Daly, TA Pedley (eds), Current Practice of Clinical Electroencephalography (2nd ed). New York: Raven, 1990;269.
4. Niedermeyer E. Abnormal EEG Patterns: Epileptic and Paroxysmal. In E Niedermeyer, F Lopes da Silva (eds), Electroencephalography: Basic Principles, Clinical Applications, and Related Fields (3rd ed). Baltimore: Williams & Wilkins, 1993;217.
5. Hauser WA, Annegers JF, Kurland LT. Indicence of epilepsy and unprovoked seizures in Rochester, Minnesota, 1935–1984. Epilepsia 1993;34:453.
6. Giuliani G, Terziani S, Senigaglia AR, et al. Epilepsy in an Italian community as assessed by a survey for prescriptions of antiepileptic drugs: epidemiology and patterns of care. Acta Neurol Scand 1992;85:23.
7. Hauser WA, Kurland LT. The epidemiology of epilepsy in Rochester, Minnesota, 1935–1967. Epilepsia 1975;16:1.
8. Loiseau J, Loiseau P, Duche B, et al. A survey of epileptic disorders in southwest France: seizures in elderly patients. Ann Neurol 1990;27:232.
9. Luhdorf K, Jensen LD, Plesner AM. Etiology of seizures in the elderly. Epilepsia 1986;27:458.
10. Scheuer ML, Cohen J. Seizures and epilepsy in the elderly. Neurol Clin 1993;11:787.
11. Obrist WD. Problems of Aging. In A Redmond (ed), Handbook of Electroencephalography and Clinical Neurophysiology (Vol. 6A). Durham, NC: Duke University Press, 1976;275.
12. Obrist WD, Busse EW. The Electroencephalogram in Old Age. In WP Wilson (ed), Applications of Electroencephalography. Durham, NC: Duke University Press, 1965;185.
13. Pedley TA, Miller JA. Clinical Neurophysiology of Aging and Dementia. In R Mayeux, WG Rosen (eds), The Dementias. New York: Raven, 1983;31.
14. Lindsley, DB. Electrical potentials of the brain in children and adults. J Gen Psychol 1938;19:285.
15. Brazier MAB, Finesinger JE. Characteristics of the normal electroencephalogram. I. A study of the occipital cortical potentials in 500 normal adults. J Clin Invest 1944;23:303.
16. Otomo E. Electroencephalography in old age: dominant alpha rhythm. Electroencephalogr Clin Neurophysiol 1966;21:489.
17. Harner RN. EEG Evaluation of the Patient with Dementia. In DF Benson, D Blumer (eds), Psychiatric Aspects of Neurologic Disease. New York: Grune & Stratton, 1975;63.

18. Smith MC. Neurophysiology of aging. Semin Neurol 1989;9:68.
19. Mundy-Castle AC, Hurst LA, Beerstecher DM, Prinsloo T. The electroencephalogram in the senile psychoses. Electroencephalogr Clin Neurophysiol 1954;6:245.
20. Obrist WD. The electroencephalogram of normal aged adults. Electroencephalogr Clin Neurophysiol 1954;6:235.
21. Hubbard O, Sunde D, Goldensohn ES. The EEG in centenarians. Electroencephalogr Clin Neurophysiol 1976;40:407.
22. Wang HS, Busse EW. EEG of healthy old persons—a longitudinal study. I. Dominant background activity and occipital rhythm. J Gerontol 1969;24:419.
23. Katz RI, Horowitz GR. Electroencephalogram in the septuagenarian: studies in a normal geriatric population. J Am Geriatr Soc 1982;3:273.
24. Matejicek M. The EEG of the aging brain. A spectral analytic study [abstract]. Electroencephalogr Clin Neurophysiol 1981;51:51.
25. Nakano T, Miyasaka M, Ohtaka T, Mori K. A follow-up study of automatic EEG analysis and the mental deterioration in old age [abstract]. Electroencephalogr Clin Neurophysiol 1982;54:27.
26. Roubicek J. The electroencephalogram in the middle-aged and the elderly. J Am Geriatr Soc 1977;25:145.
27. Oken BS, Kaye JA. Electrophysiologic function in the healthy, extremely old. Neurology 1992;42:519.
28. Giaquinto S, Nolfe G. The EEG in the normal elderly: a contribution to the interpretation of aging and dementia. Electroencephalogr Clin Neurophysiol 1986;63:540.
29. Duffy FH, Albert MS, McAnulty G, Garvey AJ. Age-related differences in brain electrical activity of healthy subjects. Ann Neurol 1984;16:430.
30. Andermann K, Stoller A. EEG patterns in hospitalized and nonhospitalized aged [abstract]. Electroencephalogr Clin Neurophysiol 1961;13:319.
31. Obrist WD, Bissell LF. The electroencephalogram of aged patients with cardiac and cerebral vascular disease. J Gerontol 1955;10:315.
32. Christian W. Das Elektrenkephalogramm im hoheren Lebensalter. Nervenarzt 1984;55:517.
33. Pollock VE, Schneider LS, Lyness SA. EEG amplitudes in healthy, late middle-aged and elderly adults: normality of the distributions and correlations with age. Electroencephalogr Clin Neurophysiol 1990;75:276.
34. Otomo E, Tsubaki T. Electroencephalography in subjects sixty years and over. Electroencephalogr Clin Neurophysiol 1966;20:77.
35. Verdeaux G, Verdeaux J, Turmel J. Étude statistique de la fréquence et de la réactivité des électroencéphalogrammes chez les sujets agés. Can Psychiatr Assoc J 1961;6:28.
36. Mundy-Castle AC. An analysis of central responses to photic stimulation in normal adults. Electroencephalogr Clin Neurophysiol 1953;5:1.
37. Kellaway P. An Orderly Approach to Visual Analysis: Parameters of the Normal EEG in Adults and Children. In DD Daly, TA Pedley (eds), Current Practice of Clinical Electroencephalography (2nd ed). New York: Raven, 1990;139.
38. Gibbs EL, Lorimer FM, Gibbs FA. Clinical correlates of exceedingly fast activity in the electroencephalogram. Dis Nerv Syst 1950;11:323.
39. Kugler J. Fast EEG activity in normal people of advanced age [abstract]. Electroencephal Clin Neurophysiol 1983;56:678.
40. Celesia GG. EEG and event-related potentials in aging and dementia. J Clin Neurophysiol 1986;3:99.
41. McAdam W, Tait AC, Orme JE. Initial psychiatric illness in involutional men. III. J Ment Sci 1957;102:819.
42. Mundy-Castle AC. Theta and beta rhythm in the electroencephalograms of normal adults. Electroencephalogr Clin Neurophysiol 1951;3:477.
43. Thompson LW, Wilson S. Electrocortical reactivity and learning in the elderly. J Gerontol 1966;21:45.

44. Muller HF, Schwartz G. Electroencephalograms and autopsy findings in geropsychiatry. J Gerontol 1978;33:504.
45. Silverman AJ, Busse EW, Barnes RH. Studies in the processes of aging: electroencephalographic findings in 400 elderly subjects. Electroencephalogr Clin Neurophysiol 1955;7:67.
46. Busse EW, Barnes RH, Friedman EL, Kelty EJ. Psychological functioning of aged individuals with normal and abnormal electroencephalograms. I. A study of non-hospitalized community volunteers. J Nerv Ment Dis 1956;124:135.
47. Torres F, Faoro A, Loewenson R, Johnson E. The electroencephalogram of elderly subjects revisited. Electroencephalogr Clin Neurophysiol 1983;56:391.
48. Birren JE, Butler RN, Greenhouse SW, et al (eds). Human Aging: A Biological and Behavioral Study. Washington, DC: US Govt Printing Office, PHS Publication No 986, 1963;328.
49. Obrist WD, Busse EW, Eisdorfer C, Kleemeier RW. Relation of the electroencephalogram to intellectual function in senescence. J Gerontol 1962;17:197.
50. Irving G, Robinson RA, McAdam W. The validity of some cognitive tests in the diagnosis of dementia. Br J Psychiatry 1970;117:149.
51. Silverman AJ, Busse EW, Barnes RH, et al. Studies on the processes of aging. 4. Physiologic influences on psychic functioning in elderly people. Geriatrics 1953;8:370.
52. Barnes RH, Busse EW, Friedman EL. The psychological functioning of aged individuals with normal and abnormal electroencephalograms. II. A study of hospitalized individuals. J Nerv Ment Dis 1956;124:585.
53. Thaler M. Relationships among Wechsler, Weigl, Rorschach, EEG findings, and abstract-concrete behavior in a group of normal aged subjects. J Gerontol 1956;11:404.
54. Obrist WD, Henry CE. Electroencephalographic findings in aged psychiatric patients. J Nerv Ment Dis 1958;126:254.
55. Cahan RB, Yeager CL. Admission EEG as a predictor of mortality and discharge for aged state hospital patients. J Gerontol 1966;21:248.
56. Meyer JS, Waltz AG. Relationships of Cerebral Anoxia to Functionality and Electroencephalographic Abnormality. In H Gastaut, JS Meyer (eds), Cerebral Anoxia and the Electroencephalogram. Springfield, IL: Thomas, 1961;307.
57. Obrist WD, Sokoloff L, Lassen NA, et al. I. Relation of EEG to cerebral blood flow and metabolism in old age. Electroencephalogr Clin Neurohysiol 1963;15:610.
58. Sulg I. The quantitated EEG as a measure of brain dysfunction. Scand J Clin Lab Invest 1969;(Suppl 109)23:155.
59. Ingvar DH, Gustafson L. Regional cerebral blood flow in organic dementia with early onset. Acta Neurol Scand 1970;(Suppl 43)46:42.
60. Harvald B. EEG in old age. Acta Psychiatr Scand 1958;33:193.
61. Turton EC. The EEG as a diagnostic and prognostic aid in the differentiation of organic disorders in patients over 60. J Ment Sci 1958;104:461.
62. Obrist WD, Busse EW, Henry CE. Relation of electroencephalogram to blood pressure in elderly persons. Neurology 1961;11:151.
63. Obrist WD. Cerebral Ischemia and the Senescent Electroencephalogram. In E Simonson, McGavack TH (eds), Cerebral Ischemia. Springfield, IL: Thomas, 1964;71.
64. Kooi KA, Guvener AM, Tupper CJ, Bagchi BK. Electroencephalographic patterns of the temporal regions in normal adults. Neurology 1964;14:1029.
65. Busse EW, Barnes RH, Silverman AJ, et al. Studies of the process of aging: factors that influence the psyche of elderly persons. Am J Psychiatry 1954;110:897.
66. Mundy-Castle AC. Central Excitability in the Aged. In HT Blumenthal (ed), Medical and Clinical Aspects of Aging. New York: Columbia University Press, 1962;575.
67. Gibbs FA, Gibbs EL. Atlas of Electroencephalography (2nd ed). Vol 3. Reading,

MA: Addison-Wesley, 1964.

68. Harner RN. EEG Evaluation of the Patient with Dementia. In DF Benson, D Blumer (eds), Psychiatric Aspects of Neurologic Disease. New York: Grune & Stratton, 1975;63.

69. Drachman DA, Hughes JR. Memory and the hippocampal complexes. III. Aging and temporal EEG abnormalities. Neurology, 1971;21:1.

70. Bruens JH, Gastaut H, Giove G. Electroencephalographic study of the signs of chronic vascular insufficiency of the Sylvian region in aged people. Electroencephalogr Clin Neurophysiol 1960;12:283.

71. Niedermeyer E. The electroencephalogram and vertebrobasilar artery insufficiency. Neurology 1963;1:412.

72. Maynard SD, Hughes JR. A distinctive electrographic entity: bursts of rhythmical temporal theta. Clin Electroencephalogr 1984;15:145.

73. Brody H. Organization of the cerebral cortex. III. A study of aging in the human cerebral cortex. J Comp Neurol 1955;102:511.

74. Brody H. Structural changes in the aging nervous system. Interdis Topics Gerontol 1970;7:9.

75. Katz RI, Horowitz GR. Sleep-onset frontal rhythmic slowing in a normal geriatric population [abstract]. Electroencephalogr Clin Neurophysiol 1983;56:27.

76. Ehlers CL, Kupfer DJ. Effects of age on delta and REM sleep parameters. Electroencephalogr Clin Neurophysiol 1989;72:118.

77. Miles LE, Dement WC. Sleep and aging. Sleep 1980;3:119.

78. Prinz PM, Peskind ER, Vitaliano PP, et al. Changes in the sleep and waking EEGs of non-demented and demented elderly subjects. J Am Geriatr Soc 1982;30:86.

79. Blois R, Feinberg I, Gaillard JM, et al. Sleep in normal and pathological aging. Experientia 1983;39:551.

80. Reynolds CF III, Kupfer DJ, Taska LS, et al. Sleep of healthy seniors: A revisit. Sleep 1985;8:20.

81. Webb WB. Disorders of aging sleep. Interdis Topics Gerontol 1987;22:1.

82. Bliwise DL. Normal Aging. In MH Kryger, WC Dement (eds), Principles and Practices of Sleep Medicine. Philadelphia: Saunders, 1989;24.

83. Wauquier A, Van Sweden B. Aging of core and optional sleep. Biol Psychiatry 1992;31:866.

84. Gibbs FA, Gibbs EL. Atlas of Electroencephalography. Methodology and Controls (2nd ed). Vol 1. Reading, MA: Addison-Wesley, 1951.

85. Feinberg I, Kodresko RL, Heller N. EEG sleep patterns as a function of normal and pathological aging in man. J Psychiatr Res 1967;5:107.

86. Guazzelli M, Feinberg I, Aminoff G, et al. Sleep spindles in normal elderly: Comparison with young adult patterns and relation to nocturnal awakening, cognitive function and brain atrophy. Electroencephalogr Clin Neurophysiol 1986;63:526.

87. Wright EA, Gilmore RL. Features of the geriatric EEG: age-dependent incidence of POSTS. Clin Electroencephalogr 1985;16:11.

88. Van Sweden B, Wauquier A, Niedermeyer E. Normal Aging and Transient Cognitive Disorders in the Elderly. In E Niedermeyer, F Lopez da Silva (eds), Electroencephalography: Basic Principles, Clincal Applications, and Related Fields (3rd ed). Baltimore: Williams & Wilkins, 1993;329.

89. Naquet R, Louard C, Rhodes J, Vigouroux M. À propos de certaines décharges paroxystiques du carrefour temporo-pariéto-occipital: Leur activation par l'hypoxie. Rev Neurol (Paris) 1961;105:203.

90. Westmoreland BF, Klass DW. A distinctive rhythmic EEG discharge of adults. Electroencephalogr Clin Neurophysiol 1981;51:186.

91. Miller CR, Westmoreland BF, Klass DW. Subclinical rhythmic EEG discharge of adults (SREDA): further observations. Am J EEG Technol 1985;25:217.

92. Westmoreland BF. Benign EEG Variants and Patterns of Uncertain Clinical Significance. In DD Daly, TA Pedley (eds), Current Practice of Clinical

Electroencephalography (2nd ed). New York: Raven, 1990;243.

93. White JC, Langston JW, Pedley TA. Benign epileptiform transients of sleep: clarification of the small sharp spike controversy. Neurology 1977;27:1061.

94. Chartrian GE, Shaw CM, Leffman H. The significance of periodic lateralized epileptiform discharges in EEG. An electrographic, clinical and pathological study. Electroencephalogr Clin Neurophysiol 1964;17:177.

95. Holmes GL. The electroencephalogram as a predictor of seizures following cerebral infarction. Clin Electroencephalogr 1980;11:83.

96. Bladin CF, Johnston PJ, Alexandrov AV, Norris JW. Poststroke seizures [abstract]. Ann Neurol 1993;34:288.

97. Ehle AL, Johnson PC. Rapidly evolving EEG changes in a case of Alzheimer's disease. Ann Neurol 1977;1:593.

98. Muller HF, Kral VA. The electroencephalogram in advanced senile dementia. J Am Geriatr Soc 1967;15:415.

99. Engel J Jr. Seizures and Epilepsy. Philadelphia: FA Davis, 1989;340.

13

Diagnostic Methods II: Imaging Studies

Robert Zimmerman

INTRODUCTION

The role of imaging (magnetic resonance imaging [MRI] and computed tomography [CT]) in the evaluation of patients with seizure disorders has been the topic of many publications during the past several years, usually with an emphasis on the detection of the epileptogenic focus in young patients with intractable seizures.[1-3] In these candidates for seizure control surgery—that is, young patients with intractable seizures—the lesions are usually small and often located in the temporal lobes. They are rarely detected using CT, and only occasionally using MRI when routine imaging sequences are used. This has led to the development of MRI pulse sequences that can detect these subtle processes (e.g., low-grade gliomas, focal neuronal dysplasias, and mesial temporal sclerosis) with greater frequency. For instance, the introduction of fast-spin echo sequences (which can reduce image acquisition time by a factor of 16) has made it possible to obtain thin-section (3 mm or less), high-resolution, high-contrast images of the temporal lobes in as few as 4 minutes. In the past, images of this quality required more than 30 minutes to obtain (during which the patient had to remain motionless) and were impractical in the majority of cases. With these high-resolution sequences, it is possible to detect subtle abnormalities associated with mesial temporal sclerosis, including cortical thinning; focal dilatation of the temporal horn, choroidal fissure, or parahippocampal sulci; and focal gliosis. An additional benefit of the fast scanning techniques is that they allow for the performance of more sequences in each patient. Magnetic resonance spectroscopy (MRS) can be used to obtain metabolic information, potentially obviating the need for positron emission tomography (PET) in patients with epilepsy.[1]

In elderly patients, the situation is different. The diseases likely to cause seizures (e.g., infarcts, post-traumatic gliosis, primary and metastatic tumors)[4-7] are usually apparent on routine CT scans and MRI. In these patients, the challenge lies in differentiating these lesions from the findings normally or commonly encountered on cranial MRI and CT. In addition, since the therapeutic options are different in elderly patients, the implications of MRI and CT findings and therefore the indications for these examinations may also be different. This chapter reviews the indications for and choices of imaging studies, describes the "normal" appearance of the aging brain on MRI, and presents the typical imaging features of the lesions that cause seizures in elderly patients.

INDICATIONS FOR IMAGING PROTOCOLS

Imaging studies should be performed as part of the initial evaluation of new-onset or chronic recurrent seizures. The most important function of the imaging study is to detect or, more commonly, exclude treatable causes of epilepsy (e.g., subdural hematoma, tumor, or infection).[7] In most cases of epilepsy in the elderly, the cause of the seizures is identified, but no specific treatment is available or necessary. In these patients, the imaging studies still provide prognostic information regarding the patient's medical and neurologic condition, which may prove useful in planning seizure control therapy. Specialized imaging protocols (PET, MRS, high-resolution temporal lobe imaging) are indicated only if seizure surgery is contemplated.

MRI is the imaging procedure of choice in the evaluation of patients with seizures or epilepsy,[1-3] as it is superior to CT in the detection of virtually all pathologic processes except acute subarachnoid hemorrhage (SAH). CT should be used if MRI is contraindicated (e.g., in patients who have pacemakers or claustrophobia or who are clinically unstable). Contrast enhancement should be employed for both CT and MRI, as it improves detection of many lesions, in particular, meningiomas (a benign and treatable cause of seizures in the elderly). Rarely, additional imaging studies such as radionuclide exams (including PET and single-photon emission computed tomography) and angiography may prove useful for lesion characterization and surgical planning. Use of new MRI techniques, including MRS and magnetic resonance angiography (MRA), may the provide the same metabolic or angiographic information, obviating the need for these traditional studies.

NEURODEGENERATIVE DISEASES AND NORMAL AND COMMON AGE-RELATED FINDINGS

Conditions such as Alzheimer's disease, multi-infarct dementia, and chronic alcohol abuse have been linked to an increased incidence of seizures in the elderly.[8, 9] The imaging features of these conditions include atrophy and multifocal areas of abnormal intensity in the deep white matter (demyelination). These processes cannot be distinguished from the "normal" appearance of the aging brain; therefore, the diagnosis of neurodegenerative conditions and their relationship to the patients' seizures must be made with caution using all available clinical, laboratory, and imaging information. The findings that are commonly encountered in neurologically and cognitively normal elderly patients include atrophy, periventricular hyperintensity (PVH), multifocal ischemic demyelina-

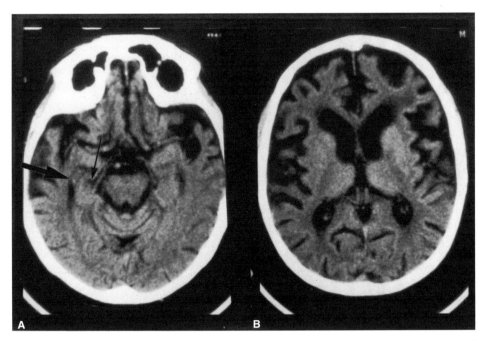

Figure 13.1 Atrophy. Computed tomography scan reveals evidence of ventricular and sulcal dilatation in this normal 81-year-old patient. Note small size of temporal horns (arrow) and choroidal fissures (small arrow).

tion, prominent perivascular spaces of Virchow-Robin (VR spaces), and loss of gray matter or white matter contrast.[10–17]

Atrophy is defined as cerebral volume loss and is manifested on CT scans and MRI by dilatation of the ventricles and sulci (Figure 13.1). This process is encountered in virtually all elderly patients, but there is a poor correlation between neurologic and mental status and qualitative assessment of the extent of atrophy in individual patients. Quantitative measures of ventricular and sulcal volumes on CT scans and MRI correlate somewhat better with objective assessments of cognitive function. Thus, it is appropriate to interpret CT and MRI studies as "normal for age" when mild ventricular and sulcal dilatation are found in elderly patients.[13, 14, 18]

Recently, it has been reported that Alzheimer's disease may be suspected when dilatation of the temporal horns, parahippocampal sulcus, and choroidal fissure[18] are detected, reflecting the anatomic distribution of this disease (Figure 13.2). In "normal," or age-appropriate, atrophy, the temporal horns and adjacent sulci and fissures are relatively small when compared with the remainder of the lateral ventricles and convexity sulci (see Figure 13.1). Another finding reported in Alzheimer's disease is rapid progression of atrophy, particularly of the temporal lobes.[18] This is in striking contrast to the situation in normal elder-

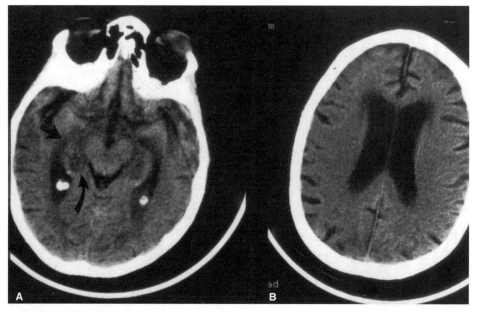

Figure 13.2 Alzheimer's disease. Generalized ventricular and sulcal dilatation are present. Note disproportionate dilatation of the temporal horns (arrow) and parahippocampal sulci (curved arrow).

ly patients in whom serial CT scans and MRI reveal little or no progression of atrophy on scans obtained over intervals of up to 10 years.

PVH is a phenomenon that was identified early in the exploration of MRI.[12] A halo of hyperintensity is seen around the lateral ventricles on long TR/intermediate TE (e.g., 2,500/40) proton-density (PD) MRI (Figures 13.3 and 13.4). PVH is the result of increased water in the periventricular white matter and was initially thought to represent transependymal resorption of cerebral spinal fluid (CSF) in patients with hydrocephalus. It quickly became apparent, however, that some degree of PVH is present in most patients and that it becomes increasingly prevalent and prominent with age. PVH does not indicate the presence of hydrocephalus or white matter infarction. Histologic studies demonstrate only myelin pallor.[11, 15] PVH is a manifestation of the normal transependymal flow of interstitial water into the ventricles. Since the brain has no lymphatic system, interstitial water is reabsorbed by diffusing along white matter tracts to the ventricular lining, where it is secreted as CSF (approximately 15% of CSF is normally produced by the ependymal lining) and recycled into the vascular system via the pacchionian granulations. In elderly patients, interstitial water is increased due to small areas of vascular damage, resulting in increased PVH.[12, 17]

Perhaps the most striking discovery of the early clinical explorations of cranial MRI was that elderly patients often have multifocal hyperintensity in supraten-

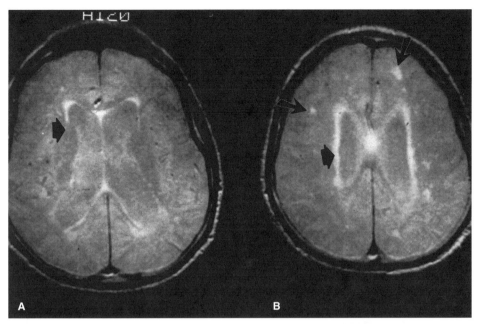

Figure 13.3 Periventricular hyperintensity. On proton-density magnetic resonance imaging in a 74-year-old man, a hyperintense halo surrounds the lateral ventricles (short arrows). A few foci of white matter hyperintensity ("unidentified bright objects") are also present (long arrows).

torial white matter on PD and T2-weighted images.[10] The foci are predominantly periventricular (most often near the atria) and irregular in contour (see Figures 13.3, 13.4, and 13.5). In severe cases, the foci become confluent, merging with the PVH to produce patchy or diffuse white matter hyperintensity, often in association with subcortical and pontine lesions (see Figure 13.4). The process was initially thought to represent demyelination secondary to white matter infarction. These MRI findings matched the pathologic features of subcortical atherosclerotic encephalopathy (Binswanger's disease), a rare cause of dementia in elderly hypertensive patients. It quickly became apparent, however, that most patients with these lesions neither have dementia nor focal neurologic dysfunction, and the foci were dubbed "UBOs" (unidentified bright objects) by William Bradley.[10] Epidemiologic studies subsequently documented a strong correlation between the presence of UBOs and evidence of generalized atherosclerosis and hypertension.[11, 13, 14] Several postmortem histology and MRI studies have demonstrated that UBOs represent a spectrum of changes ranging from myelin pallor (leukoaeriosis) through ischemic demyelination to frank lacunar infarction, which produces focal hypointensity on T1-weighted images and hyperintensity on T2-weighted images.[11, 13–15, 17]

UBOs are important in patients with seizures, as they may mimic or obscure acute infarcts and small neoplastic masses such as metastases (Figure

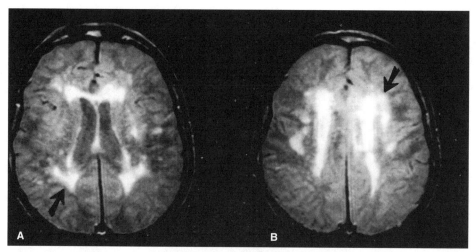

Figure 13.4 White matter hyperintensity ("unidentified bright objects") and periventricular hyperintensity. On proton-density magnetic resonance imaging in this 72-year-old woman, patchy foci of white matter hyperintensity are present (arrows), and they coalesce with the broad band of periventricular hyperintensity surrounding the ventricular system.

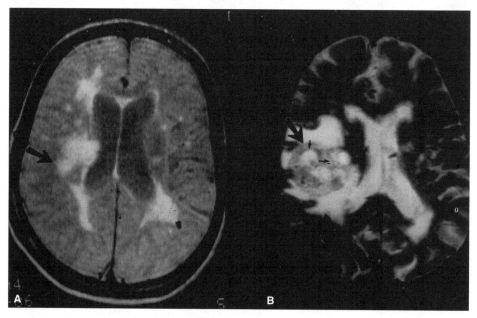

Figure 13.5 Glioma mimicking white matter hyperintensity ("unidentified bright objects"). Initial magnetic resonance imaging (A) reveals multiple "unidentified bright objects" and extensive periventricular hyperintensity in this 69-year-old woman. One "unidentified bright object" (arrow) is seen on a subsequent T2-weighted image 9 months later (B) to be a heterogeneous mass (arrow) with zones of necrosis (small arrows) and surroundings edema (curved arrow). At surgery, a malignant glioma was discovered.

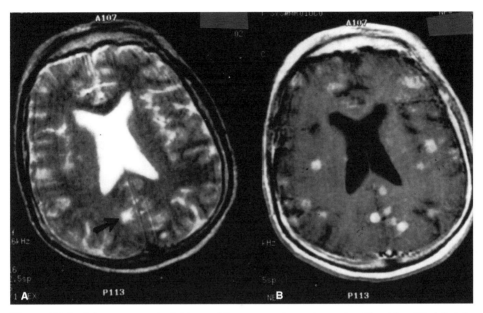

Figure 13.6 Metastases mimicking white matter hyperintensity ("unidentified bright objects"): value of contrast. Unenhanced T2-weighted image (A) in a 66-year-old patient with lung carcinoma and seizures reveals a single "unidentified bright object" (arrow). T1-weighted image after contrast administration (B) reveals multiple, small, solid enhancing masses (hyperintense) typical of metastases.

13.6). Contrast-enhanced scans are useful, as foci of ischemic demyelination never enhance. Small, subacute white matter infarcts occasionally enhance, whereas tumors, in particular metastases, virtually always enhance (Figure 13.7).

Dilatation of the VR spaces (see Figure 13.5) is another cause of focal hyperintensity in the brain on T2-weighted images, which was first discovered in the late 1980s with the advent of high-field (1.5T) MRI scanners.[16] As arteries and veins extend into and out of the brain from the subarachnoid space, they are surrounded by CSF. These small spaces became visible as scan resolution improved and were initially thought to be UBOs. These "lesions" are different from UBOs in that they are isointense to CSF on all sequences, more regular in size and contour, and are located in slightly different areas of the brain. The typical foci are hypointense to brain on T1-weighted images, isointense (and therefore invisible) on PD, and hyperintense on T2-weighted sequences. They are round or oval when used on axial images but appear more curvilinear when seen in coronal or sagittal plane, reflecting the course of the vessels they surround. VR spaces are routinely identified in patients of all ages in the inferior basal ganglia surrounding the lateral aspects of the anterior commissure within the anterior perforated substance (so named for the lenticulostriate arteries that

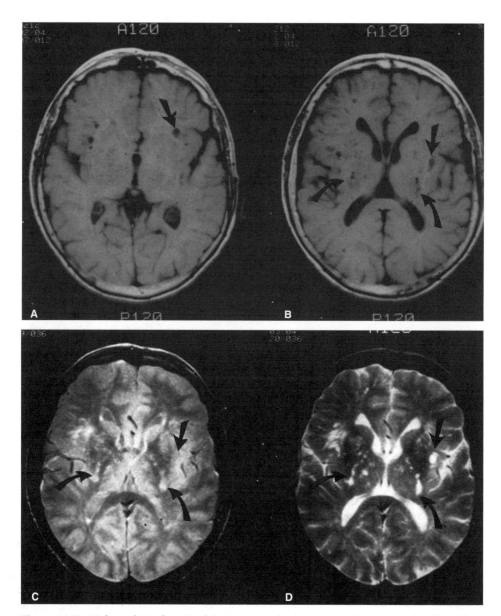

Figure 13.7 Enlarged Virchow-Robin spaces and white matter hyperintensity ("uniden-tified bright objects"). Multiple foci of hypointensity on T1-weighted images (A and B), isodensity and hyperintensity on proton-density magnetic resonance imaging (C), and hyperintensity on T2-weighted imaging (D) are identified. Foci that are isointense to cere-brospinal fluid (straight arrows) on all sequences are VR spaces. Foci that are hypo/isoin-tense on T1-weighted images and hyperintense on proton-density magnetic resonance images and T2-weighted images are areas of gliosis and demyelination ("unidentified bright objects") secondary to ischemia or infarction (curved arrows).

penetrate the brain at this level). Occasionally, these basal VR spaces may be quite large and asymmetric, mimicking mass lesions such as low-grade astrocytoma or arachnoid cyst. The location and intensity of these foci, their typical ovoid shape, and the absence of edema and mass effect allows for correct diagnosis. Prominent VR spaces are also seen in the convexity subcortical white matter and mesencephalon, where they may be mistaken for UBOs when only T2-weighted images are evaluated. The correct identification of convexity and stem VR spaces is facilitated when axial T1-weighted sequences and PD are performed. These convexity VR spaces increase in size with age (internal atrophy) and therefore are more frequently detected in elderly patients.

Finally, MRI scans in elderly patients often demonstrate poor differentiation between cortical gray and subcortical white matter on T2-weighted scans. In young and middle-aged adults, cortical gray matter is visualized as a thin rim of mild hyperintensity (light gray) relative to the adjacent darker white matter.[17]

CEREBROVASCULAR DISEASE

The most common cause of seizures in the elderly is cerebrovascular disease. Infarction,[19–21] hypertensive hemorrhage,[22] congophylic angiopathy,[23] venous thrombosis,[24] vascular malformations, and SAH[25] all may produce seizures, and in a minority of cases, epilepsy may develop (10%).[19–21] Seizures usually arise weeks to months after the ictus, and thus the results of MRI and CT scans do not affect acute treatment. Occasionally, seizures occur acutely and, rarely, may be the only finding heralding an acute vascular event. In these cases, the CT and MRI results are used to direct therapy.

Bland infarction occurs as a result of atherosclerotic occlusion (usually at the origin of the internal carotid artery), embolism (cortical branches of the middle or posterior cerebral arteries), or hypertension (deep gray matter and brain stem). Infarcts most commonly produce seizures when they are large (multilobar) or hemorrhagic.[21] Large infarcts are well seen on CT[26] but are detected earlier on MRI (6 hours using MRI versus 24 hours using CT),[27, 28] allowing for more timely intervention via anticoagulant therapy or clot lysis (e.g., direct infusion of streptokinase into the occluded artery). In addition, MRI can demonstrate major arterial occlusions,[27] dissections,[29] and subtle reperfusion hemorrhage not seen on CT.[30]

Characteristic imaging features of infarction allow for accurate diagnosis in the vast majority of cases.[26–28] Infarcts produce combined cytotoxic and vasogenic edema, which primarily involves cortex, deep gray matter, or both in the distribution of the occluded vessel(s). Edema associated with neoplastic and inflammatory lesions is vasogenic and tends to spare the gray matter while extending along white matter tracts without regard for vascular territories.

When diagnosis is in doubt, serial studies over short intervals will resolve the dilemma. Infarction has a unique temporal course, with rapid development followed by slower regression of edema, mass effect, and enhancement. Thus, studies obtained only hours or days apart will show dramatic changes in the

Table 13.1 Appearance (intensity) of hemorrhage on computed tomography (CT) and magnetic resonance imaging (MRI)

	0–12 Hrs	12 Hrs– 4 Days	4–7 Days	7–14 Days	14–28 Days	>28 Days
CT	+	++	+++	+/0	0/-	---
T1-weighted MRI	0/+	-	++	+++	++	+/0
Proton-density MRI	++	-	-+	++2	+++[b]	++[b]
T2-weighted MRI	++	---	--/0	++[b]	+++[b]	++[b]
T2[a]	-	---	--	-/+[b]	++[b]	++[b]

Note: Intensity is relative to normal gray matter.
+++ = marked hyperintensity (white); ++ = moderate hyperintensity; + = mild hyperintensity; 0 = isointensity; - = mild hypointensity; -- = moderate hypointensity; --- = marked hypointensity (black).
[a]Gradient echo sequence.
[b]Hypointense rim seen at margin of hematoma.

first few days after an acute infarct, and, in the subacute and healing phases (>10 days), distinct evidence of evolution and resolution is detected on studies performed at 3-day to 1-week intervals. By contrast, highly malignant tumors produce no obvious changes on scans obtained at weekly intervals (with the exception of lymphoma in immunocompromised patients). Acute infections (meningitis, abscess, encephalitis) cause progressive changes that are not as rapid as acute infarcts (weekly rather than daily).

The presence of hemorrhage increases the risk of seizures (25%) and epilepsy.[21] On both CT scans and MRI, the appearance of hemorrhage varies with time. The imaging features of hemorrhage are complex and beyond the scope of this discussion.[31, 32] A summary of these features is provided in Table 13.1. In general, MRI is superior to CT in detecting hemorrhage except in acute SAH secondary to ruptured aneurysm.[31–34] Hemorrhagic infarcts are usually embolic, with hemorrhage occurring several days after the onset of symptoms when flow is reestablished in damaged vessels (reperfusion).

Hypertensive cerebral vascular disease is a common cause of intracranial hemorrhage.[22] It tends to involve the small proximal perforating branches of the carotid and basilar arteries and thus occurs mainly in the supratentorial deep gray matter (basal ganglia and thalami) brain stem and cerebellum. The hypertensive hemorrhages are usually round or oval when small and become more irregular in contour as they enlarge.

Congophylic (or amyloid) angiopathy[23] is a variant of atherosclerotic cerebrovascular disease in which amyloid is deposited in small vessel walls (not related to systemic amyloidosis), leading to excessive vascular fragility (Figure 13.8). It occurs in patients older than 65 years of age, in whom it is the most common cause of lobar hemorrhage. Congophylic angiopathy produces multiple hemorrhages in the same location and in different areas of the brain. Smaller bleeds may be silent and precede large symptomatic hemorrhage, producing

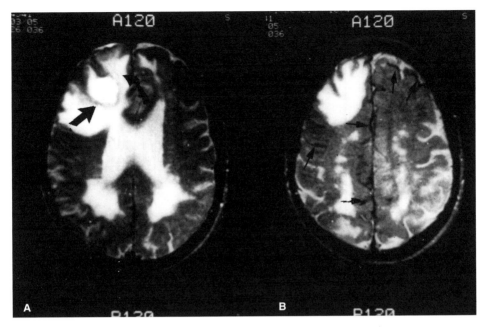

Figure 13.8 Congophylic angiopathy. T2-weighted image reveals a large subacute hematoma in the right frontal lobe (straight arrow) with surrounding edema (curved arrow). Focal cortical and curvilinear superficial areas of hypointensity represent hemosiderin deposition from prior subclinical episodes of hemorrhage elsewhere in the brain (small arrows).

idiopathic seizures. CT will detect large acute hemorrhage but not small prior bleeds. MRI will document both recent and old hemorrhages (foci of hypointensity in parenchyma and meninges due to hemosiderin deposition). Clinical findings and MRI and CT findings may mimic neoplasm when there is recurrent hemorrhage in the same location.

Cerebral venous thrombosis (CVT)[24] may present with seizures as a result of acute subcortical hemorrhagic infarction or venous hypertension with chronic ischemia (Figure 13.9). Since seizures occur during the active (acute or chronic) phase of the disease rather than as a consequence of a prior event, the patient can benefit from primary treatment such as systemic anticoagulation or direct endovascular clot lysis.

CVT is difficult to diagnose. The patient may present with an acute stroke-like ictus (often accompanied by seizures), with a rapidly progressive course having features that mimic infection, or with a slow, incremental picture suggestive of neoplasm. These protean clinical manifestations are dependent on a number of factors, including location (e.g., superior sagittal sinus, transverse sinus, deep veins, or cortical veins), extent of thrombosis, adequacy of collateral venous drainage, and chronicity of process. Conditions that produce increased

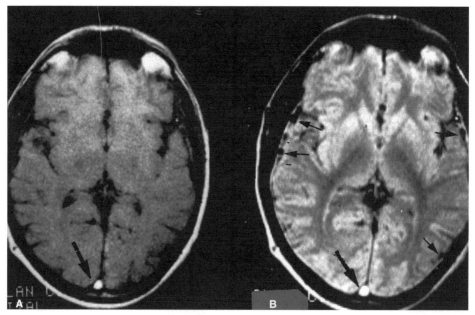

Figure 13.9 Chronic venous thrombosis. T1-weighted image (A) and a proton-density magnetic resonance image (B) reveal increased signal in the superior sagittal sinus (arrows) indicative of thrombosis (note appearance of the same structure on other images in this presentation (e.g., see Figure 13.7A). Prominent collateral cortical veins are identified along the convexities (small arrows).

blood viscosity, hypercoaguable states, or both may lead to the development of CVT in the elderly (e.g., hematopoietic disorders, neoplasms, dehydration, meningitis).

Because CVT has such variable clinical features, the correct diagnosis is often entertained only after imaging studies reveal evidence of this disorder. Before the advent of MRI, the diagnosis of CVT was difficult because the CT findings were often subtle or nonspecific. One or more subcortical hemorrhages, diffuse swelling, nodular enhancing densities on the surface of the brain and along the tentorium and falx (collateral draining veins), and filling defects within dural venous sinuses ("empty delta sign") are identified, but each finding is seen in a minority of patients. Thus, MRA is required in most cases to confirm the diagnosis of CVT.

The diagnosis of CVT has been greatly facilitated by MRI, since the effects of the thrombosis (hemorrhage, edema, and generalized swelling) are more easily detected using this procedure. The thrombosed veins and the collateral venous channels are better seen and characterized on MRI than on CT scans.[24] The patent collateral veins and the thrombosed venous structures can be directly visualized because of the unique MRI features of flowing blood. Most commonly, there is no intraluminal signal (flow void) on the MRI due to the movement of protons within the flowing blood during image acquisition. Thus, the presence of a signal equal to or greater than adjacent brain is highly suggestive of thrombosis. There are circumstances when normal flow does produce intraluminal signal (flow-related enhancement on T1-weighted scans and rephrasing on T2-weighted scans) but, with experience, these can be distinguished from occlusions based on the appearance of the vessels on multiple sequences. The recent advent of MRI angiography has further facilitated the diagnosis of CVT, replacing conventional angiography in virtually all cases.

Underlying vascular anomalies such as aneurysms, atriovenous malformations (AVMs), venous angiomas, and cavernous angiomas, may present with SAH and parenchymal hemorrhage.[25] Acute aneurysmal SAH is the one entity better seen on CT than on MRI.[31–34] The diffuse, unclotted blood in the subarachnoid space produces subtle intensity changes on MRI that are not as the dramatic as the density changes encountered on CT. Aneurysms, AVMs, and venous angiomas may be directly visualized on MRI, MRA, and less often on CT, but conventional angiography is necessary to confirm the diagnosis and for surgical planning. Cavernous angiomas are angiographically occult but produce typical MRI features of small areas of intense recurrent hemorrhage, often in the brain stem or cerebellum.[25]

TRAUMA

Seizures and epilepsy are most commonly the consequence of prior parenchymal damage and may occur many years after the traumatic episode.[4–7] Hemorrhagic contusions and frank hematomas go on to produce foci of gliosis, cystic encephalomalacia, and hemosiderin deposition, which act as seizure foci in approximately 10% of patients with significant head trauma.

Acute extra-axial hematomas (subdural and epidural) rarely produce seizures without underlying brain damage, whereas seizures occur in approximately 5% of patients with chronic subdural hematomas.[35] MRI is superior to CT in detecting all extra-axial hematomas because of multiplanar imaging and absence of artifact from adjacent bone.[36] SAH is usually seen in association with larger more consequential hemorrhages (e.g., hemorrhagic contusions). SAH as an isolated or predominant finding in head trauma is rare (<10%) and implies rupture of a major artery.

NEOPLASTIC AND INFLAMMATORY LESIONS

With neoplastic and inflammatory lesions, the disease process causing the seizures is active and progressive. Therapy (if available) is required, even though seizures will often persist after successful treatment of the underlying lesion. MRI and CT are used in determining the extent of the lesion and its likely histology. MRI is superior to CT in virtually all of these conditions. Contrast administration will aid in identification and characterization of the

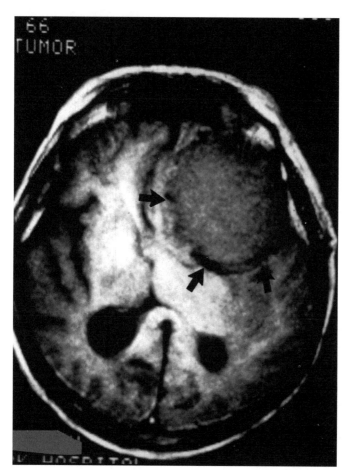

Figure 13.10 Meningioma. T1-weighted image reveals a large left convexity sharply marginated superficial mass that is isointense to gray matter. Note nodular hypointensity at the margin of the lesion (arrows) representing displaced cortical veins that form a cleavage plane between the mass and the brain.

lesions. In young patients with intractable seizures, the most common lesions are chronic, low-grade, intrinsic tumors of glial origin (e.g., astrocytoma, oligodendroglioma, and ganglioglioma).[1, 2] In elderly patients, the lesions commonly encountered include meningioma, high-grade glioma, and metastatic disease.[37]

Meningiomas are benign extra-axial tumors that are most commonly encountered in elderly patients (Figure 13.10). Most are amenable to at least partial resection, and prognosis is excellent. On CT scans and MRI, the lesions are discrete masses with relatively smooth borders. The presence of a cleavage plane between the tumor and the brain (produced by spinal fluid, vessels, or the cortical gray matter) is the most reliable sign that a mass is a extra-axial and therefore a meningioma. A flat, long border along a dural surface is indicative of meningioma, but this contour can be seen in discrete superficial cortical masses (e.g., metastases and low-grade gliomas). Meningiomas are usually homogeneously isodense to hyperdense on CT (focal hyperdensity reflects calcification). They are relatively isointense to brain on all MRI pulse sequences. Vasogenic edema is usually present and may be extensive. Small lesions without edema may be difficult to detect on unenhanced CT and MRI. Intense enhancement after contrast administration on both CT scans and MRI renders the tumor more visible and, with multiplanar MRI, allows for excellent assessment of the relationship between the tumor and adjacent brain. A tongue of enhancement is often seen extending away from the tumor on MRI. This "dural tail" is a characteristic but not pathognomonic finding in meningiomas and represents dural reaction with or without tumor extension. Tumor vascularity and its relationship to important venous structures may be ascertained with MRA, obviating the need for conventional angiography.

Gliomas (see Figure 13.6) in older patients are more likely to be of a higher grade (e.g., anaplastic astrocytoma and glioblastoma multiforme) and therefore carry with them a poor prognosis. Surgery, radiation, and chemotherapy are all used, but long-term survival is rare. Gliomas are usually large and irregular, with necrosis and cyst formation producing multilocular irregular, poorly marginated ring-enhancing lesions on MRI and CT scans.[37] The degree of enhancement correlates roughly with tumor grade, but absence of enhancement is not a reliable sign of benignity. Surrounding vasogenic (white matter) edema is variable and produces mass effect. The tumor typically infiltrates into the adjacent brain, where it is indistinguishable from the peritumoral edema. Occasionally, the tumor is purely infiltrative and appears as an area of vasogenic edema without an enhancing core. In these cases, the lesion may be mistaken for encephalitis or infarction. Hemorrhage and calcification produce hyperdensity on CT scans and variable intensity on MRI (both marked hypointensity and hyperintensity may be encountered depending on the pulse sequence, type of calcification, or age of hemorrhage). Less commonly, smooth-walled ring lesions (mimicking metastases and abscesses) and discrete homogeneous nonenhancing masses without edema (representing or mimicking low-grade gliomas) are encountered.

Metastatic foci may also present with seizures.[37] Absolute distinguishing features from gliomas and abscesses do not exist, but metastases are more often multiple, small, solid, or uniformly cystic than gliomas (see Figure 13.7).

Hemorrhage is common in lesions such as melanoma, renal, and thyroid metastases and may be seen in lung and breast cancer as well. The hemorrhage will usually obscure the underlying lesion. Contrast administration is necessary to identify small lesions (<1 cm), as these tumors are often isodense (on CT) and isointense (on MRI) to the brain, with little or no surrounding edema (see Figure 13.7). Enhanced scans are also necessary to distinguish between neoplastic and ischemic foci in the white matter.

Lymphoma (primary or secondary) has a predilection for the deep gray (basal ganglia and thalamus) and white matter (corpus callosum). It produces relatively solid, uniformly enhancing masses with mild edema and a tendency to spread along the ependyma.

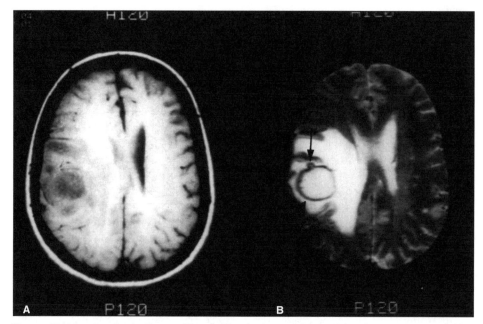

Figure 13.11 Cerebral abscess. T1-weighted (A) and T2-weighted (B) images reveal a well defined, smooth-walled ring lesion with surrounding edema in the right frontal lobe. The capsule is well seen as a hypointense ring on the T2-weighted image (arrow). Note small satellite lesion at anterior margin of the capsule (small arrow).

Infections are uncommon but often treatable causes of seizures in the elderly.[38] Prognosis is directly related to timeliness of intervention; therefore, early recognition and diagnosis based on imaging criteria have a dramatic effect on outcome. Pyogenic abscesses, viral encephalitis, meningitis, and extra-axial empyemas may all present with seizures. Systemic signs of infection such as fever and leukocytosis are helpful clues to diagnosis but may be absent in some cases.[38]

Pyogenic abscesses (Figure 13.11) have a stereotypical clinical course that correlates well with their pathologic and radiographic appearance.[38–40] Patients have evidence of a rapidly growing mass (seizures, focal deficits, obtundation) with or without (30%) systemic signs of infection. Pathologically, the acute cerebritis stage lasts approximately 5 days, with ill-defined areas of edema containing polymorphonucleocytes and viable bacteria. This is followed by the chronic cerebritis stage (5–10 days), during which most patients become symptomatic. There is central coalescence of necrotic debris and peripheral vascular proliferation, leading to macrophage and fibroblast infiltration at the edge of the necrotic cavity. By 2 weeks, this peripheral zone has developed into the unique fibrogliotic capsule of an acute abscess, which walls off the infection. If untreated, the capsule will thicken and may calcify, but eventually the abscess will rupture, usually into the ventricle.

Acute cerebritis produces vasogenic edema with a central core of vague hypointensity on T2-weighted MRI images. Over the next week, mass effect and edema progress, and a necrotic cavity surrounded by an intensely enhancing rim becomes apparent. The rim is characteristically hypointense on T2-weighted images (due to the T2 shortening effects of macrophage-produced, oxygen-free radicals), and as the late cerebritis matures into an acute abscess, this rim becomes more discrete. The capsule is of variable thickness, and there are often one or more small loculations (satellite lesions) at its margin. Metastases may have a similar appearance; however, there is usually subtle wall nodularity not seen in abscesses, and the extent of edema is more variable. Rapid progression occurs (much faster than with malignant neoplasms) if the abscess is not promptly treated. With appropriate surgical and antibiotic therapy, complete lesion regression and resolution will take place over a 6-month period.

Viral encephalitis[41] is most commonly caused by herpes simplex, which gains access to the brain via direct spread from the nasopharynx or via reactivation of latent virus in the gasserian ganglion (fifth nerve) at the base of the middle cranial fossa. It produces poorly confined edema and petechial hemorrhage, which extends across gray and white matter of the temporal and frontal lobes. Initially, the disease is unilateral but, if unchecked, will spread to the opposite hemisphere. Rapid treatment (<3 days) with acyclovir results in excellent clinical recovery. MRI is superior to CT in the early detection of this disorder, but treatment is usually started empirically based on clinical features. Edema and swelling of the temporal lobe and insular cortex that terminate abruptly at the external capsule are detected. More extensive involvement of the ipsilateral frontal and contralateral temporal lobe is seen as the disease progresses. Nonherpetic, sporadic, viral encephalitis produces diffuse white matter edema and swelling and is difficult to distinguish from vasogenic edema and infiltrative gliomas.

Acute bacterial and viral meningitis, when uncomplicated, produce no significant abnormalities on CT scans, whereas on MRI, meningeal enhancement may be seen.[38, 42] The complications of meningitis, including venous thrombosis and hydrocephalus, are best detected on enhanced MRI.

Granulomatous meningitis (e.g., tuberculosis) commonly produces abnormalities, including basal cistern enhancement, hydrocephalus, and deep infarction due to periarterial spread.[38] Subdural empyemas are rare but potentially fatal infections because of their propensity to produce retrograde cortical venous thrombosis. They are usually the result of direct spread from infected sinuses or mastoid air cells. The empyemas are small extra-axial fluid collections that are much more easily detected by MRI than by CT.[43]

Debilitated and immunocompromised patients may develop opportunistic infections (e.g., norcardiosis, aspergillosis, actinomycosis). Multiple, ill-defined lesions with minimal edema are typically seen and usually mistaken for metastases.[38]

Even if a mass is successfully treated, the patient may experience seizures as a result of residual damage to the brain or treatment (surgery, radiation, chemotherapy). This will obviously be a greater problem in more benign diseases such as meningioma and infection but may also complicate the course of partially or unsuccessfully treated malignant tumors.

REFERENCES

1. Jack CR. Epilepsy: surgery and imaging. Radiology 1993;189:635.
2. Hauser WA. Seizure disorders: the changes with age. Epilepsia 1992;33(Suppl 4):6.
3. Bronen RA. Epilepsy: the role of MR imaging. AJR Am J Roentgenol 1992; 159:1165.
4. Dam AM, Fugslang-Fredeiksen A, Svarre-Olson U, et al. Late-onset epilepsy: etiologies, types of seizures, and value of clinical investigation, EEG and computerized tomography scan. Epilepsia 1985;26:227.
5. Lopez JLP, Lonzo J, Quintana F, et al. Late onset epileptic seizures. Acta Neurol Scand 1985;72:380.
6. Luhdorf K, Jensen LK, Plesner AM. Etiology of seizures in the elderly. Epilepsia 1986;27:458.
7. Hauser WA, Hersdorffer U. Risk Factors. In Epilepsy: Frequency Causes and Consequences. Demos, 1990;53.
8. Shorvon SD. Late Onset Seizures and Dementia: A Review of the Epidemiology and Aetiology. In MR Trimble, EH Reynolds (eds), Epilepsy, Behavior and Cognitive Function. New York:Wiley, 1988;187.
9. Rovner BW, Folstein MF. Alzheimer's disease research at Johns Hopkins. Md Med J 1990;39:399.
10. Bradley WG, Waluch V, Brandt-Zawadski M, et al. Patchy periventricular white matter lesions in the elderly: a common observation during NMR imaging. Noninvasive Med Imag 1984; 1: 35-41.
11. Awad IA, Spetzler RF, Hodak JA, et al. Incidental subcortical lesions in the elderly. 1. Correlation with age and cerebral vascular risk factors. Stroke 1986;27:1090.
12. Zimmerman RD, Fleming CA, Lee BCP, et al. Periventricular hyperintensity as seen by magnetic resonance: prevalence and significance. AJNR Am J Neuroradiol 7;1986:13.
13. Drayer BP. Imaging of the aging brain. Part I. Normal findings. Radiology 1988;166:785.
14. Drayer BP. Imaging of the aging brain. Part II. Pathological conditions. Radiology 1988;166:797.
15. Boyko OB, Alston SR, Burger PC. Neuropathologic and post mortem MR imaging correlation of confluent periventricular white matter changes in the aging brain. Radiology 1989;173:86.
16. Heier LA, Bauer CJ, Schwartz L, et al. Large Virchow-Robin spaces: MR-clinical correlation. AJNR Am J Neuroradiol 1989;10:929.
17. Heier LA. White matter disease in the elderly: vascular etiologies. Neuroimaging Clin North Am 1992;2:441.
18. de Leon MJ, Golomb J, George AE, et al. Radiologic prediction of Alzheimer's disease: atrophic hippocampal formation. AJNR Am J Neuroradiol 1993;14:897.
19. Olsen TS, Hogenhaven H, Thage O. Epilepsy after stroke. Neurology 1987;37:1209.
20. Kotila M, Waltimo O. Epilepsy after stroke. Eplipesia 1992;33:495.
21. Lancman ME, Golimstok A, Norscini J, et al. Risk factors for developing seizures after a stroke. Epilepsia 1993;344:141.
22. Gokaslan ZL, Narayan RK. Intracranial hemorrhage in the hypertensive patient. Neuroimaging Clin North Am 1992;2:171.

23. Cosgove GR, Leblanc R, Moagher-Villemure K, et al. Cerebral amyloid angiopathy. Neurology 1985;35:625.
24. Zimmerman RD, Ernst RJ. Neuroimaging of cerebral venous thrombosis. Neuroimaging Clin North Am 1992;2:463.
25. Lownie SP. Intracranial hemorrhage in aneurysms and vascular malformations. Neuroimaging Clin North Am 1992;2:195.
26. Weingarten K. Computed tomography of cerebral infarction. Neuroimaging Clin North Am 1992;2:409.
27. Bryan RN, Levy LN, Wilcott MR, et al. Diagnosis of acute cerebral infarction: comparison of CT and MR imaging. AJNR Am J Neuroradiol 1991;12:611.
28. Yuh WTC, Crain MR. Magnetic resonance imaging of acute cerebral ischemia. Neuroimaging Clin North Am 1992;2:421.
29. Sue DE, Brandt-Zawodski MN, Chance J. Dissection of the cranial arteries of the neck: correlation of MRI with arteriography. Neuroradiology 1992;34:273.
30. Weingarten K, Filippi C, Zimmerman RD, et al. Detection of hemorrhage in acute cerebral infarction: evaluation with spin-echo and gradient-echo MRI. Clin Imaging 1994;18:43.
31. Zimmerman RD, Heier LA, Snow RB, et al. Acute intracranial hemorrhage: intensity changes on sequential MR scans at 0.5T. AJNR Am J Neuroradiol 1988;9:47.
32. Bradley WG. MR appearance of hemorrhage in the brain. Radiology 1993;189:15.
33. Ogawa T, Inugami A, Shimosegawa E, et al. Subarachnoid hemorrhage: evaluation with MR imaging. Radiology 1993;186:345.
34. Atlas SW. MR imaging is highly sensitive for acute subarachnoid hemorrhage...not! Radiology 1993;186:319.
35. Rubin G, Rappaport ZH. Epilepsy in chronic subdural hematoma. Acta Neurochir (Wien) 1993;123:39.
36. Kelly AB, Zimmerman RD, Snow RB, et al. Head trauma: comparison of MR and CT experience in 100 patients. AJNR Am J Neuroradiol 1988;9:699.
37. Masters LA, Zimmerman RD. Imaging of supratentorial tumors in adults. Neuroimaging Clin North Am 1993;3:649.
38. Zimmerman RD, Weingarten K. Evaluation of Intracranial Inflammatory Disease by CT and MRI. In WH Theodore (ed), Frontiers in Clinical Neuroscience 1988;4:75.
39. Haimes AB, Zimmerman RD, Morgello S, et al. MR imaging of brain abscesses. AJNR Am J Neuroradiol 1989;10:279.
40. Zimmerman RD, Weingarten K. Neuroimaging of cerebral abscesses. Neuroimaging Clin North Am 1991;1:1.
41. Jordan J, Enzmann DR. Encephalitis. Neuroimaging Clin North Am 1991;1:17.
42. Harris TM, Edwards MK. Meningitis. Neuroimaging Clin North Am 1991;1:39.
43. Weingarten K, Zimmerman RD, Becker RD, et al. Subdural and epidural empyemas: MR imaging. AJNR Am J Neuroradiol 1989;10:81.

14

Cognitive and Adjustmental Consequences of Seizures and Antiepileptic Drugs in the Elderly

Carl B. Dodrill

INTRODUCTION

There is no neuropsychological area of epilepsy known to this author that is more neglected than the neuropsychological study of the elderly. A review of the area reveals not a single data-based paper dealing with either the cognitive consequences of seizures or with the effects of antiepileptic drugs in the elderly. This finding is consistent with the results of a recent review.[1] Thus, there is literally no literature to review that presents previous studies in the area.

One must first inquire as to why so few neuropsychological investigations have been done with the elderly. The primary reason appears to be that these patients are infrequently referred for neuropsychological evaluations. This may be especially true if the patients have epilepsy alone rather than seizures as an accompaniment of another ongoing neurologic disorder. This author reviewed his own database, which had arisen from 23 years of neuropsychological testings. Of approximately 2,685 patients with epilepsy who received complete neuropsychological evaluations during this time, only 18 (0.67%) had confirmed epilepsy and were at least 60 years of age at the time of testing.

This infrequency of neuropsychological evaluations in the elderly is apparently typical across the United States. The present author informally polled the neuropsychologists at six other epilepsy centers across the country and asked about the commonness of neuropsychological evaluations at their centers of patients with epilepsy who were at least 60 years of age. The typical response was "rare," "unusual," or "only very occasionally." The neuropsychologist at one center thought he may see as many as one such patient per month, but all other responses obtained indicated far less common assessments of the elderly. In general, it appears that most epilepsy centers have only a small group of patients with confirmed epilepsy within this age range on whom neuropsychological evaluations have been accomplished.

The information just presented is in marked contrast to the availability of neuropsychological data on all other age groups. The reasons for this cannot be stated with precision, but they appear to include the following: (1) fewer referrals of the elderly from community physicians to epilepsy centers, (2) greater numbers of deaths in epilepsy than in the general population, and (3) fewer referrals of the elderly within epilepsy centers for neuropsychological evaluations. The last reason is evidently due to several factors, including the almost complete absence of a need of neuropsychological evaluations for job placements, a perception that such individuals are beyond the age of surgical interest, the exclusion from at least some drug studies, and the general belief that little can be done cognitively at this point in the life of the patient that would justify the amount of effort and time required to complete a battery of tests. The result of all these factors is that few complete neuropsychological evaluations are obtained with this age group.

Even without specific psychological testing data to confirm cognitive losses in elderly patients with epilepsy, there is certainly evidence to suggest that this might well be present. Gastaut et al.[2] reported that secondarily generalized epilepsy of late onset was associated with cerebral atrophy. Also, a greater sensitivity to the adverse effects of antiepileptic drugs might be expected in the elderly, including cognitive dulling, memory problems, and behavioral difficulties.[1] Even apart from epilepsy and its treatment, the process of aging results in adverse changes in cognitive abilities, which have been documented for many years.[3] Magnetic resonance image (MRI) scanning has now made it possible to evaluate pathologic changes in the brain in normal aging. In a recent study, for example, documented hippocampal atrophy in approximately one-third of neurologically normal adults who were 55–88 years of age.[4] Furthermore, it is now evident that cognitive impairment can be detected by systematic clinical ratings in up to 30% of elderly inpatients with medical (non-neurologic) conditions and that at least half of this is missed in routine medical workups.[5] Overall, there is ample reason to suspect that cognitive problems might be commonly found in elderly patients with epilepsy.

In view of the complete lack of directly relevant literature in the area, the author has chosen to present the original data available to him in order to meet the following objectives in at least a preliminary way: (1) to set the stage for the neuropsychological study of elderly individuals with epilepsy by describing their seizure-related characteristics in comparison with younger adults with epilepsy; (2) to present the cognitive, emotional, and psychosocial characteristics of elderly individuals with epilepsy along with any evidence for the cognitive effects of seizures and antiepileptic drugs; and (3) to compare the findings of elderly individuals with epilepsy with those of elderly patients with brain-related disorders who do not have epilepsy and also with those of healthy, age-comparable controls.

AGE-RELATED SEIZURE HISTORY CHARACTERISTICS

A definitive epidemiologic study of the age-related characteristics of epilepsy such as that recently published by Hauser et al.[6] is clearly beyond the scope of the present investigation. It is desirable, however, to include some basic seizure information on the samples to be reported here to facilitate comparison with other studies, particularly with respect to variables of special relevance to psychological investigations. Furthermore, except for normal controls described later, all patients included in the present report were those who had been referred for neuropsychological evaluations and who were able to complete all or nearly all of a full battery of tests. This may have created a bias in patient selection not found in other studies.

In the investigations reported here, "elderly" patients with epilepsy are identified as those who were 60 years of age or older at the time of their evaluations. To identify these people, the author reviewed his entire neuropsychology database of approximately 2,685 patients with epilepsy. Of these, he identified 236 patients ages 20–29 years, 45 patients ages 40–49 years, and 18 patients ages 60 years or older. All of these people had confirmed epilepsy, along with detailed, seizure-related information, and all had extended neuropsychological evaluations using the Neuropsychological Battery for Epilepsy.[7] This group of tests includes the Halstead-Reitan Neuropsychological Battery[8] the Minnesota Multiphasic Personality Inventory (MMPI), and the Washington Psychosocial Seizure Inventory[9] and typically requires approximately 7–10 hours for administration in the elderly age group.

Descriptive information on the three groups of patients with epilepsy is presented in Table 14.1. This table shows that certain basic descriptive variables (years of education, sex, handedness) are very much the same across the groups. Seizure type is also similar, as is the proportion of people with seizure disorder etiologies that are known versus unknown. When etiology is known, however, it is variable across the age groups, with a greater proportion of trauma in the youngest group (20%) than in the middle group (9%) or the eldest group (6%). On the other hand, vascular disorders as causes of seizures were found much less commonly in the youngest group (1%) and in the middle group (4%) than in the eldest group (28%). This is consistent with previously published research from a number of different centers as recently reviewed,[1] and the sample seems similar in neurologic history to groups previously reported in the literature.

Table 14.1 provides additional information of interest. Age at onset of seizures is clearly much more advanced in the eldest group. This has clear implications for studies of the type reported here, since physical development, psychological development, and socialization have long since been completed before the typical elderly person with epilepsy experienced the first seizure. Indeed, only one (6%) of the 18 elderly people with epilepsy experienced their first seizure before age 6 years, and only four (22%) before age 21 years. The parallel figures for the group of patients in their 40s were 20% and 60%, and for the patients in their 20s the numbers were 21% and 87%, respectively. Only one elderly patient had experienced seizures consistently from childhood to time of evaluation, whereas many of the patients in the other groups (and especially the youngest group) had this experience. All of these findings are clearly favorable for elderly individuals with epilepsy relative to their younger counterparts.

Table 14.1 Descriptive information on three groups of patients with epilepsy

Variable		Patient Group in Years			Statistic (p Level)
		Age 20–29	Age 40–49	Age 60–71	
N		236	45	18	
Age	Mean	24.28[a]	43.16[a]	63.89[a]	$F = 133.22$ (.0000)
	SD	2.92	2.61	3.46	
Education	Mean	12.15	11.76	12.61	$F = 0.82$ (.4419)
	SD	2.47	2.73	2.79	
Sex	Males	130	15	10	Fisher's exact (0.255)
	Females	106	30	8	
Handedness	Right	204	41	17	Fisher's exact (.5601)
	Left	32	4	1	
Seizure type					$\chi^2 = 9.79$ (.1336) (partial alone versus all generalized alone versus partial + generalized versus other)
SPS alone		3	1	1	
SPS + generalized tonic-clonic		21	4	3	
CPS alone		32	9	4	
CPS + generalized tonic-clonic		82	17	7	
Absence alone		0	1	0	
Absence + generalized tonic-clonic		17	1	0	
Generalized tonic-clonic alone		38	9	3	
Other combinations		43	3	0	
Etiology					Fisher's exact (.8403) (known versus unknown)
Unknown		124	24	11	
Trauma		47	4	1	
Infection		29	3	0	
Birth/congenital		10	2	0	
Vascular		3	2	5	
Tumor		4	1	0	
Other known		19	9	1	

Table 14.1 (continued)

Age at onset	Mean	12.13[a]	19.13[a]	42.67[a]	F = 18.61 (.0000)
	SD	7.08	13.29	21.37	
Duration of seizures	Mean	12.14[a, b]	23.56[a]	21.22[b]	F= 15.57 (.0000)
	SD	6.93	13.44	21.12	
Total seizures in last 30 days	Mean	6.74	2.85	5.17	F = 1.37 (.2561)
	SD	10.30	3.54	14.31	
Years of seizure control	Mean	1.43	1.42	4.46	F = 2.54 (.0814)
	SD	3.04	5.39	14.35	
Percentage of years in life without seizures	Mean	41.56[a]	46.94	19.19[a, b]	F = 6.35 (.0021)
	SD	26.27	29.98	26.29	
Number of years on medications for seizures	Mean	9.82[a]	19.14[a]	15.07	F = 6.52 (.0018)
	SD	6.55	12.81	17.60	
Number of medications at testing	Mean	1.93[a]	2.07[b]	1.39[a, b]	F = 4.21 (.0158)
	SD	0.87	0.86	0.78	

SD = standard deviation; CPS = complex partial seizures; SPS = simple partial seizures.
Note: F statistics are from one-way analysis of variance using ranked data. For each variable, subject groups having superscripts containing single letters (a or b) are statistically significantly different from each other (P <.05, Newman-Keuls procedure). For example, in the variable "Number of medications at testing" the first and third groups are statistically different as shown by the fact that the superscripts for each of these groups contains the common letter a. Also, the second and third groups are statistically different as shown by their superscripts, which contain the common letter b. The first and second groups are not statistically different, as they do not have a common letter in their superscripts.

Additional information in Table 14.1 pertains to the question of seizure control. No differences were found across the groups in terms of numbers of seizures for the 30 days before testing. Number of years with complete control of seizures was greater in the elderly patients than in the other groups, but this did not reach statistical significance in part because of substantial variability in the more elderly group, even with ranked data. It is nevertheless believed that there likely is a practical difference here because several patients had a large number of seizure-free years but could not make an estimate as to their number, as they could not recall their histories 30–60 years previously. A derived variable was computed, however, which was the number of years with seizures divided by the patient's age multiplied by 100. This percentage of years in one's entire life with seizures was markedly lower for elderly patients (19%) than for either patients in their 20s (42%) or patients in their 40s (47%). Thus, it is clear that seizures have been a problem for a much smaller proportion of the elderly patients lives than for younger patients. These findings are consistent with those of Scheuer and Cohen,[1] who reported relatively lower rates of seizures in elderly patients with epilepsy.

A final comment concerning seizures pertains to lifetime histories of generalized tonic-clonic seizures. Information on this variable was examined in detail for the more elderly group. It was discovered that 12 of the 18 patients had at least one such attack but that only four patients (22%) had histories of more than five convulsions in their lifetime. This is far less than the 100 or more generalized tonic-clonic attacks associated by some investigators[10, 11] with cognitive impairment or significant emotional and psychosocial problems.[12] Consequently, it is not believed that seizures themselves likely had a significant impact on functioning in this group of elderly patients.

With respect to medication, elderly patients did not differ from the two younger groups with respect to how long they had taken medications, even though the two younger groups differed from each other. At the time of testing, however, they were taking fewer antiepileptic drugs than patients in either of the other two groups (see Table 14.1).

All of the above findings indicate that elderly patients with epilepsy have seizure disorders that are significantly different from those of younger patients in several important respects. Except for an increased incidence of cerebrovascular disease, the differences are all favorable for the elderly patient with epilepsy.

PSYCHOLOGICAL CHARACTERISTICS OF ELDERLY PATIENTS WITH EPILEPSY

We now turn to the second objective of this chapter, which is to describe the cognitive, emotional, and psychosocial characteristics of our sample of elderly patients with epilepsy.

The first column of figures in Table 14.2 gives data on the intellectual and cognitive abilities of elderly patients with epilepsy. All patients had been administered the complete Wechsler Adult Intelligence Scale-Revised (WAIS-R) or the Wechsler Adult Intelligence Scale (with adjustment to WAIS-R intelligence quotient values as specified in the WAIS-R manual). Data were analyzed by means of one-way ANOVA with the Newman-Keuls procedure to evaluate differences between groups. Intellectually, on the WAIS-R, it is clear that this group is within the average range with respect to both verbal and visual-spatial skills. This is fully 10 points higher than the intellectual level of a sample of 840 younger patients also evaluated at our facility.[13]

Neuropsychological abilities were evaluated by means of the Neuropsychological Battery for Epilepsy.[7] Especially good scores for this age of patient were obtained in the areas of verbal memory (Wechsler Memory Scale [WMS] Logical Memory) and motor speed (finger tapping). The poorest scores were found on measures of visual-spatial memory (Tactual Performance Test [TPT] Memory, TPT Localization, WMS Visual Reproduction) and on indicators of attention and concentration (Stroop 3, tonal memory). Intermediate scores were found on perceptual skills and problem solving. Overall, indicators

Table 14.2 Cognitive and adjustmental information on three groups of older patients (epileptic, neurologic [nonepileptic], and normal control)

		Patient Group			F Statistic (p level)
Variable		Epileptic	Neuro-logic	Control	
WAIS-R					
Verbal IQ	Mean	99.82	101.30	113.33	3.19 (.0531)
	SD	13.79	10.41	16.01	
Performance IQ	Mean	94.06[a]	98.20	106.50[a]	4.49 (.0182)
	SD	10.27	11.21	10.54	
Full-scale IQ	Mean	97.35[a]	99.30[b]	111.08[a, b]	4.35 (.0204)
	SD	12.31	8.12	14.71	
Neuropsychological Battery for Epilepsy					
Stroop 1 (reading speed)	Mean	106.33	113.31	90.92	3.12 (.0551)
	SD	48.82	25.92	13.04	
Stroop 2-1 (interference)	Mean	228.06	189.15	176.50	2.40 (.1038)
	SD	73.21	73.21	54.26	
WMS verbal memory (number correct)	Mean	17.67	17.69	22.25	2.20 (.1240)
	SD	6.49	5.39	6.25	
WMS visual memory (number correct)	Mean	6.83	6.54	8.92	2.19 (.1257)
	SD	3.15	3.10	3.00	
Perceptual exam (total errors)	Mean	13.06[a]	19.38[a, b]	8.00[b]	4.24 (.0214)
	SD	14.96	15.86	7.05	
Name writing, total (letters/sec)	Mean	0.78	0.89	0.98	2.19 (.1248)
	SD	0.25	0.32	0.19	
Category test (total errors)	Mean	65.35	54.08	63.50	1.04 (.3615)
	SD	20.42	17.04	22.13	
TPT, total time (minutes)	Mean	30.52	32.94	21.87	1.69 (.1968)
	SD	16.82	18.13	11.54	
TPT memory (blocks recalled)	Mean	4.89[a]	2.17[b]	7.67[a, b]	8.16 (.0011)
	SD	2.17	2.65	1.56	
TPT localization (blocks located)	Mean	1.39[a]	2.31[b]	3.67[a, b]	8.32 (.0010)
	SD	1.24	1.65	1.56	
Seashore rhythm (number correct)	Mean	24.18[a]	23.77[b]	26.17[a ,b]	4.26 (.0212)
	SD	3.54	5.46	5.91	
Tonal memory (number correct)	Mean	17.65	19.00	22.42	1.31 (.2805)
	SD	7.62	7.85	5.60	
Finger tap, total (taps/10 sec)	Mean	88.11	81.85	83.00	0.49 (.6183)
	SD	13.40	21.87	12.73	
Trail making B (secs)	Mean	110.72	120.92	89.83	0.59 (.5600)
	SD	58.24	64.67	24.14	
Aphasia screening (total errors)	Mean	3.83[a]	3.92[b]	1.67[a, b]	4.26 (.0209)
	SD	4.18	3.97	1.59	
Constructional dyspraxia (rating)	Mean	1.39	1.38	0.75	2.75 (.0763)
	SD	0.98	0.65	0.75	

Table 14.2 (continued)

Variable		Epileptic	Neuro-logic	Control	F Statistic (p level)
			Patient Group		
Summary: Halstead	Mean	0.72[a]	0.72[b]	0.53[a, b]	4.78 (.0138)
Impairment Index	SD	0.21	0.21	0.16	
Summary: percentage of	Mean	68.78[a]	63.92[b]	46.50[a, b]	6.75 (.0030)
tests outside normal	SD	15.67	22.98	15.47	

SD = standard deviation; WAIS-R = Wechsler Adult Intelligence Scale-Revised; WMS = Wechsler Memory Scale; TPT = Tactual Performance Test.
Note: F statistics are from one-way analysis of variance using ranked data. For each variable, subject groups having superscripts containing single letters (a or b) are statistically significantly different from each other ($P < .05$, Newman-Keuls procedure). For example, in the perceptual exam variable, the epileptic and neurologic groups are statistically different from each as shown by the common letter a in their superscripts. The neurologic and control groups are shown as statistically different from each other by the common letter b. However, the epileptic and control groups are not statistically different from each other, as shown by the absence of a common letter in their superscripts.

(Halstead Impairment Index, percentage of scores outside normal limits on the Neuropsychological Battery for Epilepsy) showed that approximately 70% of the tests were performed outside normal limits. Only approximately 45–55% would be expected to be performed in this range based on aging factors alone.[8] Thus, only mild deficiencies were noted on the neuropsychological measures overall.

The MMPI was administered to provide an index of emotional functioning, and the average profile is presented in Figure 14.1. This average profile shows that, although in general elderly patients with epilepsy do not demonstrate substantial psychiatric disturbance, they are mildly depressed. They are also a little more tense and anxious than is desirable, and they are somewhat more focused on somatic problems than would normally be expected, even for individuals their age. The slightly increased score on the Sc (schizophrenia) scale is not remarkable, as elevations of this degree are common for patients with epilepsy generally due to the characteristics of their seizures (e.g., having spells during which they knew what was going on around them but could not respond, experiencing feelings of distorted reality, etc.). Overall, the MMPI was consistent with that of patients with epilepsy tested at our facility.[14]

Psychosocial adjustment was evaluated by means of the Washington Psychosocial Seizure Inventory.[9] This 132-item, quality-of-life measure evaluates psychosocial functioning in epilepsy with respect to seven areas. It also contains an overall functioning scale and three validity scales. The profile for the group of elderly patients is presented in Figure 14.2. As with the MMPI, higher scores indicate more problems. On the far right, the areas of profile elevation are indicated with the following approximate interpretations: area 1—no problems; area 2—questionable problems or slight difficulties; area 3—definite problems; area 4—marked psychosocial concerns. A limited elevation on the Emotional Adjustment Scale was consistent with the MMPI in pointing to mild discouragement, tension,

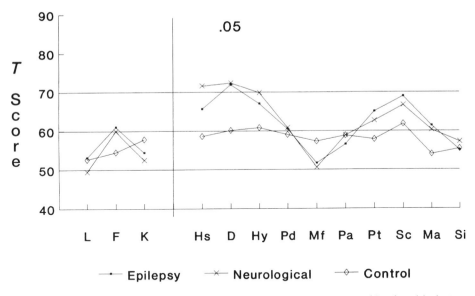

Figure 14.1 Minnesota Multiphasic Personality Inventory average profiles for elderly (age 60 years and older) groups: epilepsy, neurologic nonepileptic, normal control. (L = lie scale; F = infrequency scale; K = K scale; Hs = hypochondriasis; D = depression; Hy = conversion hysteria; Pd = psychopathic deviate; Mf = masculinity-feminity; Pa = paranoia; Pt = psychasthenia; Sc = schizophrenia; Ma = hypomania; Si = social introversion.)

and anxiety. The patients also reported that their seizures were of some concern to them, although they did not appear to be overwhelmed by them. The overall profile points to only a few psychosocial concerns rather than major difficulties in any area. It is similar to that of profiles from many places across the United States, except that there are fewer vocational and financial difficulties.[15] At least for the vocational area, this would appear to be entirely reasonable for this age group.

We now turn to the possible effects of medications on cognition and adjustment in the elderly. Sixteen of the 18 elderly epilepsy patients were taking one or more medications for epilepsy, and serum level data were complete on 14 cases. Eight patients were on monotherapy (five were taking phenytoin; two were taking carbamazepine; one was taking phenobarbital), and eight were on polytherapy (three were taking phenytoin and primidone; two were taking phenytoin and phenobarbital; two were taking carbamazepine and valproate; one was taking carbamazepine and mephenytoin). Average serum levels were as follows (µg/ml): phenytoin, 12.0; carbamazepine, 8.7; phenobarbital, 25.2; primidone, 8.8; valproate, 66.0; and mephenytoin, 17.4. Of the 24 serum levels obtained, only one (a phenytoin level of 20.1) was considered to be even slightly above the therapeutic range. All the data on medications are simultaneously considered and the pattern of deficiencies on the neuropsychological tests examined, and it does not

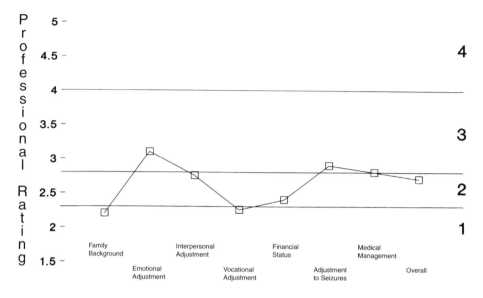

Figure 14.2 Washington Psychosocial Seizure Inventory average profile for elderly (ages 60–71 years) patients with epilepsy.

appear likely that medications had a significant adverse impact on cognition or adjustment. For example, tests of motor speed are often affected by the drugs used here,[16] but finger tapping was among those tasks best performed.

COMPARISON OF EPILEPSY WITH OTHER ELDERLY SUBJECT GROUPS

Thirteen patients 60–70 years of age or older were identified who had brain-related disorders other than epilepsy. They averaged 64.54 years of age and 13.08 years of education. There were 10 men and three women. Twelve were right-handed. Diagnoses for this group were as follows: Seven had cerebrovascular disease, two had trauma, one had a tumor, one had anoxia, one had cerebral atrophy, and one had a movement disorder.

Twelve control adults ages 60–74 years were identified whose neurologic histories were totally normal. They had never had any type of central nervous system disorder or problem at any point in life and had never had a seizure. All had volunteered to be part of research studies, and they were from the community in general rather than from any medical group or clinic. They averaged 67.08 years of age and had an average of 12.92 years of education. There were eight men and four women. All were right-handed.

Table 14.2 presents a comparison of the three elderly groups on cognitive measures. A perusal of this table reveals that the control group routinely performed better than the other two groups. This, of course, was entirely expected, but it was observed that the differences reached statistical significance less than half the time. This was unexpected, particularly in view of previous results with the same neuropsychological tests with younger patients, in which all variables attained high levels of statistical significance.[7] An informal review of comparable data for younger individuals with neurologic conditions other than epilepsy (neurologic cases) and younger control cases revealed greater differences than those shown here. Thus, our younger patients with epilepsy are relatively worse off in comparison with normal controls than our elderly patients with epilepsy.

A major reason for the conclusion just reached is that our normal control group showed significant aging effects by the time they were in their mid 60s. Even though intelligence quotient scores held well because they are age-corrected, scores on the other neuropsychological tests with younger neurologically normal individuals were substantially better than those of the elderly individuals in good health who were examined here.[7] Thus, normal aging apparently reduced the discrepancy in cognitive functioning between normal individuals and patients with neurologic conditions including epilepsy. This agrees with a recent study that concluded that hippocampal atrophy probably exists in one-third of normal elderly adults.[4]

Another conclusion evident from the data presented in Table 14.2 is that the cognitive deficits found in epilepsy were by no means peculiar to it. On the contrary, whenever the group with epilepsy performed statistically more poorly than the normal controls, the neurologic group also performed statistically more poorly, and the epilepsy group did not perform reliably better or worse than the neurologic group. The only exception was the perceptual examination, in which the neurologic group performed worse than the group with epilepsy. In general, the epilepsy and neurologic groups were highly similar in performance.

Finally, emotional and personal adjustment as evaluated by the MMPI showed only mildly increased depression and an emphasis on somatic concerns in both the epilepsy and the general neurologic groups (see Figure 14.2). The profiles for the neurologic and epilepsy groups are in fact remarkably similar. These data raise the possibility that it is the presence of brain-related disorders that is to be associated with the limited degree of emotional concern expressed here. Whether or not epilepsy is present does not appear to be a key point in distinguishing these people from healthy controls.

CONCLUSIONS

For various reasons, very little study has been completed on the cognitive and adjustmental impacts of seizures and antiepileptic drugs in the elderly with epilepsy. Although the results of the present study with its small number of elderly patients with epilepsy are tentative, they raise the possibility that their seizure disorders may not be as disabling as those of younger individuals with epilepsy. The elderly patients with epilepsy do not appear functionally different from age-comparable neurologic patients without epilepsy. Therefore, the possibility is raised that the primary problem is not the seizures at all, but instead the underlying neurologic difficulty that brought the seizures on. Cognitive effects of both seizures and antiepileptic drugs did not appear to be of importance in this sample. Especially in view of the increasing elderly population in the United States, all of these tentative conclusions deserve serious research attention in the future.

Acknowledgments
Appreciation is expressed to the physicians who referred the elderly and neurologic cases for neuropsychological evaluations, including George A. Ojemann, Linda M. Ojemann, Mark Sumi, Alan J. Wilensky, Robert J. Wilkus, H. Richard Winn, and Mark Yerby.

REFERENCES

1. Scheuer ML, Cohen J. Seizures and epilepsy in the elderly. Neurol Clin North Am 1993;11:787.
2. Gastaut H, Pinsard N, Genton P. Electroclinical Correlations of CT Scans in Secondary Generalized Epilepsies. In R Canger, F Angeleri, JK Penry (eds), Advances in Epileptology: XIth Epilepsy International Symposium. New York: Raven, 1980;45.
3. Lindenberger U, Mayr U, Kliegl R. Speed and intelligence in old age. Psychol Aging 1993;8:207.
4. Golomb J, de Leon MJ, Kluger A, et al. Hippocampal atrophy in normal aging. Arch Neurol 1993;50:967.
5. Ardern M, Mayou R, Feldman E, Hawton K. Cognitive impairment in the medically ill: how often is it missed? Int J Geriatr Psychiatry 1993;8:929.
6. Hauser WA, Annegers JF, Kurland LT. Incidence of epilepsy and unprovoked seizures in Rochester, Minnesota, 1935–1984. Epilepsia 1993;34:453.
7. Dodrill CB. A neuropsychological battery for epilepsy. Epilepsia 1978;19:611.
8. Heaton RK, Grant I, Matthews CG. Comprehensive Norms for an Expanded Halstead-Reitan Battery. Odessa, FL: Psychological Assessment Resources, 1991.
9. Dodrill CB, Batzel LW, Queisser HR, Temkin N. An objective method for the assessment of psychological and social problems among epileptics. Epilepsia 1980;21:123.
10. Dodrill CB. Correlates of generalized tonic-clonic seizures with intellectual, neuropsychological, emotional, and social function in patients with epilepsy. Epilepsia 1986;27:399.
11. Lennox WG, Lennox MA. Epilepsy and Related Disorders. Boston: Little, Brown, 1960.
12. Dodrill CB, Batzel LW. Interictal behavioral features of patients with epilepsy. Epilepsia 1986;27(Suppl 2):64.
13. Dodrill CB. Interictal cognitive aspects of epilepsy. Epilepsia 1992;33(Suppl 6):7.
14. Dodrill CB. Neuropsychological aspects of epilepsy. Psychiatr Clin North Am 1992;15:383.
15. Dodrill CB, Breyer DN, Diamond MB, et al. Psychosocial problems among adults with epilepsy. Epilepsia 1984;25:168.
16. Duncan JS, Shorvon SD, Trimble MR. Effects of removal of phenytoin, carbamazepine, and valproate on cognitive function. Epilepsia 1990;31:584.

15

Clinical and Epidemiologic Study of Status Epilepticus in the Elderly

Robert J. DeLorenzo

INTRODUCTION

Status epilepticus (SE) is recognized as a major medical and neurologic emergency that requires immediate treatment to prevent significant morbidity and mortality.[1-8] The acute medical management of SE has been reviewed.[2, 6, 7, 10-12] It has been recommended that standard protocols for treatment be developed in advance in medical centers and clinical practice facilities to have a treatment plan ready for immediate use and, thus, facilitate the rapid initiation of treatment of this condition.[2, 3] Despite advances in treatment, SE is still associated with a significant morbidity and mortality that can be diminished only by developing a better understanding of the pathophysiology of this condition and new insights into more effective treatment.[9]

It has been difficult to study SE because of its complex clinical presentations.[5] Individuals with epilepsy represent a considerable "at-risk" population for developing SE, but the majority of SE cases occur in acute medical and neurologic illnesses.[5] Initial epidemiologic studies of SE[4, 5] have indicated that approximately 50,000–150,000 cases of SE occur annually in the United States. Thus, the relative frequency of occurrence of SE and its combined morbidity and mortality demonstrate the need for further study of this important neurologic condition.

Studies from the Medical College of Virginia (MCV) Epilepsy Research Center[9] in Richmond, Virginia, used a sophisticated statistical analysis of a large SE patient population to develop clinical predictive indicators of outcome for mortality in SE. Seizure duration, specific etiologies, and age were shown to be reliable predictive indicators of outcome.[9] Sex, race, and certain other etiologies were found not to be factors that significantly affect morbidity and mortality. In addition, it has been demonstrated that electrophysiologic monitoring with evoked potentials[13] and electroencephalography[14] (EEG) may also be of predictive value. Analysis of this large population of patients should provide an outcome scale to assist in identifying high-risk patients, thus providing a focus for future studies aimed at improving outcome.

The elderly population has been identified in these initial studies[4, 9] as having the highest mortality. Age has been clearly established as a predictive

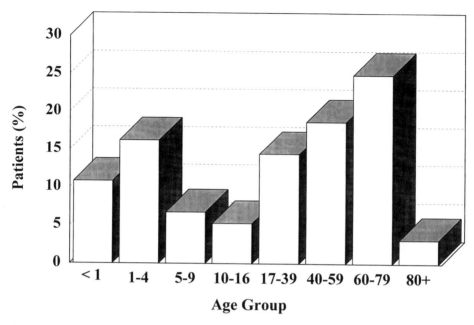

Figure 15.1 Age distribution of status epilepticus cases in the Medical College of Virginia Status Epilepticus database. The data are represented as the percent of patients in each age group. The total number of patients in the study was 611.

indicator for a poor outcome in SE,[9] and initial evidence indicated that SE was common in the aging population.[4, 5] Thus, evaluating SE in the elderly population may provide important insights into this condition and offer possible strategies for new treatment initiatives.

Previous Studies of Status Epilepticus in the Elderly

Previous studies[4, 5, 9] demonstrated that the number of SE cases in a large patient population increases with advancing age. A large proportion of adult patients in most clinical studies of SE was represented by patients in the later decades, as summarized in Figure 15.1. In addition, mortality was found to increase with age and also to be statistically associated with poor outcome in SE.[9] Thus, SE was shown to be a major clinical condition of the elderly.

The elderly are uniquely susceptible to SE because they are more prone to medical illness that may lead to increased seizure frequency. There is, however, little clinical information on the clinical presentations, etiologies, and outcomes of SE in the elderly population. The current study was initiated to provide a prospective analysis of a large, hospital-based group of elderly patients with SE.

Features of this analysis along with initial estimates of incidence and epidemiology are presented.

Epidemiology of Status Epilepticus

The MCV Epilepsy Research Center has initiated a large prospective population-based study of SE.[4] This patient database is being used to develop epidemiologic information on the clinical presentation, incidence, and prognosis of patients with SE. The advantage of this type of study is that it allows a more complete picture of the presentation of SE in the natural setting.

Using this database, we have collected validated data on the presentation of SE over a 2-year period from 1989 to 1991. Patients identified in this study have been documented to live within the zip code localities of the city of Richmond. Careful validation of each SE case in this database further established a representative presentation of this condition in the population.

The number of cases of SE presenting per 100,000 individuals per year in the city of Richmond was defined as the incidence of SE. Approximately 47 cases of SE per 100,000 individuals occur per year in the Richmond community. However, at least double this incidence, 93 per 100,000, occurred in the elderly population, demonstrating that the elderly represent a high-risk population for developing SE. The pediatric population, 1 month to 16 years of age, had an incidence of 56 per 100,000 per year. Young adults from the ages of 16 years to 60 years had an incidence of 29 per 100,000. These results demonstrate that the lowest incidence of SE occurred in the young adult group. The pediatric population had a slightly increased incidence of SE compared with the total Richmond population, whereas the elderly population was clearly the highest-risk group, with an incidence twice that of the general population.

The elderly population was further subdivided into age groups of 60–69 years, 70–79 years, and 80+ years for further study (Figure 15.2). The high incidence of SE in the overall elderly age group, 93 per 100,000, was seen in each of the later decades (see Figure 15.2). The highest incidence of 100 per 100,000 individuals per year was reached in the 70–79 age group.

These data represent the first population-based incidence values for SE in the elderly population. This incidence value, however, is significantly underestimated. Only patients who meet the strict definition of SE[9] established by the International Classification of Seizure Disorders[15] were accepted into this study. When the diagnosis could not be rigorously established, patients were excluded from the database. If the diagnosis of SE was suspected by clinical history but could not be proved, the cases were omitted. In addition, although the validation rate for the MCV Hospital was at least 90%, the ascertainment of cases in the community hospitals in Richmond often could not be obtained above 30–40%. If the incidence data were corrected for these underestimates, the incidence of SE in the elderly would be significantly higher. Thus, the incidence of SE in the elderly probably exceeds the verified value of 93 per 100,000 individuals per year.

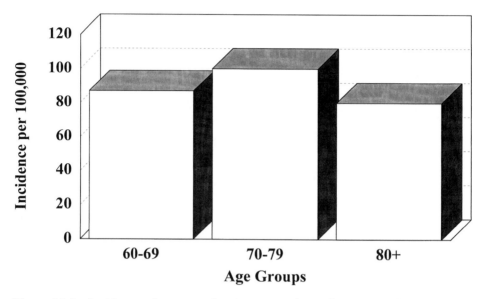

Figure 15.2 Incidence of status epilepticus in Richmond, Virginia, for the 60–69, 70–79, and 80+ age groups. The data represent the number of status epilepticus cases per year per 100,000 individuals in the Richmond city limits as verified by address. The data were collected during a 2-year period from 1989 to 1991.

A PROSPECTIVE DATABASE FOR STATUS EPILEPTICUS

To study the presentation of SE in the elderly, a large prospective clinical database was used. We identified 171 patients with SE ages 60 years and older who presented to MCV from July 1, 1989, to June 30, 1994. Thus, for the purpose of this study, the elderly patient was defined as a patient 60 years of age or older. SE was defined using the International Classification of Epileptic Seizure definition of SE.[15] This definition states that SE is any seizure lasting for a duration of 30 minutes or longer or intermittent seizures lasting for 30 minutes or longer from which the patient does not regain consciousness as described in our previous reports.[9]

The case history and charts of potential SE patients were identified and reviewed by the MCV SE Research Team (SERT) to determine if each case satisfied the formal definition of SE.[15] The SERT consisted of a group of scientists, nurses, and clinicians who evaluated on a weekly basis all cases presenting to the study. Patients with SE presenting to the MCV Hospital emergency department or on the inpatient service in the hospital were brought to the attention of the SERT in fewer than 4–5 hours. SERT members were on call 24 hours a day, 7 days a week to be able to respond to each new case of SE in a prospective,

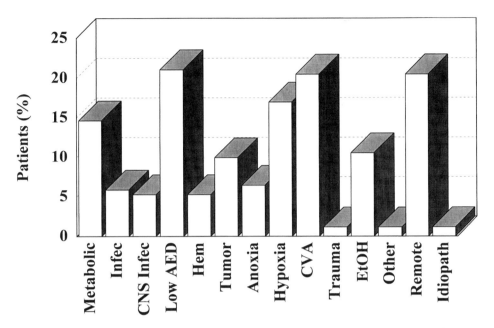

Figure 15.3 Etiology of elderly patients with status epilepticus. The data give the percent of patients in each etiology group for the elderly database ($n = 171$). Multiple etiologies were included for some patients. Etiology groups are defined in the text. (Metabolic = metabolic disorders; Infec = systemic infection; CNS Infec = central nervous system infection; Low AED = low serum levels of antiepileptic drugs; Hem = central nervous system hemorrhage; CVA = cerebrovascular accident; EtOH = alcohol withdrawal; Remote = remote symptomatic conditions; Idiopath = idiopathic [no definable etiology].)

timely manner.[4, 9] The onset of SE was documented by observations of witnesses or paramedics in the nonhospital setting and by nursing or physician observations in SE cases presenting in the hospital. Approximately 86% of the reported SE cases were validated and satisfied the definition of SE. The remaining patients had to be excluded because the SERT could not rigorously establish the diagnosis based on the formal definition.

For each SE case, the medical records were carefully reviewed during the hospitalization or immediately after discharge. A form entry data collection system was completed on each patient and included the following information: detailed seizure history, demographic data, electrophysiologic data, immediate precipitating etiology of SE, previous medical or neurologic history, laboratory studies, outcome, and hospital course. A time line for each SE event was established to evaluate duration of SE and time to recovery or death. In this study, mortality was defined as alive or dead within 30 days of the cessation of SE.

Etiology of SE was defined as the immediate precipitating cause as described previously.[9] The following etiologies were observed (Figure 15.3):

Table 15.1 Remote symptomatic etiologies of status epilepticus

Etiology	Number of Patients
Old cerebral hemorrhage	1
Old cerebral infarction	29
Old cerebral trauma	2

low antiepileptic drug serum levels, cerebrovascular accidents (CVAs), alcohol withdrawal, no identifiable etiology (idiopathic), metabolic disorders (metabolic, hypoxia, anoxia, tumor, trauma), central nervous system (CNS) infection, systemic infection, CNS hemorrhage, remote symptomatic, and other. Medical conditions that were not directly the cause of SE or previous medical conditions that were not related to the initiation of SE were not considered acute etiologies. These conditions were classified as remote symptomatic. Table 15.1 gives the etiologies of the remote symptomatic group. The vast majority of remote symptomatic cases were CVAs, comprising 29 of the 32 remote symptomatic etiologies. The other three etiologies were two cases of trauma and one case of hemorrhage. Unknown SE represented patients who had no identifiable immediate precipitating cause for SE. Alcohol withdrawal SE was defined as SE caused by documented withdrawal of alcohol or alcohol-related complications. Lowered antiepileptic drugs was defined as a case of SE due to documented cessation of anticonvulsant medication in a patient with previous epilepsy. The other group was composed of one case of drug overdose and one case of a congenital malformation. Hypoxia, CVA, tumor, metabolic conditions, and trauma were defined as significant causes of SE, using standard clinical criteria for these precipitating events.[9]

Seizure types in SE were defined as partial, generalized, or secondarily generalized, based on standard International Classification of Seizure types and types of SE as defined by the International League Against Epilepsy.[15] Statistical analysis was conducted using standard well established procedures.[9]

Status Epilepticus in the Elderly

The age distribution of the 611 patients analyzed prospectively in the MCV Hospital database is shown in Figure 15.1. The distribution was bimodal, with a decline after the first years of life followed by a gradually progressive increase from age 40 years to the later decades. Patients older than 60 years of age represented at least 40% of the patients in the database. These results were consistent with the findings of our epidemiologic study[4] indicating that the elderly have an increased incidence of SE compared with the general population.

The mortality for SE in this series for each age group is shown in Figure 15.4. As described in our retrospective data,[4, 9] there was a marked increase in mortality from SE with age, particularly in those older than 60 years. Thus, SE

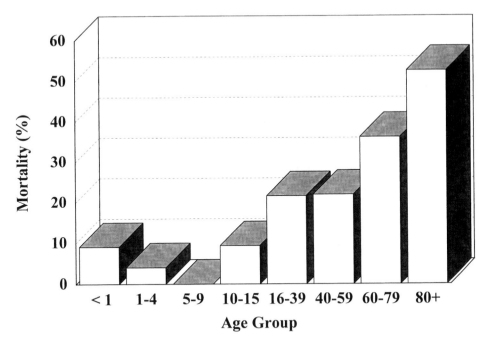

Figure 15.4 Mortality for each age group in the Medical College of Virginia population. The data present the percent mortality for each age subgroup.

in the elderly is of particular concern, as there are both an increased number of patients who have SE and an increased mortality because of it (see Figures 15.1 and 15.4).

Demographics of Status Epilepticus in the Elderly

The elderly patients in this study represented 171 patients in the MCV database prospectively collected from 1989 to 1994. The mortality for this population and percent of patients is shown in Figure 15.5 for the age groups 60–70 years, 70–80 years, and 80+ years. The percent of patients in the elderly population in the three decades from age 60 years to 80 years decreased with age; however, the mortality gradually increased to 50% for patients in the 80+ age group (see Figure 15.5).

The distribution of males and females in the elderly population was 52% and 48%, respectively. There were essentially no differences in the number of males and females presenting with SE older than age 60. The race distribution of white versus nonwhite patients was 31% and 69%, respectively. The higher percentage of nonwhite patients in the database reflected the inner city demographics of the city of Richmond and was comparable to the proportions of white and nonwhite citizens in the city of Richmond.

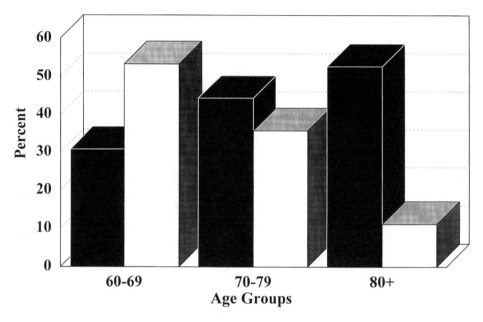

Figure 15.5 Number of patients (white) and mortality (black) for age group subdivisions in the elderly in the Medical College of Virginia study. The data give the percent of patients in the population and present mortality for each group ($n = 171$).

Etiologies of Status Epilepticus in the Elderly

The etiologies of SE in this study are shown in Figure 15.3. The major etiologies, each representing at least 15% of the population of patients used in the study, included CVA, hypoxia, remote symptomatic causes, low serum levels of anticonvulsant drugs, and metabolic disorders. Etiologies representing 5–10% of the patients included systemic infection, CNS infection, CNS hemorrhage, tumors, anoxia, and alcohol withdrawal. The mortalities for each etiology are presented in Figure 15.6. Anoxia in the elderly was associated with at least a 90% mortality. Metabolic disorders, systemic infections, CNS infections, hemorrhages, tumors, hypoxia, CVAs, and trauma were associated with at least a 30% mortality. Low serum levels of antiepileptic drugs, alcohol withdrawal, and idiopathic etiologies had mortalities of less than 6%. Remote symptomatic causes had a mortality of 14%. The "other" group had only two patients with etiologies of drug overdose and a congenital malformation. Both of these patients died. These results indicate that most of the specific etiologies associated with SE in the elderly were associated with a significant mortality.

The remote symptomatic category was composed primarily of cases with a history of previous CVA (see Table 15.1). This etiology represented at least 20% of the patients and, in combination with acute CVA, represented

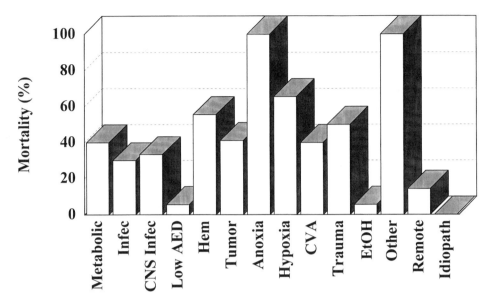

Figure 15.6 Etiology and mortality of elderly patients in the Medical College of Virginia study. The data show the percent mortality for each etiologic subgroup. (Metabolic = metabolic disorders; Infec = systemic infection; CNS Infec = central nervous system infection; Low AED = low serum levels of antiepileptic drugs; Hem = central nervous system hemorrhage; CVA = cerebrovascular accident; EtOH = alcohol withdrawal; Remote = remote symptomatic conditions; Idiopath = idiopathic [no definable etiology].)

at least 40% of the patients in the elderly series. Thus, CVA, acutely or remotely, was the major cause of SE in the elderly. The basic mechanisms that lead to the development of SE after cerebrovascular accidents is an area that needs further investigation.

Seizure Types in Status Epilepticus in the Elderly

The distribution of seizure types for SE in the elderly is shown in Figure 15.7. Partial, partial with secondary generalized, and generalized seizure types represented 29%, 45%, and 26% of the elderly SE patients, respectively. These data demonstrated that 74% of the SE cases in the elderly began with a partial seizure. The mortality associated with each major seizure type is shown in Figure 15.8. The highest mortality, 49%, was observed for the generalized seizure type. Partial and partial with secondary generalized seizures were associated with mortalities of 30% and 36%, respectively.

Further breakdown of the partial and generalized seizure types observed in this study are shown in Figure 15.9. Partial SE was subdivided into simple partial, simple partial with loss of consciousness, complex partial, and com-

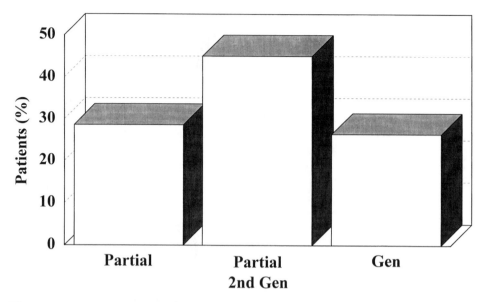

Figure 15.7   Major status epilepticus seizure types in the elderly. The data give the percent of partial, partial with secondary generalization, and generalized seizure types (*n* = 171).

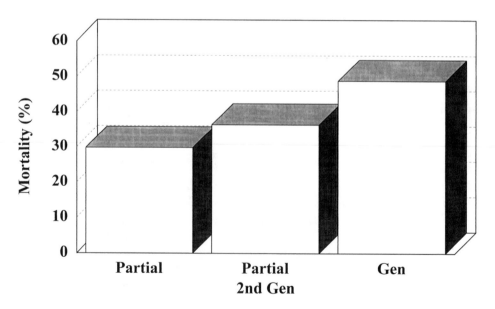

Figure 15.8   Status epilepticus seizure type and mortality in the elderly. The data show the percent mortality for each status epilepticus seizure type (partial, partial with secondary generalization, and generalized seizure types; *n* = 171).

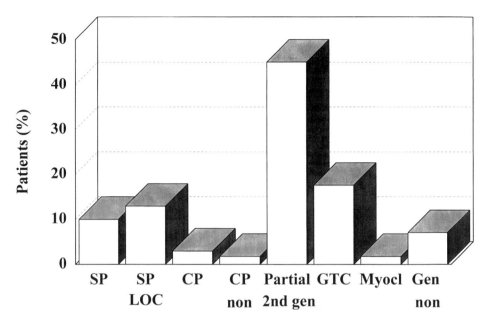

Figure 15.9 Subclassification of status epilepticus seizure types in the elderly. The data give the percent of patients with each status epilepticus seizure type ($n = 171$). (SP = simple partial; SP LOC = simple partial with loss of consciousness; CP = complex partial; CP Non = complex partial nonconvulsive; Partial 2nd gen = partial with secondary generalization; GTC = generalized tonic-clonic; Myocl = myoclonic; Gen non = generalized nonconvulsive.)

plex partial nonconvulsive seizures. Generalized SE was further divided into partial with secondary generalization, generalized tonic-clonic, myoclonic, and generalized nonconvulsive seizures. The majority of elderly patients presented with partial with secondary generalized tonic-clonic and generalized tonic-clonic seizures (see Figure 15.9). A significant number of patients, however, demonstrated simple partial, simple partial with loss of consciousness, and generalized nonconvulsive seizures. Generalized absence SE was not observed in this population.

Approximately 10% of the patients had classic simple partial seizures. More than 13% of the patients had focal motor seizures but were unconscious during the focal motor seizure activity. As the loss of consciousness in these patients was considered to be related to a secondary medical condition, these seizures were classified as simple partial with loss of consciousness rather than complex partial seizures. Although these cases could also be classified as complex partial seizures, we believe they represented a unique subgroup of patients who were unconscious and developed a simple partial seizure. Thus, we kept this category as a separate group. Patients who were

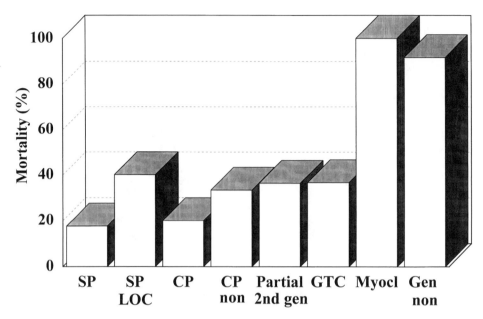

Figure 15.10 Mortality of subclasses of status epilepticus seizure types in the elderly. The data present the percent mortality for each seizure type ($n = 171$). (SP = simple partial; SP LOC = simple partial with loss of consciousness; CP = complex partial; CP non = complex partial nonconvulsive; Partial 2nd gen = partial with secondary generalization; GTC = generalized tonic-clonic; Myocl = myoclonic; Gen non = generalized nonconvulsive.)

unconscious and had focal electrographic SE discharges without corresponding clinical seizure activity were classified as having complex partial nonconvulsive SE. SE that initiated with a partial seizure that then secondarily generalized to a tonic-clonic seizure represented the largest percent of patients in the elderly population. The SE elderly cases that presented with partial followed by secondarily generalized seizures may represent seizure types developing from focal brain injury such as CVA. Myoclonic SE represented only 2% of the SE cases in the elderly. Generalized nonconvulsive SE was observed in 7% of the patients. Cases of nonconvulsive SE were primarily diagnosed by EEG criteria in comatose patients. This group of SE patients is often underdiagnosed in medical centers that do not routinely perform EEGs on all comatose patients.

Mortalities by seizure types are shown in Figure 15.10. The highest mortality was associated with myoclonic SE in the elderly. This category of seizures in the elderly had a mortality of 100%. Generalized nonconvulsive SE was also associated with a mortality of at least 90%. The majority of subclasses of SE were associated with mortalities between 30% and 40%. The lowest mortalities were seen with simple partial and complex partial SE.

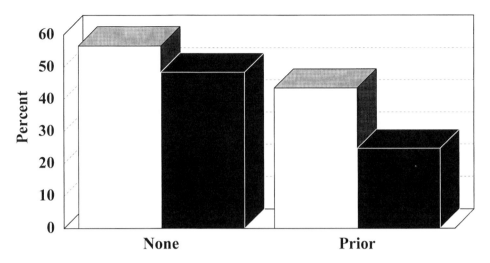

Figure 15.11 Number of elderly patients and mortality of elderly patients with or without a prior seizure history. The data give the percent of patients (white) and mortality (black) for elderly patients with (Prior) or without (None) a previous seizure history (*n* = 171).

Prior Seizure History and Status Epilepticus

A previous seizure history has been thought to play a major role in the development of SE.[4, 5, 9, 16] Thus, we investigated the seizure history of the 171 elderly patients in this study. Figure 15.11 presents the number of patients with and without a previous seizure history. The majority of elderly SE patients (56%) had no previous seizure history. Patients with no previous seizure history had a much higher mortality than those with a history of seizures (48% and 25%, respectively). Thus, a previous seizure history was associated with a significantly lower mortality.

The predisposition of the elderly to develop systemic metabolic diseases and CVA made them more susceptible to developing SE. The higher mortality associated with some of these etiologies of SE (see Figure 15.6) may partially account for the higher mortality associated with patients without a previous seizure history. Furthermore, a previous seizure history included all patients with low antiepileptic drug levels. This etiologic group represented at least 20% of the patients in the population, approximately half of the previous seizure history group. The low mortality of the group with low levels of antiepileptic drugs (see Figure 15.6) contributed to the low mortality in the previous seizure history group. These results demonstrate that a previous seizure history in an elderly SE patient is associated with a lower mortality. Further evaluation of seizure history as a predictive indicator of mortality in SE may provide new insights into developing a predictive outcome scale for SE.[9]

CONCLUSIONS

The results of this investigation indicate that SE is a major clinical concern in the elderly population. Epidemiologic studies in the Richmond database show that elderly patients have almost twice the incidence of developing SE compared with the general population. Thus, the elderly represent the major high-risk group for developing SE.

This study demonstrates that the mortality rate of SE in the elderly is at least 30%. The 80+ age group has a mortality of at least 50%. In addition, specific etiologies and seizure types were also clearly associated with increased mortality. Thus, etiology could contribute to the increased SE mortality in the elderly. Further investigation of the causes of this increased mortality in the elderly needs to be initiated.

Results from this initial study of SE in the elderly indicate that SE in this population requires additional study. Further research on SE in the elderly population may provide important insights into preventing the high mortality and morbidity of SE in this age group. The relationship of CVAs and initiation of SE also needs further evaluation, since CVAs represent the major etiology of SE in the elderly.

Acknowledgments
This chapter was written with the assistance and input of the epilepsy research team at the Medical College of Virginia Epilepsy Research Center. The contributions of Drs. A. Towne, J. Boggs, and D. Ko in analyzing cases and in coordinating the database were greatly appreciated. The data management assistance of C. Fortner and R. Boyle also greatly contributed to this research effort. Carolyn Cole's assistance with the preparation of the manuscript was greatly appreciated. This research effort was supported by the Medical College of Virginia Epilepsy Research Center (PO2 NS25630) to R.J. DeLorenzo and by the Sophie and Nathan Gumenick Neuroscience and Alzheimer's Research Fund.

REFERENCES

1. Aminoff NJ, Simon RP. Status epilepticus: causes, clinical features and consequences in 98 patients. Am J Med 1980;69:657.
2. DeLorenzo RJ. Status epilepticus: concepts in diagnosis and treatment. Semin Neurol 1990;2:396.
3. DeLorenzo RJ. Status Epilepticus. In Current Therapy in Neurologic Disease-3. Philadelphia: BC Decker, 1990;47.
4. DeLorenzo RJ, Towne AR, Pellock JM, Ko D. Status epilepticus in children, adults and the elderly. Epilepsia 1992;33(Suppl 4):14.
5. Hauser WA. Status epilepticus: epidemiology considerations. Neurology 1990;40(Suppl 2):9.
6. Leppik IE. Status epilepticus. Clin Ther 1985;7:272.
7. Leppik IE. Status epilepticus. Neurol Clin 1986;4:633.
8. Lowenstein DH, Alldredge BK. Status epilepticus at an urban public hospital in the 1980s. Neurology 1992;43:483.

9. Towne AR, Pellock JM, Ko D, DeLorenzo RJ. Determinants of mortality in status epilepticus. Epilepsia 1994;5:27.
10. Delgado-Escueta AV, Wasterlain CG, Treiman DM, Porter RJ. Management of Status epilepticus. N Engl J Med 1982;36:1337.
11. Dodson WE, DeLorenzo RJ, Pedley TA, et al. The treatment of convulsive status epilepticus: recommendation of the Epilepsy Foundation of America's working group on status epilepticus. JAMA 1993;270:854.
12. Treiman DM. Status Epilepticus. In Current Therapy of Neurologic Disease-2. Philadelphia: BC Decker, 1987;38.
13. Sgro JA, Jaitly R, DeLorenzo RJ. Conventional and rapid evoked potential in patients with status epilepticus. Epilepsy Res 1993;15:149.
14. Jaitly R, Sgro JA, Towne AR, DeLorenzo RJ. A prospective study of prolonged (24 hr) EEG monitoring in a large population of status epilepticus patients. Neurology 1994;44(Suppl. 2):172.
15. Gastaut H. Classification of Status Epilepticus. In AV Delgado-Escueta, CG Wasterlain, DM Treiman, RJ Porter (eds), Status Epilepticus: Mechanisms of Brain Damage and Treatment. New York: Raven, 1983;15.
16. Hauser WA, Hesdorffer DC. Epilepsy: Frequency, Causes and Consequences. New York: Demos, 1990.

16

Status Epilepticus in the Elderly: Nosology and Therapy

David M. Treiman, Patti D. Meyers, and Nancy Y. Walton

Status epilepticus (SE) is a complication of both chronic epilepsy and acute insult to the brain. SE occurs most frequently in children and in elderly adults. In adults, it appears that the peak occurrence is in the two decades between 60 years and 80 years of age. Therefore, it is worth asking whether SE has any different characteristics in the elderly population compared with younger adults. In this chapter, generalized convulsive status epilepticus (GCSE) is primarily focused on because it is by far the most common and dangerous type of SE. Also discussed are two other forms of SE that are particularly common in the elderly: de novo absence SE and the syndrome of confusional SE with periodic epileptiform discharges.

SE is defined as two or more epileptic seizures without full recovery of neurologic function between seizures or as more or less continuous clinical or electrical seizure activity persisting for more than 30 minutes, whether or not consciousness is impaired.[1] From this definition, it is apparent that any type of epileptic seizure, if it lasts long enough or recurs frequently enough, can be considered SE.[2] GCSE is now recognized to be a dynamic disorder with a range of behavioral and electrical characteristics that vary between the beginning and end of an episode.[3] GCSE may exhibit paroxysmal or continuous tonic-clonic motor activity (which may be symmetric or asymmetric and overt or subtle) that is associated with marked impairment of consciousness and bilateral (but frequently asymmetrical) ictal discharges on the electroencephalogram (EEG). Typically, GCSE starts as a series of overt generalized convulsions separated by periods of coma, during which time there may be partial but incomplete recovery of neurologic function before the next seizure occurs. If GCSE is allowed to continue without treatment or is inadequately treated, there is a gradual conversion from overt convulsive movements to increasingly subtle motor manifestations of the seizures. Ultimately, the patient may progress to a state of profound coma with only mild twitching movements of the extremities, trunk, or face or nystagmoid jerks of the eyes. This is what Treiman et al.[4] called subtle GCSE; the diagnosis can be made only by observing ictal discharges on the EEG.

Just as there is evolution from overt to increasingly subtle motor manifestations during the course of untreated or undertreated GCSE, there is also a predictable sequence of progressive EEG changes if GCSE is allowed to progress over a period of time.[5] Initially, discrete electrographic seizures are seen accompanying discrete overt convulsions. On the EEG, these seizures have the characteristics of typical isolated generalized convulsions. If GCSE persists, the discrete seizures begin to merge and exhibit a waxing and waning of frequency and amplitude and sometimes a degree of spread from the primary focus. Ultimately, the waxing and waning ictal discharges become continuous, with relatively little variation in amplitude, frequency, or distribution. Subsequently, the continuous activity is punctuated by periods of relative flattening that lengthen as the ictal discharges get shorter until, finally, the EEG contains periodic epileptiform discharges on a relatively flat background (PEDs). This sequence of EEG changes in GCSE in humans has also been observed in six experimental rat models of SE.[6, 7]

Recognition that GCSE is a dynamic state with different clinical and electrical presentations depending on the stage of the episode of status has allowed us to study how other parameters, such as treatment response, outcome, and age, relate to the stage of the episode.

METHODS

In this chapter, we present preliminary data from an ongoing Veterans Administration (VA) Cooperative Study (CSP #265) that is comparing four intravenous treatment regimens in the initial management of GCSE in the adult. The treatment groups consist of phenytoin (18 mg/kg), diazepam (0.15 mg/kg) followed by phenytoin (18 mg/kg), phenobarbital (15 mg/kg), and lorazepam (0.1 mg/kg). Sixteen VA medical centers and six affiliated university hospitals have participated in this study. Patients with overt GCSE and subtle GCSE are separated into two groups. Success at stopping status is verified by EEG as well as clinical observation. Data discussed in this chapter are from the first 452 patients included in the study. To determine the influence of age on the various parameters to be discussed, patients were divided into those younger than 65 years of age and those 65 years of age and older.

Results

Figure 16.1 shows the number of SE cases by age decade, for both subtle and overt GCSE presentation. These data are broken into the number of patients younger than 65 years of age and the number of those 65 and older in Table 16.1 and show no difference in presentation distribution between these two age groups.

The distribution of different categories of etiology by age group for overt and subtle cases is shown in Table 16.2. Overt and subtle presentations were associated with a different etiologic distribution, with remote neurologic etiologies occurring more frequently with overt presentation and life-threatening medical conditions and cardiopulmonary arrest occurring more frequently with subtle presentation. Significant differences between the age groups were found

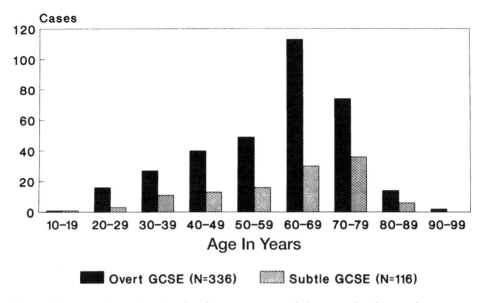

Figure 16.1 Incidence by decade of overt versus subtle generalized convulsive status epilepticus.

Table 16.1 Distribution of overt and subtle generalized convulsive status epilepticus by age group

	<65 Years	*>65 Years*
Overt GCSE	181 (75%)	155 (73%)
Subtle GCSE	60 (25%)	56 (27%)
Total	241	211

GCSE = generalized convulsive status epilepticus.

with acute neurologic etiologies in the overt cases (more frequent in the elderly patients), life-threatening medical conditions in the subtle cases (more frequent in the younger patients), and drug toxicity in overt cases (more frequent in the younger patients).

There were no significant differences between the age groups in distribution of the initial ictal EEG pattern for either the overt or subtle cases. These distributions are shown in Figures 16.2 and 16.3 (patients with only postictal EEG patterns were not included). We also found no difference in response to treatment in the two age groups for either overt or subtle cases. These distributions are shown in Figures 16.4 and 16.5.

Table 16.2 Distribution of etiologic categories by age group for subtle and overt presentation[a]

	Overt Presentation		Subtle Presentation	
	<65 Years (N = 178)	≥65 Years (N = 146)	<65 Years (N = 56)	≥65 Years (N = 54)
Acute neurologic insult	37 (21%)	47 (32%)[b]	20 (36%)	19 (35%)
Life-threatening medical condition	52 (29%)	50 (34%)	40 (71%)[b]	23 (43%)
Status post cardiopulmonary arrest	14 (8%)	10 (7%)	23 (41%)	21 (39%)
Remote neurologic insult	130 (73%)	99 (68%)	14 (25%)	24 (44%)
Alcohol withdrawal	6 (3%)	8 (5%)	1 (2%)	0 (0%)
Drug toxicity	17 (10%)[b]	4 (3%)	3 (5%)	2 (4%)

[a]Number of cases is followed by percentage in parentheses. The total percentage within each age group is >100 because patients may have had more than one etiologic factor.
[b]$P < .05$.

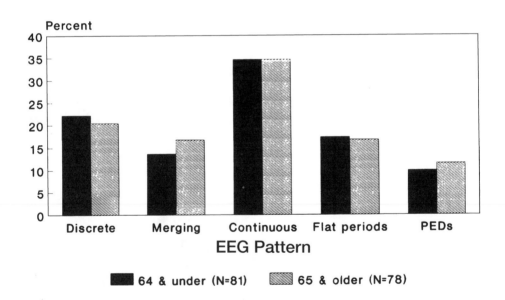

Figure 16.2 Effect of age on the electroencephalographic pattern in overt generalized convulsive status epilepticus before first treatment.

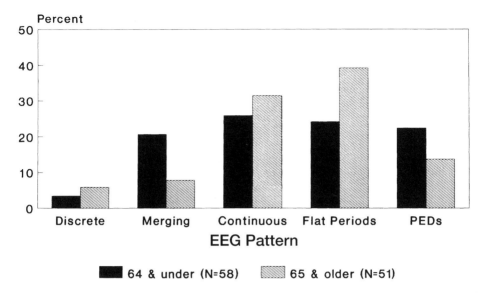

Figure 16.3 Effect of age on the electroencephalographic pattern in subtle generalized convulsive status epilepticus before first treatment.

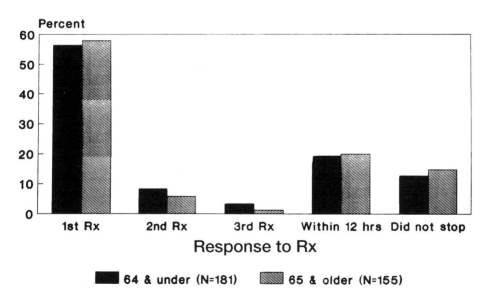

Figure 16.4 Effect of age on treatment success in overt generalized convulsive status epilepticus.

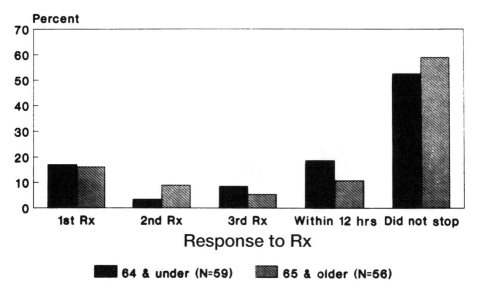

Figure 16.5 Effect of age on treatment success in subtle generalized convulsive status epilepticus.

Table 16.3 Outcome 30 days after treatment of generalized convulsive status epilepticus for overt and subtle cases, by age group*

	Overt Presentation		Subtle Presentation	
	<65 Years (N = 181)	≥65 Years (N = 154)	<65 Years (N = 56)	≥65 Years (N = 56)
Discharged from hospital	115 (64%)	61 (40%)	8 (14%)	3 (5%)
Still hospitalized	27 (15%)	39 (25%)	15 (27%)	12 (21%)
Dead	39 (22%)	54 (35%)	33 (59%)	41 (73%)

*Number of cases is followed by percentage in parentheses. Overall difference in distribution is statistically significant, $P < .0001$.

Elderly patients had significantly poorer prognoses, as measured by outcome 30 days after treatment of the status episode. These data are shown in Table 16.3 for both overt and subtle cases. Elderly patients also were more likely to suffer from cardiovascular or respiratory distress during GCSE, as shown in Table 16.4. Antiepileptic drug-induced hypotension was more common in the elderly patients, as shown in Table 16.5.

Table 16.4 Frequency of cardiovascular and respiratory distress during protocol treatment drug infusions by age group

	<65 Years	≥65 Years
Cardiovascular distress	(n = 241)	(n = 211)
	97 (46%)	85 (35%)*
Respiratory distress	(n = 240)	(n = 209)
	27 (11%)	39 (19%)*

*P < .05.

Table 16.5 Effect of age on antiepileptic drug–induced hypotension

	<65 Years (N = 188)	≥65 Years (N = 155)
Pretreatment systolic BP (mean)	141.3 mm Hg	138.1 mm Hg
BP with treatment	17.7%	25.5%*
BP drop >20%	44.7%	60.0%
BP drop >33%	17.6%	34.2%

BP = blood pressure.
*P < .01.

DISCUSSION

There have been few other studies of SE in the elderly. The observations that peak occurrence of GCSE in this adult study occurs between 60 years and 80 years of age and that acute neurologic insult is a more common cause in the 65 and older age group are consistent with observations reported by Sung and Chu.[8] These authors studied 342 patients who had their first seizure after the age of 60 years. One hundred two (29%) had SE. Cerebrovascular disease (35%) was the leading cause of SE, followed by head trauma (21%). Overall mortality in the SE patients (defined as death within 1 month of the episode of SE) was 35%. We also observed a 30-day mortality of 35% in our overt GCSE patients older than 64 years old (see Table 16.3). The occurrence of antiepileptic drug-induced hypotension in elderly patients during the treatment of SE has been described previously by Cranford et al.[9] and Walton.[10]

Our study did not include patients with two other presentations of SE that are especially common in elderly adults: de novo absence SE and the syndrome of confusional SE with periodic epileptiform discharges.

Absence SE in the adult occurs in three groups of people: (a) individuals with childhood onset primary generalized epilepsy that persists into adulthood, (b) individuals with a past history of childhood primary generalized epilepsy in whom absence SE occurs after a long seizure-free period (frequently many years), and (c) de novo absence SE in individuals with no prior history of epilepsy. More than 80 cases of de novo absence SE in the adult have been reported, mostly in elderly patients. Sixty-four were summarized in a recent review.[11] The mean age was 62 years. Many of these cases had a history of psychiatric illness, and most episodes occurred after withdrawal from benzodiazepines or psychotropic drugs. As with absence SE in patients with primary generalized epilepsy, behavior during the SE episode of de novo absence SE may range from extremely subtle behavioral changes (generally the patient is described as being unusually quiet and lacking initiative) to catatonia and profound stupor. The EEG typically exhibits diffuse bilaterally symmetric spike-wave discharges of 1- to 4-Hz frequency. Intravenous benzodiazepines are almost always effective at normalizing both the patient's behavior and the EEG. Episodes do not recur unless there are other episodes of drug withdrawal.

Confusional SE with periodic epileptiform discharges is a disorder characterized by recurrent and prolonged episodes of confusion associated with periodic, sometimes lateralized, periodic epileptiform discharges on the EEG. Normalization of behavior and the EEG coincide. Terzano et al.[12] described seven such cases in detail in patients older than age 60 years and concluded that this condition may represent a peculiar form of nonconvulsive SE in the elderly.

Both disorders can be easily confused with other confusional states of psychiatric or organic etiology. This possibility emphasizes the importance of EEG evaluation of any patient in an unexplained confusional state, especially an elderly psychiatric patient.

SUMMARY AND CONCLUSION

GCSE, at least in an acute hospital setting, is most common in adults between the ages of 60 years and 80 years. In an ongoing VA Cooperative Study of the treatment of SE, nearly one-half of the patients are 65 years of age or older. When the elderly (age 65 years and older) and younger (younger than age 65 years) groups are compared, there are relatively few differences in etiology, nature of the clinical or electrical presentation, or response to treatment. Outcome is poorer in the elderly age group. Cardiovascular distress is seen somewhat more often in the elderly age group, as are respiratory complications.

Large differences between the overt and subtle presentation groups were seen. This suggests that it is not age but rather the severity of the episode of status and its underlying etiology that are the principal determinants of responsiveness to treatment and outcome in GCSE.

Two other presentations of SE occur most commonly in elderly adults: de novo absence SE and confusional SE with periodic epileptiform discharges. Both may cause mild alterations of behavior and, without EEG tracings, may be difficult to differentiate from other causes of confusion.

Acknowledgments
Appreciation is expressed to the Department of Veterans Affairs Status Epilepticus Study Group.

REFERENCES

1. Treiman DM, Delgado-Escueta AV. Status Epilepticus. In RA Thompson, JR Green (eds), Critical Care of Neurological and Neurosurgical Emergencies. New York: Raven, 1980;53.
2. Gastaut H. Classification of status epilepticus. Adv Neurol 1983;34:15.
3. Treiman DM. Generalized convulsive status epilepticus in the adult [review]. Epilepsia 1993;34(Suppl 1):2.
4. Treiman DM, DeGiorgio CM, Salisbury S, et al. Subtle generalized convulsive status epilepticus. Epilepsia 1984;25:653.
5. Treiman DM, Walton NY, Kendrick C. A progressive sequence of electroencephalographic changes during generalized convulsive status epilepticus. Epilepsy Res 1990;5:49.
6. Lothman EW, Bertram EH, Bekenstein JW, et al. Self-sustaining limbic status epilepticus induced by 'continuous' hippocampal stimulation: electrographic and behavioral characteristics. Epilepsy Res 1989;3:107.
7. Handforth A, Treiman DM. A new, non-pharmacologic model of convulsive status epilepticus induced by electrical stimulation: behavioral/electroencephalographic observations and response to phenytoin and phenobarbital. Epilepsy Res 1994;19:15.
8. Sung C-Y, Chu N-S. Status epilepticus in the elderly: etiology, seizure type and outcome. Acta Neurol Scand 1989;80:51.
9. Cranford RE, Leppik IE, Patrick B, et al. Intravenous phenytoin: clinical and pharmacokinetic aspects. Neurology 1978;28:874.
10. Walton NY. Systemic effects of status epilepticus in the geriatric patient. Nurs Home Med 1995; [in press].
11. Thomas P, Beaumanoir A, Genton P, et al. 'De novo' absence status of late onset: report of 11 cases. Neurology 1992;42:104.
12. Terzano MG, Parrino L, Mazzucchi A, et al. Confusional states with periodic lateralized epileptiform discharges (PLEDs): a peculiar epileptic syndrome in the elderly. Epilepsia 1986;27:446.

IV

Antiepileptic Drugs:
Characteristics and
Interactions in the Elderly

17

Commonly Used Antiepileptic Drugs: Age-Related Pharmacokinetics

James Cloyd

A large and rapidly increasing number of the elderly, particularly those older than age 75 years, are taking antiepileptic drugs (AEDs).[1, 2] Treating elderly patients with AEDs is complicated by age-related changes in hepatic, renal, and gastrointestinal function, which alter pharmacokinetics. Illnesses commonly experienced by the elderly have additional effects on AED pharmacokinetics. As shown in Figure 17.1, elderly patients receiving AEDs also take a large number of other medications.[2] The interactions resulting from multiple drug therapy affect the pharmacokinetics of the interacting medications and can produce clinically significant alterations in response.

AGE-RELATED CHANGES IN PHYSIOLOGY: EFFECT ON ANTIEPILEPTIC DRUG PHARMACOKINETICS

Age-related changes in physiology can affect absorption, distribution, metabolism, and elimination. Changes in gastrointestinal function can either increase or decrease bioavailability depending on the drug, but there is insufficient information to assess their practical significance on either rate or extent of AED absorption.[3]

Age-related alterations in serum proteins have a significant effect on total serum concentrations of highly bound AEDs such as carbamazepine, phenytoin, and valproic acid. Total serum drug concentration represents the concentration bound to serum proteins and the unbound, or free, concentration. The ratio of unbound to total concentration is the free fraction.

$$\text{Free fraction} = \frac{\text{Unbound concentration}}{\text{Total concentration}}$$

Total serum drug concentration correlates well with therapeutic and toxic response when protein binding is stable or the fraction of drug bound is relatively low (less than 75%). Unbound drug concentration, which is in direct equilibrium with the concentration at the site of action, often better correlates

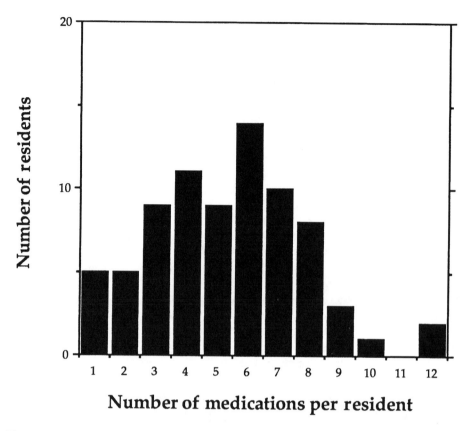

Figure 17.1 Maintenance medications in elderly residents taking antiepileptic drugs.

with response when protein binding of highly bound drugs (75%) is altered.[4] For restrictively cleared drugs, increases or decreases in free fraction will alter the steady-state total concentration but usually do not affect unbound concentration, which is determined by drug clearance.[5] By age 65 years, many individuals have low normal albumin or are frankly hypoalbuminemic.[6] Albumin concentration may be further reduced by conditions such as malnutrition, renal insufficiency, and rheumatoid arthritis.[7] As the serum albumin level declines, there is a greater likelihood of a decrease in drug binding. The alpha$_1$-acid glycoprotein (AAG) concentration increases with age; further elevations occur during pathophysiologic stress, such as stroke, heart failure, trauma, infection, myocardial infarction, surgery, arthritis, and chronic obstructive pulmonary disease.[7] When the concentration of AAG increases, binding of weakly alkaline and neutral drugs can increase.[8] This has the effect of causing higher *total* serum drug concentrations.

Age-related reductions in liver volume, hepatic blood flow, and glomerular filtration rate are responsible for a decline in drug elimination in the elderly.[9, 10] Phase I reactions (oxidation, reduction, and hydroxylation) are apparently affected to a greater extent than phase II reactions (glucuronidation, acetylation, and sulfation).[11] A gradual, age-related, highly variable decline in P-450 metabolism, equivalent to 1% per year after age 40 years, has been observed.[12] Declines in drug-metabolizing capacity result in a reduction in drug clearance. Renal function, as measured by glomerular filtration rate, also decreases approximately 1% per year beginning at age 40 years.[10]

Clearance for most AEDs is affected by protein binding and intrinsic metabolizing capacity (intrinsic clearance) of unbound drug. The amount of drug absorbed, free fraction, and intrinsic clearance determine steady-state total drug concentrations:

$$\text{Drug concentration} = \frac{(\text{Dose})(\text{Fraction absorbed})}{(\text{Free fraction})(\text{Intrinsic clearance})}$$

In contrast, steady-state unbound drug concentration for most AEDs is determined only by the amount of drug absorbed and intrinsic clearance; changes in protein binding do not affect unbound concentration[5]:

$$\text{Unbound drug concentration} = \frac{(\text{Dose})(\text{Fraction absorbed})}{(\text{Intrinsic clearance})}$$

These pharmacokinetic relationships predict that age-associated changes in protein binding affect total serum concentrations of highly bound AEDs such as carbamazepine, phenytoin, and valproic acid. Age-associated changes in phase I reactions predict increase unbound drug concentration. As shown in Figure 17.2, decreases in both protein binding and intrinsic clearance predict lower total and higher unbound concentration. Decreases in hepatic drug-metabolizing capacity and renal function result in reduced clearance and, thus, lower doses to maintain desired unbound serum concentration.

ANTIEPILEPTIC DRUG PHARMACOKINETICS IN THE ELDERLY

Few reports on AED pharmacokinetics in the elderly have been published despite the theoretical effects of age-related physiologic changes on drug disposition and the widespread use of AEDs in the elderly. These studies generally involve single-dose evaluations in a small number of the "young elderly" subjects—that is, individuals 65–74 years old. Table 17.1 summarizes the available information on AED pharmacokinetics in the elderly.

Carbamazepine itself is bound 65–85% to a combination of albumin and AAG, whereas its active metabolite, carbamazepine-10,11-epoxide, is bound to a lesser extent to the same proteins.[13] There are no studies on car-

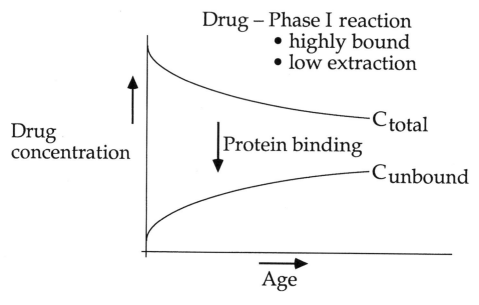

Figure 17.2   Effect of age-related physiologic changes on pharmacokinetics.

bamazepine protein binding in the elderly. Only two reports describe carba-mazepine elimination pharmacokinetics in the elderly. Hockings et al. gave a single dose of carbamazepine to young and elderly volunteers and found no differences in disposition.[14] In contrast, Cloyd et al. found that carba-mazepine clearance averaged 40% less in seven elderly patients, compared with 12 younger patients: 41.0 ± 19.6 versus 71.4 ± 35.8 ml/hr/kg, respec-tively (P = .055).[2]

There are no studies to date that characterize the pharmacokinetics of fel-bamate in elderly patients. Felbamate weakly binds to serum proteins and, in younger patients, its elimination is approximately 50% renal and 50% oxidative hepatic metabolism.[15] It is likely that elderly patients require smaller dosages given less frequently.

Gabapentin displays saturable absorption and low protein binding and undergoes renal elimination.[16] Absorption occurs through an enzyme-mediated, active-transport system that can become saturated with standard doses.[17] It is not known if transport capacity declines with age. Gabapentin clearance, how-ever, does decline by 30–50% in elderly subjects and is linearly correlated with creatinine clearance.[16] Assuming gabapentin bioavailability is similar to that observed in younger adults, elderly patients will require 30–50% smaller doses given less frequently.

Lamotrigine is rapidly absorbed, weakly bound to plasma protein (55%) and extensively metabolized via conjugation with glucuronic acid.

Table 17.1 Antiepileptic drug pharmacokinetics in elderly and younger adults[a]

Drug	Protein Binding (%) Elderly	Protein Binding (%) Younger Adults	Half-Life (hrs) Elderly	Half-Life (hrs) Younger Adults	Apparent Clearance (ml/hr/kg) Elderly	Apparent Clearance (ml/hr/kg) Younger Adults	Route of Elimination Elderly and Younger Adults	Effect on Dosage in Elderly Patients
Carbamaze-pine	NA	75–85 albu-min and alpha$_1$-acid gly-coprotein	NA	12–24[b]	41.0 ± 19.6[b] ml/hr/kg	50–100[b] ml/hr/kg	Hepatic oxidation; undergoes auto-induction	Elevations in the alpha$_1$-acid glycoprotein con-centration could increase total concentrations Dosage requirements reduced much as 40%
Felbamate	NA	25–35	NA	13–23	NA	30 ± 8 ml/hr/kg	50% Hepatic oxi-dation; renal	Dosage adjustments may be necessary in elderly patients
Gabapentin	NA	<10	NA	5–8	125 ml/min	225 ml/min	Renal	Elderly patients with diminished renal func-tion may need a decrease in dose
Lamotrigine	NA	55	31 hrs	29	NA	41.9 ± 10.3 ml/min	Hepatic-glucuro-nide conjugation	Dosage adjustment may not be necessary since conjugation reactions are only slightly dimin-ished
Phenobarbital	NA	45–50	NA	75–126	NA	3.7 ± 0.7 ml/hr/kg	45–65% Hepatic; renal	Dosage adjustments may be necessary

Table 17.1 (continued)

| Drug | Protein Binding (%) | | Half-Life (hrs) | | Apparent Clearance (ml/hr/kg) | | Route of Elimination | Effect on Dosage in Elderly Patients |
	Elderly	Younger Adults	Elderly	Younger Adults	Elderly	Younger Adults	Elderly and Younger Adults	
Phenytoin	80–93	87–93	At 15 mg/liter, half-life is 40–60 hrs	At 15 mg/liter, half-life is 20–40 hrs	$K_m = 5.8 \pm 2.3$ mg/liter $V_{max} = 5.5 \pm 1.9$ mg/kg/day	$K_m = 6.3$ mg/liter $V_{max} = 8.5$ mg/kg/day	Hepatic	Initial dosage 3–4 mg/kg Subsequent increases should be small (<10% of dose)
Primidone	NA	<20	12.1 ± 4.6	5–19	34.8 ± 9.0 ml/hr/kg	20–80 ml/hr/kg	40–60% Renal; hepatic	Renal clearance of PRM, PB and PEMA reduced Dosage may need to be reduced in patients with decreased renal function
Valproic acid	87–95	90–95	11–17	9–18	Clearance of unbound drug is 60–100 ml/hr/kg	Clearance of unbound drug is 90–140 ml/hr/kg	Hepatic oxidation and glucuronidation	40–50% Decrease in dosage based on unbound clearance data

NA = information not available for elderly patients; PRM = primidone; PB = phenobarbital; PEMA = phenylethylmalonamide.
[a]Values for patients on monotherapy; data from references.
[b]After autoinduction.

Theoretically, lamotrigine dosing and dosing frequency are less likely to be altered in elderly patients, since advanced age has little apparent effect on conjugation reactions. One study found that the half-life of lamotrigine in 12 elderly subjects was similar to that observed in younger adults: 31 versus 29 hours, respectively.[18]

Phenobarbital and primidone are weakly bound to plasma protein. In younger adults, renal excretion eliminates approximately 50% of both drugs, with the remainder undergoing oxidative metabolism. Total body clearance of phenobarbital is reduced in the elderly, but the extent has not been well defined.[19] The effect of aging on other pharmacokinetic parameters has not been established, but it is likely that the elimination half-life of phenobarbital is prolonged, which would extend the time to reach steady state after initiation of therapy or changes in maintenance doses. A lower than usual initial maintenance dose is recommended in the elderly. Martines et al. found primidone clearance and half-life were similar for elderly and younger adult patients.[20] There was a 30% decline in primidone renal clearance, but this did not reach statistical significance. Serum concentrations for both phenobarbital and phenylethylmalonamide, another active metabolite, were higher in the elderly patients.

Phenytoin is slowly absorbed, extensively bound to serum albumin, and eliminated via a saturable cytochrome P-450 enzyme. A number of studies have reported reduced binding in the elderly.[21-25] Phenytoin metabolism as measured by V_{max} also declines with age. In a group of patients ages 60–79 years, V_{max} was reduced on average by 20%, whereas K_m remained unchanged.[26] The usually recommended starting dose of 300 mg/day may be too large for many elderly patients. Furthermore, the elderly patient's reduced capacity to metabolize phenytoin results in very large changes in serum concentrations when even small increases are made in the maintenance dose (Figure 17.3). Initial doses of 3–4 mg/kg are more likely to result in concentrations within the proposed therapeutic range. If an adjustment in dose is indicated, only small increases, on the order of 10% or less, should be made. Phenytoin elimination half-life, which increases with concentration, is prolonged in elderly patients. Using mean V_{max} and K_m values for an elderly group, the elimination half-life ranges from 40 to 60 hours at a concentration of 15 mg/liter. Decreases in protein binding may result in lower total concentrations, whereas decreases in V_{max} may result in higher unbound concentrations.

Valproic acid protein binding and metabolism are reduced in the elderly.[27, 28] Several studies have found that valproic acid mean free fraction is approximately 50% greater and mean unbound clearance was 40% less in elderly subjects compared with younger adults. The net effect of altered protein binding and unbound (intrinsic) clearance is that total concentrations are similar, but unbound concentrations are greater in elderly patients given the same dose as younger patients.

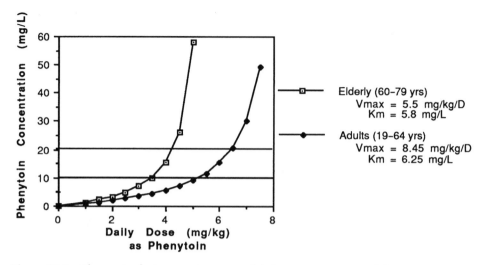

Figure 17.3 Phenytoin dosing requirements: elderly versus younger adults.

ANTIEPILEPTIC DRUG PHARMACODYNAMICS IN THE ELDERLY

Age-related changes in central nervous system anatomy and physiology appear to alter the response to some drugs. Studies have shown that elderly individuals are more sensitive to the sedative and cognitive effects of benzodiazepines as compared with younger adults with similar unbound drug concentrations.[29, 30] These findings suggest that the maximum tolerated AED concentration may be lower in elderly patients, resulting in a more narrow therapeutic range (Figure 17.4).

CONCLUSION

Elderly patients require smaller doses given less frequently to maintain desired unbound AED concentrations. Serum concentrations at the upper limits of proposed AED therapeutic ranges may more frequently cause side effects. Measurement of unbound concentration may be useful in situations in which altered protein binding is suspected or in which response (either therapeutic or toxic) does not correlate with total drug concentration. Studies involving patients, particularly those older than age 75 years, are needed to further characterize the pharmacokinetics, metabolism, efficacy, and safety of AEDs in the elderly.

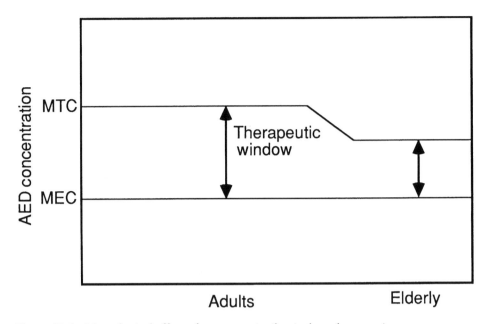

Figure 17.4   Hypothetical effect of age on antiepileptic drug therapeutic ranges.

REFERENCES

1. Hauser WA, Annegers JF, Kurland LT. Prevalence of epilepsy in Rochester, Minnesota, 1940–1980. Epilepsia 1991;32:429.
2. Cloyd JC, Lackner TE, Leppik IE. Antiepileptics in the elderly: pharmacoepidemiology and pharmacokinetics. Arch Fam Med 1994;3:589.
3. Dawling S, Crome P. Clinical pharmacokinetic considerations in the elderly: an update. Clin Pharmacokinet 1989;17:236.
4. Levy RH, Schmidt D. Utility of free level monitoring of antiepileptic drugs. Epilepsia 1985;26:199.
5. MacKichan JJ. Influence of Protein Binding and the Use of Unbound (Free) Drug Concentrations. In WE Evans, JJ Schentag, JJ Jusko (eds), Applied Pharmacokinetics: Principles of Therapeutic Drug Monitoring (3rd ed). Vancouver, WA: Applied Therapeutics, 1992;1.
6. Greenblatt DJ. Reduced serum albumin concentrations in the elderly: a report from the Boston Collaborative Drug Surveillance Program. J Am Geriatr Soc 1979;27:20.
7. Wallace SM, Verbeeck RK. Plasma protein binding of drugs in the elderly. Clin Pharmacokinet 1987;12:41.
8. Tiula E, Neuvonen PJ. Antiepileptic drugs and alpha-1 acid glycoprotein. N Engl J Med 1982;307:1148.
9. Woodhouse KW, Wynne HA. Age-related changes in liver size and hepatic blood flow: the influence on drug metabolism in the elderly. Clin Pharmacokinet 1988;15:287.
10. Rowe JW, Andres R, Tobin JD, et al. The effect of age on creatinine clearance in men: a cross-sectional and longitudinal study. J Gerontol 1976;31:155.
11. Woodhouse KW, James OF. Hepatic drug metabolism and aging. Br Med Bull 1990;46:22.

12. Vestal RE, Norris AH, Tobin JD, et al. Antipyrine metabolism in man: influence of age, alcohol, caffeine and smoking. Clin Pharmacol Ther 1975;18:425.
13. MacKichan JJ, Duffner PK, Cohen ME. Salivary concentrations and plasma protein binding of carbamazepine and carbamazepine 10,11-epoxide in epileptic patients. Br J Clin Pharmacol. 1981;12:31.
14. Hockings N, Moody APJ, Davidson AVM, Davidson DLW. The effects of age on carbamazepine pharmacokinetics and adverse effects. Br J Clin Pharmacol 1986;22:725.
15. Graves NM. Felbamate. Ann Pharmacother 1993;27:1073.
16. Richens A. Clinical Pharmacokinetics of Gabapentin. In D Chadwick (ed), New Trends in Epilepsy Management: The Role of Gabapentin. London: Royal Society of Medicine Services, 1993.
17. Stewart BH, Kugler AR, Thompson PR, Bockbrader HN. A saturable transport mechanism in the intestinal absorption of gabapentin is the underlying cause of the lack of proportionality between increasing dose and drug levels in plasma. Pharm Res 1993;10;276.
18. Peck AW. Clinical pharmacology of lamotrigine. Epilepsia 1991;32(Suppl 2):9.
19. Eadie MJ, Lander CM, Hooper WD, Tyrer JH. Factors influencing plasma phenobarbitone levels in epileptic patients. Br J Clin Pharmacol 1977;4:41.
20. Martines C, Gatti G, Sasso E, et al. The disposition of primidone in elderly patients. Br J Clin Pharmacol 1990;30:607.
21. Patterson M, Heazelwood R, Smithhurst B, Eadie MJ. Plasma protein binding of phenytoin in the aged: in-vivo studies. Br J Clin Pharmacol 1982;13:423.
22. Hayes MJ, Langman MJS, Short AH. Changes in drug metabolism with increasing age. II: phenytoin clearance and protein binding. Br J Clin Pharmacol 1975;2:73.
23. Umstead GS, Morales M, McKercher PL. Comparison of total, free, and salivary phenytoin concentrations in geriatric patients. Clin Pharm 1986;5:59.
24. Drinka PJ, Miller J, Voeks SK, Hamel P. Phenytoin binding in a nursing home. J Geriatr Drug Ther 1988;3:73.
25. Edwards GB, Culbertson VL, Andresen GB, Rhodes PJ. Free phenytoin concentrations in geriatrics. J Geriatr Drug Ther 1988;3:97.
26. Bauer LA, Blouin RA. Age and phenytoin kinetics in adult epileptics. Clin Pharmacol Ther 1982;31:301.
27. Perucca E, Grimaldi R, Gatti G, et al. Pharmacokinetics of valproic acid in the elderly. Br J Clin Pharmacol 1984;17:665.
28. Bauer LA, Davis R, Wilensky A, et al. Valproic acid clearance: unbound fraction and diurnal variation in young and elderly adults. Clin Pharmacol Ther 1985;37:697.
29. Castleden CM, George CF, Marcer D, Hallett C. Increased sensitivity to nitrazepam in old age. BMJ 1977;1:10.
30. Cook PJ, Flanagan R, James IM. Diazepam tolerance: effect of age, regular sedation and alcohol. BMJ 1984;289:351.

18

Commonly Used Antiepileptic Drugs: Age-Related Efficacy

L. James Willmore

Management of epilepsy in the elderly requires the accurate classification of seizures, a thorough neurologic assessment to define etiology, and a comprehensive assessment of the patient's health and living situation. Treatment with an antiepileptic drug (AED) requires understanding the general health of the patient and the nature of all medications being given to the patient by other physicians. Effective management also requires communication with the spouse, any adult children, or the caregivers to be sure all understand goals of treatment, medication side effects, and monitoring strategies. All need to have realistic expectations regarding seizure control and understand the need to try drugs in sequence. Concomitant illness such as neurologic, psychiatric, or cardiac disorders will require individualization of plans and instructions.

TREATMENT PLANNING

Challenges to treatment of the elderly include concomitant diseases; polypharmacy with accompanying drug interactions; and changes in body physiology that alter drug absorption, protein binding, metabolism, and drug elimination.

Administration of any medication to an elderly patient is complicated by both complex and specific pharmacokinetics, mandatory polypharmacy, concomitant illness, and unusual sensitivity to drug effects with a narrowing of the therapeutic range of drugs. Elderly patients with declining intellectual function, motor impairment, or altered sensory function may be especially susceptible to dose-related central nervous system side effects of AEDs. Multifactorial decline in mental function may be accentuated by drug-induced delirium or intensifying underlying dementia. Drug-induced delirium is a common problem in the elderly. Declining memory and intellect has an impact on compliance by causing failure to follow prescription instructions.

PHARMACOKINETICS

The effect of a drug on a target organ is determined by the drug concentration at the site of action. Both seizure control and toxic effects are determined by the quantity of circulating free drug not bound by plasma proteins that is in equilibrium with brain water. Commonly available methods for monitoring serum levels of AEDs measure total drug levels. Although monitoring total plasma levels provides useful information in younger patients, the elderly are a challenge because of common pertubations that occur in the process of aging. Measurement of total serum concentration of a drug is best used when the drug is not highly protein-bound or when the ratio of unbound drug to free drug is stable over a range of concentrations. Phenytoin (PHT), valproate (VPA), and carbamazepine (CBZ) are highly bound to protein. Any changes that alter protein binding could influence the amount of the active agent available to exert a physiologic effect.

Changes in the quantity of free drug in plasma water available for penetration into the neuropil occur with a decline in the amount of circulating albumin or with the occupation of drug binding sites by hormones or by metabolites, as occurs in renal disease. Reduction in protein-binding sites will displace the drug, causing increases in the free fraction. An increase in circulating free drug has several consequences. First, a greater quantity of drug is available to develop equilibrium with neural extracellular water, causing dose-related neurologic toxicity. Second, presentation of more unbound drug to the hepatocyte will increase the metabolism of the total amount of drug, leading to the need for increased dose of drug to maintain the free level within the therapeutic range.

Common physiologic changes in the elderly include reduced hepatic blood flow, decreased liver volume,[1] and changes in the concentration of circulating plasma proteins.[2, 3] Elderly patients have reduced levels of serum albumin and increases in alpha$_1$-acid glycoprotein (AAG).[4] AAG is a reactant serum protein.[5] Circulating serum levels of AAG increase with physiologic stress associated with diseases such as cerebral infarction, cardiac failure, infection, surgical procedures, and obstructive pulmonary diseases. Levels of AAG are also increased normally with increased age. Hepatic enzyme induction caused with some AEDs also will increase levels of AAG. AAG binds weakly alkaline and neutral drugs. The total serum levels of drugs so affected will increase, but unbound drug levels will remain unchanged.[6] Levels of albumin are reduced by alterations in hepatic metabolism, concomitant illness, and social problems such as malnutrition.

SPECIFIC DRUGS

Phenytoin

PHT is a weak organic acid, poorly soluble in water, and available as free acid and as a sodium salt. Absorption occurs in the intestines. The peak concentration occurs at 3–12 hours after administration. Approximately 90% of PHT is protein-bound. The drug is eliminated by metabolic transformation, mostly via parahydroxylation. The elimination kinetics of PHT are nonlinear. The drug is metabolized by hepatic enzymes that are capacity-limited. This system is saturated at serum concentrations of 8–10 µg/ml. Thus, the half-life of the drug increases with higher plasma concentrations. Gastrointestinal (GI) absorption is altered both by physiologic changes in the elderly and by medications that change GI motility. The usual maintenance dose is 4–6 mg/kg/day. Because of saturation kinetics, dose changes must be made with care. The 30-mg preparation containing the sodium salt of PHT is best, but the 50-mg scored tablet of the acid may be used as well for fine-dose adjustment. Remember, the acid contains 8% more active drug and may cause a disproportionate saturation. The most important factor in alteration of PHT steady state is interaction with other drugs.[7, 8]

Because of the saturation kinetics of PHT, small changes in the maintenance dose will produce large changes in the total serum concentration. Since 300 mg/day of phenytoin would produce a serum level of 15 μg/ml in a 70-kg patient, increasing the dose by 10% to a total dose of 330 mg/day will increase the concentration by 67% to a level of 25 mg/ml, causing clinical toxicity.[9] This effect has resulted in the recommendation that the initial dose of PHT in the elderly be adjusted to 3 mg/kg to anticipate this process, with dose adjustments of 10 mg/day.[10]

In addition to changes in protein binding, PHT metabolism in the elderly is reduced.[4, 11–13] The deceased V_{max} associated with aging will cause saturation of enzyme sites at lower total concentrations than would occur in younger adults.[14–17] Hence, careful changes in dose, relying on 30-mg capsules as well as the 100-mg capsules, is of importance. Keep in mind that the 100-mg capsule contains 92 mg of phenytoin sodium. Since the total plasma level of drug does not correlate well with the concentration of phenytoin reaching brain water, it is best to monitor free levels and adjust doses accordingly. Renal dysfunction or disease alters PHT binding.[18] Measurement of free levels should improve monitoring in patients with complicating diseases. Investigators have determined that achieving a blood level of 15 μg/ml of phenytoin in an elderly patient would require administration of 79% of the total daily dose that would be used in a younger adult.

Valproate

Age-related changes in pharmacokinetics of VPA should be anticipated because of the high percentage of drug that is protein-bound.[14] VPA is a branched-chain carboxylic acid that may be metabolized either through mitochondrial mechanisms or via cytoplasmic enzymes. Dehydrogenation of VPA results in the accumulation of 2-en, 3-en, and 4-en-VPA compounds. The 4-en metabolites are highest in infants, and levels decline with age. The 2-en compound has anticonvulsant potency.[19, 20] VPA binds to albumin at high- and low-affinity sites. This binding is saturable; hence, the free fraction increases with dose. One study measured clearance of unbound drug in young adult and elderly volunteers. The time to peak concentration and the maximum total plasma concentration after a single oral dose of VPA were similar, yet the unbound fraction of drug was significantly higher in the elderly subjects. Younger adults had 6.4% drug unbound to protein, whereas the unbound fraction in the elderly was 10.7%.[21] Total drug clearance was similar for both age groups. In another study,[22] serum elimination half-life was 14.7 hours in elderly, whereas it was 7.2 hours in younger subjects. Furthermore, the volume of distribution for VPA was significantly larger in the elderly: 0.19 liter/kg versus 0.13 liter/kg in the younger patients.

As with PHT, clinical response to treatment, development of side effects, and measurement of free levels are important in treating elderly patients with VPA.

Carbamazepine

CBZ is insoluble in aqueous solutions, behaving as a neutral lipophilic substance.[23] CBZ is biotransformed, forming CBZ-10,11-epoxide.[24, 25] The epoxide is formed at the 10,11 double bond of the azepine ring, catalyzed by the hepatic monoxygenases.[26] The epoxide is hydrated by the microsomal epoxide hydrolase.[9] Because of the problem with solubility, GI absorption of CBZ is both slow and unpredictable.[27] Peak plasma levels occur at 4–8 hours of ingestion; hence, multiple dosing is required.[23]

Elimination of CBZ follows dose-dependent kinetics. Although the single-dose half-life ranges from 18 hours to 55 hours, the half-life in most adults is 6–12 hours. The elimination of CBZ varies greatly with age.[27, 28] CBZ also is involved in problematic drug interactions with other AEDs and with various other medications as well. Since CBZ induces its own metabolism, any drug that increased the quantity of P-450 enzymes will cause a fall in CBZ blood levels. Inhibition of the activity of epoxide hydrolase, as occurs with concomitant administration of VPA, will increase the quantity of the epoxide.[29] Both CBZ and the epoxide have effects as anticonvulsants.[30, 31]

Initiation of therapy with CBZ usually requires starting with 200 mg/day, increasing the dose by 200 mg each week until the best therapeutic response is obtained. Maximum induction of metabolism occurs at 3–4 weeks after the initiation of treatment.[32] The usual monotherapy dose of CBZ is 10 mg/kg/day, but if the patient is being treated with comedication, a dose of 15–20 mg/kg/day may be required.[23]

CBZ is bound both to albumin and to AAG at 65–85% of the total drug. CBZ-10-11 epoxide is also protein-bound, but by a lesser percentage.[33] Fluctuations in levels of circulating albumin and AAG will influence the amount of both compounds present in plasma water for brain penetration, but assays for the epoxide and free carbamazepine are not available routinely. Single-dose studies failed to reveal any age-specific significant differences. CBZ clearance may be reduced by approximately 40% in the elderly when compared with younger adults, however.[33] Management of patients treated with CBZ requires correlation of plasma levels with clinical response and close attention to the development of any side effects.[23]

CBZ has few toxic effects. Most are concentration-dependent or idiosyncratic. Diplopia is a common concentration-dependent effect that is useful for clinical titration. Nystagmus and ataxia can occur.[34, 35] The most severe reactions alter hematopoietic, skin, and cardiovascular systems.[34] Communication with the patient and informed consent are important for successful long-term monitoring.[35] Some specific problems, such as congestive heart failure, cardiac conduction changes,[36–39] and hyponatremia, may occur.[40–43]

Phenobarbital

Little specific information is available regarding phenobarbital clearance in the elderly. The drug is not highly protein-bound. There is some evidence that clearance is reduced in the elderly. This change suggests the practical actions of using lower total daily maintenance doses and, when initiating therapy, anticipating an increase in the time to reach steady state.[44, 45]

Benzodiazepines

These compounds are used commonly in the elderly for treatment of behavioral problems. Although benzodiazepines are used less commonly for chronic treatment of seizures, acute administration is required occasionally. Diazepam is an important drug for intravenous use to terminate convulsive status epilepticus. The drug is highly protein-bound; the metabolite desmethyldiazepam is active as well. Although the free fraction of diazepam increases with age, the clearance of the unbound drug decreases, causing prolonged plasma elimination half-lives of the drug and its metabolite.[46] Lorazepam is 90% protein-bound and conjugated for elimination as a glucuronide. The free fraction of the drug and the volume of distribution increase with age, but studies of the elimination half-life are similar in the young and the elderly.[47] Although the pharmacokinetics profile of lorazepam may be somewhat more favorable than diazepam, prolonged sedation after the use of lorazepam must be considered when selecting a benzodiazepine for intravenous use to terminate convulsive status epilepticus.[48]

Pharmacodynamic effects also are important in the use of benzodiazepines in the elderly. These patients are sensitive to effects on neural function that are independent of elimination half-life, volume of distribution, and protein binding.[48, 49]

THE CHALLENGE OF POLYPHARMACY

Surveys of drug use show the elderly use a mean of seven drugs each day.[33] The most commonly used drugs by category are the psychotropics. Thyroid supplements, antacids, and medications used to treat blood pressure elevation are also widely used. Addition of an AED to an elderly patient's medical regimen requires careful review of all drugs being used. Drug interactions[50] can be assessed within the framework of the mechanism of drug clearance. Other pharmacologic effects occur that are related to protein-binding alterations, changes in renal clearance, and altered hepatic function.

Elderly patients have concomitant medical problems in addition to epilepsy. Hypertension, cardiac disease, infections, and GI disturbances all require

Table 18.1 Drugs causing increased blood levels of carbamazepine and phenytoin

Medications causing increased concentration of carbamazepine
    Cimetidine
    Isoniazid
    Propoxyphene
    Erythromycin
    Troleandomycin
    Phenytoin
    Verapamil
    Diltiazem
    Nicotinamide
    Viloxazine
    Imipramine
Medications causing increased concentration of phenytoin
    Cimetidine
    Isoniazid
    Chloramphenicol
    Chlordiazepoxide
    Disulfiram
    Halothane
    Phenylbutazone
    Propranolol

treatment. Since drugs used to treat associated illnesses may alter absorption, distribution, and metabolism of AEDs, they have an adverse impact on efficacy and increase the occurrence of adverse effects. Tables 18.1, 18.2, and 18.3 list commonly used drugs and their effects on AEDs.[23]

The AEDs may induce metabolism of other agents, resulting in a decline in the target response, and some drugs interfere with the metabolism of AEDs, causing dose-related toxicity. A complete drug inventory is important. The patient or a caregiver must bring all drugs to the office for review and recording.

Drugs with a high degree of protein binding displace AEDs, leading to decreased total levels with increase in free fractions. Calcium channel-blocking agents and both erythromycin and propoxyphene may block access to metabolic enzymes, causing marked increase in total blood levels of PHT and CBZ. Psychoactive drugs, commonly needed to manage behavioral problems in the elderly, alter AED levels or efficacy. In addition, the expected effects of a drug may be impaired if administered to a patient receiving an enzyme-inducing drug such as CBZ. Haloperidol metabolism may be enhanced by concomitant administration to a patient receiving an AED. Seizure threshold may be reduced with use of perphenazine, trifluoperazine, promazine, or chlorpromazine.

Table 18.2 Drugs causing decreased blood levels of carbamazepine and phenytoin

Medications causing decreased concentration of carbamazepine
    Phenobarbital
    Phenytoin
    Primidone
    Valproate
Medications causing decreased concentration of phenytoin
    Antacids
    Ethanol
    Nicotine
    Phenobarbital
    Phenothiazines
    Phenylbutazone
    Heparin
    Salicylates
    Valproate

Table 18.3 Mediations that may lose effectiveness or have reduced concentrations when administered with carbamazepine or phenytoin

Concentrations reduced by concomitant administration of carbamazepine
    Doxycycline
    Phenobarbital
    Phenytoin
    Warfarin
    Valproate
Concentrations or effectiveness reduced by phenytoin
    Carbamazepine
    Dicumarol
    Doxycycline
    Folic acid
    Haloperidol
    Oral contraceptives
    Theophylline
    Vitamin D

REFERENCES

1. Wynne HA, Cope LH, Mutch E, et al. The effect of age upon liver volume and apparent liver blood flow in healthy man. Hepatology 1989;9:297.
2. Wallace SM, Verbeeck RK. Plasma protein binding of drugs in the elderly. Clin Pharmacokinet 1987;12:41.
3. Greenblatt DJ. Reduced serum albumin concentrations in the elderly: a report from the Boston Collaborative Drug Surveillance Program. J Am Geriatr Soc 1979;27:20.

4. Verbeeck RK, Cardinal J-A, Wallace SM. Effect of age and sex on the plasma binding of acidic and basic drugs. Eur J Clin Pharmacol 1984;27:91.
5. Tiula E, Neuvonen PJ. Antiepileptic drugs and alpha-1 acid glycoprotein. N Engl J Med 1982;307:1148.
6. Dawling S, Crome P. Clinical pharmacokinetic considerations in the elderly. Clin Pharmacokinet 1989;17:236.
7. Kutt H. Interactions between anticonvulsants and other commonly prescribed drugs. Epilepsia 1984;25(Suppl 2):118.
8. Kutt H, Fouts JR. Diphenylhydantoin metabolism by rat liver microsomes and some of the effects of drug or chemical pretreatment on diphenylhydantoin metabolism by rat liver microsomal preparations. J Pharmacol Exp Ther 1971;176:11.
9. Bender AD, Post A, Meier JP, et al. Plasma protein binding of drugs as a function of age in adult human subjects. J Pharm Sci 1975;64:1711.
10. Bauer LA, Blouin RA. Age and phenytoin kinetics in adult epileptics. Clin Pharmacol Ther 1982;31:3010.
11. Umstead GS, Morales M, McKercher PL. Comparison of total, free, and salivary phenytoin concentrations in geriatric patients. Clin Pharm 1986;5:59.
12. Drinka PJ, Miller J, Voeks SK, Hamel P. Phenytoin binding in a nursing home geriatric patient population. J Geriatr Drug Ther 1988;3:73.
13. Hayes MJ, Langman MJS, Short AH. Changes in drug metabolism with increasing age, II: phenytoin clearance and protein binding. Br J Clin Pharmacol 1975;2:73.
14. Perucca E, Grimaldi R, Gatti G, et al. Pharmacokinetics of valproic acid in the elderly. Br J Clin Pharmacol 1984;17:665.
15. Lambie DC, Caird FI. Phenytoin dosage in the elderly. Age Ageing 1977;6:133.
16. Troupin AS, Johannessen SI. Epilepsy in the Elderly: A Pharmacologic Perspective. In DB Smith (ed), Epilepsy: Current Approaches to Diagnosis and Treatment. New York: Raven, 1990;141.
17. Bach B, Hansen JM, Kampmann JP, et al. Disposition of antipyrine and phenytoin correlated with age and liver volume in men. Clin Pharmacokinet 1981;6:389.
18. Reidenberg MM, Odar-Cederlof I, von Bahr C, et al. Protein binding of diphenylhydantoin and desmethylimipramine in patients with poor renal function. N Engl J Med 1971;285:264.
19. Loscher W, Nau H. Pharmacological evaluation of various metabolites and analogues of valproic acid: anticonvulsant and toxic potencies in mice. Neuropharmacology 1985;24:427.
20. Loscher W, Nau H, Marescaux C, Vergnes M. Comparative evaluation of anticonvulsant and toxic potencies of valproic acid and 2-en-valproic acid in different animal models of epilepsy. Eur J Pharmacol 1984;99:211.
21. Bauer LA, Davis R, Wilensky A, et al. Valproic acid clearance: unbound fraction and diurnal variations in young and elderly adults. Clin Pharmacol Ther 1985; 37:697.
22. Bryson SM, Verma N, Scott PJW, Rubin PC. Pharmacokinetics of valproic acid in young and elderly subjects. Br J Clin Pharmacol 1983;16:104.
23. Leppik IE. Metabolism of antiepileptic medication: newborn to elderly. Epilepsia 1992;33(Suppl 4):32.
24. Patsalos PN, Stephenson TJ, Krishna S, et al. Side-effects induced by carbamazepine-10,11-epoxide. Lancet 1985;2:496.
25. Schoeman JF, Elyas AA, Brett EM, Lascelles PT. Correlation between plasma carbamazepine-10,11-epoxide concentration and drug side effects in children with epilepsy. Dev Med Child Neurol 1984;26:756.
26. Riley RJ, Kitteringham NR, Park BK. Structural requirements for bioactivation of anticonvulsants to cytotoxic metabolites in vitro. Br J Clin Pharmacol 1989;28:482.
27. Morselli PL, Bossi L. Carbamazepine Absorption, Distribution and Excretion. In DM Woodbury, JK Penry, CE Pippenger (eds), Antiepileptic Drugs (2nd ed). New York: Raven, 1982;465.

28. Hockings N, Pall A, Moody APJ, et al. The effects of age on carbamazepine pharmacokinetics and adverse effects. Br J Clin Pharmacol 1986;22:725.
29. McLachlan M. Anatomic Structural and Vascular Changes in the Aging Kidney. In JFM Nunez, JS Cameron (eds), Renal Function and Diseases in the Elderly. London: Butterworths, 1987.
30. Albright PS, Bruni J. Effects of carbamazepine and its epoxide metabolites on amygdala-kindled seizures in rats. Neurology 1984;34:1383.
31. Bourgeois BFD, Wad N. Individual and combined antiepileptic and neurotoxic activity of carbamazepine and carbamazepine-10,11-epoxide in mice. J Pharmacol Exp Ther 1984;231:411.
32. Pitlick WH, Levy RH, Troupin AS, Green JR. Pharmacokinetic model to describe self-induced decreases in stedy-state concentrations of carbamazepine. J Pharm Sci 1976;65:462.
33. Cloyd JC, Lackner TE, Leppik IE. Antiepileptics in the elderly: pharmacoepidemiology and pharmacokinetics. Arch Fam Med 1994;3:589.
34. Pellock JM. Carbamazepine side effects in children and adults. Epilepsia 1987;28:64.
35. Pellock JM, Willmore LJ. A rational guide to routine blood monitoring in patients receiving antiepileptic drugs. Neurology 1991;41:961.
36. Ladefoged SD, Mogelvang JC. Total atrioventricular block with syncopes complicating carbamazepine therapy. Acta Med Scand 1982;212:185.
37. Louis S, Kutt H, McDowell F. The cardiocirculatory changes caused by intravenous Dilantin and its solvents. Am Heart J 1967;74:523.
38. Beermann B, Edhag O. Depressive effects of carbamazepine on idioventricular rhythm in man. BMJ 1978;2:171.
39. Hewetson KA, Ritch AES, Watson RDS. Sick sinus syndrome aggravated by carbamazepine therapy for epilepsy. Postgrad Med J 1986;62:497.
40. Lahr MB. Hyponatremia during carbamazepine therapy. Clin Pharmacol Ther 1985;37:693.
41. Kalff R, Houtkooper MA, Meyer JW, et al. Carbamazepine and serum sodium levels. Epilepsia 1984;25:390.
42. Soelberg Sørenson P, Hammer M. Effects of long-term carbamazepine treatment on water metabolism and plasma vasopressin concentration. Eur J Clin Pharmacol 1984;26:719.
43. Stephens WP, Coe JY, Baylis PH. Plasma arginine vasopressin concentrations and antidiuretic action of carbamazepine. BMJ 1978;1:1445.
44. Sherwin AL, Loynd JS, Bock GW, Sokolwski CD. Effects of age, sex, obesity and pregnancy on plasma diphenylhydantoin levels. Epilepsia 1974;15:507.
45. Eadie MJ, Lander CM, Hooper WD, Tyrer JH. Factors influencing plasma phenobarbitone levels in epileptic patients. Br J Clin Pharmacol 1977;4:541.
46. Greenblatt DJ, Allen MD, Harmatz JS, Shader RI. Diazepam disposition determinants. Clin Pharmacol Ther 1980;27:301.
47. Greenblatt DJ, Allen MD, Locniskar A, et al. Lorazepam kinetics in the elderly. Clin Pharmacol Ther 1979;26:103.
48. Cook PJ, Flanagan R, James IM. Diazepam tolerance: effect of age, regular sedation and alcohol. BMJ 1984;289:351.
49. Crooks J, Stevenson IH. Drug response in the elderly—sensitivity and pharmacokinetic considerations. Age Ageing 1981;10:73.
50. Pitlick WH. Antiepileptic Drug Interactions. New York: Demos, 1989.

19

New Antiepileptic Medications: Pharmacokinetic and Mechanistic Considerations in the Treatment of Seizures and Epilepsy in the Elderly

Michael J. McLean

INTRODUCTION

New antiepileptic medications (AEMs) with a variety of chemical structures are appearing in waves in the United States. Their advent raises expectations of improved seizure control for individuals of all ages with epilepsy. This is perhaps more true for the elderly, among whom the incidence of seizures and epilepsy is highest.[1] The most common seizure types with onset after 65 years of age are partial seizures with or without secondary generalization.[1] As demonstrated in the first Veterans Administration (VA) Cooperative Study,[2] 40% of patients with these seizure types were inadequately or unsatisfactorily controlled, either because of inefficacy or adverse effects. Between the two large comparative VA cooperative studies,[2, 3] the percentage of patients continuing to take carbamazepine, phenytoin, and valproate on a long-term basis was approximately equal. Switching to a second drug resulted in satisfactory control in approximately half of those failing a first AEM.[4] There are no consistent indicators of how a patient will best respond to a given AEM. Thus, to a certain extent, the physician is reduced to empiricism in the management of the clinical epilepsies.

None of the new AEMs has been tested in a head-on comparative study with other standard or novel AEMs. As part of the Food and Drug Administration (FDA) approval process, the efficacy of all the new compounds is being tested in add-on trials, and in some cases monotherapy trials, against partial seizures with or without secondary generalization and refractory to conventional AEMs. The older medications—for example, carbamazepine, phenobarbital, phenytoin, and valproate—are effective against these types of seizures in many patients. Also, the older drugs undoubtedly will remain significantly less expensive than the new AEMs. Thus, to justify selection of the new AEMs over standard medications, cost-conscious managed-care organizations and facilities involved in the care of the elderly will require that the new AEMS have a clear advantage in terms of efficacy, pharmacokinetic properties, reduced adverse effects, and reduced monitoring of plasma levels and with other laboratory tests (e.g., liver enzymes and complete blood counts). In addition, the elderly often have systemic illnesses that require treatment with multiple medications in addition to AEMs. As with the standard AEMs, knowledge of potential drug-drug interactions will be required to use new medications optimally. Fortunately, some of the new medications have simple pharmacokinetics and no significant interactions to date.

Mechanisms of epileptogenesis in the elderly are not well understood. Many elderly patients have symptomatic partial epilepsies as a result of strokes or tumors, for example. The aging brain is an ever-changing pharmacologic landscape, however. Changes in neurotransmitter systems occur progressively, including a decline in the concentration of the inhibitory transmitter γ-aminobutyric acid (GABA) and the activity of its synthetic enzyme.[5] Such changes could be epileptogenic in their own right and could explain some cryptogenic cases ultimately.[5a] Not knowing the impact of age-related factors presents a challenge for selecting AEMs on a mechanistic basis to treat seizures in the elderly.

Novel cellular mechanisms of action or combinations of actions are expected of the new AEMs. A caveat worth considering, however, is that pharmacodynamic interactions could result from new mechanisms. This is important in learning limits of the usefulness of the new AEMs. For example, benzodiazepines and barbiturates enhance GABA–activated chloride conductance. These classes of compounds have been associated with adverse behavioral effects.[6] The addition of new AEMs with GABA-enhancing mechanisms of action could potentiate the effects of the other compounds and either worsen behavior or precipitate abnormal behavior de novo. This may be especially important for elderly patients who, as a group, are often given psychotropic medications.[7] The prospect of such interactions is not restricted to the new AEMs, and learning to deal with emergent problems will come only with experience. Minimizing dose increments and rate of escalation and using the lowest effective dose of the new AEMs in monotherapy whenever possible should avoid potential adverse pharmacodynamic interactions. In the words of *The All-Knowing Mentor*, "Start low and go slow." Use of the new AEMs in monotherapy must be tempered by the fact that some of them are or will be approved initially as add-on therapy. Optimal methods of using the new compounds in the elderly probably will require years of experience in widespread clinical use. As physicians become comfortable with the first wave of new drugs, the second wave should become available over the next few years. Thus, we can expect continuing appearance of new treatment options for patients with difficult-to-control seizures. Even if their efficacy does not exceed that of the standard AEMs, new medications with few or no drug-drug interactions are likely to gain widespread acceptance in the treatment of elderly patients because they reduce the possibility of toxicity. In addition, the cost of monitoring plasma levels to guide dose adjustments, which is required to minimize the interactions, should decline. The purpose of this review is to assess pharmacokinetic properties and mechanisms of action of novel AEMs that might have particular impact in the treatment of the elderly patient. Also, this chapter might help increase understanding of how the new medications can be used along with or instead of the standard AEMs.

PERSPECTIVES ON PHARMACOKINETICS

The study of pharmacokinetics is basically the study of logistics, or how drugs reach and are maintained at their target. Tables 19.1 and 19.2 compare some of the pharmacokinetic properties of the standard and new AEMs. One of the salient differences is the greater water solubility of the newer compounds. Absorption of the older AEMs is fairly complete, but the rate of absorption can be influenced modestly by simultaneous food intake. For example, absorption of phenytoin is generally enhanced by eating.[8] Conversely, the bioavailability of the new AEMs is not adversely affected by eating. The older AEMs are, in general, hydrophobic compounds with limited aqueous solubility. As a consequence, a large proportion of the absorbed compound is transported bound to plasma proteins, especially to albumin, thus creating a potential for drug interactions. For example, valproate, which is bound in a concentration-dependent manner to plasma proteins,[9] may compete with carbamazepine[10] and non-AEMs, such as tolbutamide,[11] for binding sites. As a result of greater water solubility of some new AEMs, there is a reduced chance of interactions due to competition for protein binding sites in the blood. Standard lipid-soluble AEMs are metabolized in the liver, another site for drug-drug interactions. It is important to note that some of the new AEMs are not metabolized and consequently have fewer or no known drug-drug interactions. Excretion of AEMs in urine, either as unchanged compounds or as hepatic metabolites, is a major route of elimination of old and new AEMs. Metabolism and elimination are important aspects of AEM pharmacokinetics in the elderly because hepatic and renal function decline with age.[12, 13] Dysfunction in either of these organs may result in decreased drug clearance, increased toxicity, and more significant interactions. It will be interesting to see whether decreased clearance due to interaction at renal sites becomes a significant problem with the unmetabolized new AEMs.

PERSPECTIVES ON MECHANISMS

Most physicians who care for patients with epilepsy plumb the arcane world of the mechanist rarely, and mechanisms seldom enter their therapeutic decision-making process. In the hands of the initiate, mechanisms of action become tactics that can be allied with logistics (pharmacokinetics) in the design of a therapeutic regimen to produce a strategy of antiepileptic care. In the best of all worlds, the treating physician would go to the shelf to pick a drug or combination of drugs that specifically suppress the epileptogenic mechanism in a given patient without adverse effects. In practice, mechanisms of epileptogenesis, regional neurochemistry of the focus, and cellular mechanisms of action of AEMs are rarely understood in sufficient detail to dictate the choice of medications.

Mechanisms were not the principal determinant in the selection of the first wave of new AEMs for clinical development. Only two of the new AEMs—

Table 19.1 Selected pharmacokinetic properties of some standard antiepileptic medications

	Carbamazepine	Ethosuximide	Phenobarbital	Phenytoin	Valproate
Bioavailability (%)	~85	88–98 (animals)	80–100	~95	100
T_{max} (hrs)	6–20	1–3	6–12	4–12	1–4
Protein bound (%)	72–76	0	50	80–90	93 at 50 µg/ml, 70 at 150 µg/ml
V_d (liter/kg)	0.72–1.30	0.67–0.72	0.54–1.00	0.7–1.3	0.1–0.4
Principal metabolites	Epoxide, diol	Hydroxy compounds and glucuronides	Hydroxy, O-methyl, and N-glucoside	Hydroxy compounds	Conjugates, β-oxidation, δ-dehydrogenation (4-en toxic)
Active metabolites	Epoxide	None	None	None	2-en
Liver enzyme induction	Yes	No	Yes	Yes	No
Liver enzyme inhibition	No	No	No	No	Yes
Autoinduction	Yes	No	No	No	No
$t_{1/2}$ (hrs)	18–55 at inception; 5–26 after autoinduction	35–54	72–96	7–42	4–12
Urinary excretion (% unchanged)	2	17–38	42	<5	<7

Table 19.2 Pharmacokinetic properties of new antiepileptic medications

	Felbamate	Gaba-pentin	Lamo-trigine	Oxcarbazepine	Tiagabine	Topiramate	Vigabatrin
Bioavailability	~85	~60	~95	100	100	100	100
T_{max} (hrs)	6–20	2–3	4–12	2–4 (Monohydroxy derivative)	0.5–1.0	1.4–4.3	0.75–2.0
Protein-bound (%)	25–35	0	~55	~50 (Monohydroxy derivative)	96	<20	0
V_d (liters/kg)	~1.0	0.65–1.04	~1.1	0.3–0.8	~1.0	0.6–0.8	0.8
Principal metabolites	Hydroxy compounds, mono-carbamate	None	Glucuro-nides	Monohydroxy derivative and conjugates	5-oxo derivative	? Hydroxy compounds	None
Active metabolites	None	None	None	Monohydroxy derivative	None	None	None
Hepatic enzyme induction	No	No	No	Less than carbamazepine	No	No	No
Hepatic enzyme inhibition	Probable	No	No	No	No	No	No
Autoinduction	No	No	No	No	No	No	No
$t_{1/2}$ (hrs)	~19	5–9	~24	8–10	4.5–13.4	20–24	5–8
Urinary excretion (% unchanged)	40–50	100	10	<1 as oxcarbazepine, ~70 as monohy-droxy derivative	<2 as tiaga-bine	~85 topiramate	100

vigabatrin and tiagabine—possess specific mechanisms of action for which they were designed. These compounds augment brain concentrations of the inhibitory amino acid transmitter, GABA, and prevent GABA reuptake, respectively. Gabapentin, enigmatically, seems to be a counter example. It was designed to facilitate the transport of GABA across the blood-brain barrier by coupling GABA with a lipophilic cyclohexane moiety. So far, there is no published evidence that it increases brain GABA levels. Also, it is assumed to cross the blood-brain barrier by a saturable transport system rather than by lipophilic mechanisms. All of the other new AEMs of the first and second waves were active in animal screening models that were used to identify the old AEMs. Since all of the new AEMs had some efficacy against maximal electroshock (MES)–induced seizures, the model that gave us phenytoin, carbamazepine, and valproate, it should come as no surprise that new AEMs are effective against complex partial and secondarily generalized seizures. A jaded, if not nihilistic, view is that the new AEMs are "me too" drugs to some extent. Subtle differences in their capacity to control complex partial seizures may reflect subtle mechanistic or pharmacokinetic differences. Elaboration of powerful molecular-cloning techniques eventually may allow the deliberate engineering of compounds targeted against specific subunits of neurotransmitter receptors. Nonetheless, it will still be necessary to demonstrate uniqueness of mechanisms by comparative testing with standard AEMs in both animal models and controlled clinical studies. Until further understanding of epileptogenesis and mechanisms of action allow design of novel agents or more rational drug selection, availability of additional AEMs with overlapping spectra of efficacy increases the chances of successfully treating the individual with refractory seizures. Clinical experience will determine whether the new medications are more effective than the older ones—or, at least, sufficiently more so as to justify their cost.

Despite an incomplete grasp of the cellular mechanisms of action of any single AEM, considerable information has been derived about the effects on four naturally occurring aspects of neuronal function that can be modulated to control seizures. Effects of AEMs on voltage-sensitive sodium[14] and calcium[15, 16] channels and on GABA-[17–19] and glutamate-activated[20–23] ion channels are reviewed primarily. Less is known about AEM interactions with many biochemical processes,[24] endogenous proconvulsant[25, 26] or anticonvulsant[27–29] compounds and other neurotransmitters,[30] and ionic conductances (especially potassium). Much more will have to be known to completely account for the clinical spectra of efficacy of AEMs, both old and new.

Voltage-Sensitive Sodium Channels

Sodium influx through voltage-sensitive channels generates the upstroke of action potentials recorded from axons and somata of central neurons.[31] The operational cycle of sodium channels underlying conducted action potentials has been described by Hodgkin and Huxley.[32] In this model, channels may be in the resting, activated (conducting), or inactive state or in configuration. With depolarization, available resting channels open quickly and nearly synchronously and admit sodium ions flowing inward along their concentration gradient. Generation of sufficient current by this influx triggers the action potential. The channels inactivate spontaneously as slower conformational changes close the inner mouth of the channel. Repriming, or recovery from inactivation, occurs with time after repolarization. The number of channels available to contribute to the next action potential is determined to a large extent by the interval between spikes, that is to say, rate-dependent, and the transmembrane voltage, that is to say, voltage-dependent. At high frequencies (>150 Hz), the rate of cycling may not be fast enough for some channels to reprime. The result is that the sodium current, I_{Na}, and maximal rate of rise of action potentials (V_{max}) decrease at fast rates. Sodium channel proteins have been cloned, and sequences involved in various aspects of channel function have been identified.[14] Although kinetic parameters vary, all voltage-sensitive ion channels must go through a similar operational cycle. Kinetic models of drug interaction with different aspects of channel function have had an important impact on the development of antiepileptic and antiarrhythmic drugs.[33, 34]

Several standard AEMs bind to sodium channels, with resultant accumulation of sodium channels in the inactivated state, prolongation of refractoriness, and failure of some action potentials. Phenytoin, carbamazepine, and valproic acid all limit sustained high-frequency repetitive firing (SRF) of sodium-dependent action potentials and prolong refractoriness at concentrations that correspond to therapeutic free plasma levels.[35–37] Limitation could occur due to the effects on sodium, calcium, or potassium channels. Reduction of V_{max} suggests an effect on sodium channels. These three AEMs also reduce voltage-dependent sodium current in a use-dependent manner and slow recovery from inactivation.[38–43] Such effects on sodium channels parallel the ability of these compounds to protect against tonic hind-limb extension in the MES model in animals and may contribute to clinical efficacy against generalized tonic-clonic and partial seizures.[44]

Barbiturates[45] and benzodiazepines[46] limit SRF only at high concentrations that might be encountered in the treatment of status epilepticus, suggesting that these compounds work by other mechanisms in ambulatory patients. Ethosuximide does not block SRF.[37] Other compounds, including local anesthetics[47] and tricyclic antidepressants,[48] act at voltage-sensitive sodium channels, yet they are not useful clinically as antiepileptics.

Sodium channel block by standard AEMs has several important characteristics. First, the effect is concentration-dependent. Sometimes, very high concentrations are necessary to demonstrate an effect on sodium channels in vitro. This could result from either low affinity for sodium channels or technical conditions. The *N*-methyl-D-aspartate (NMDA) channel-blocking compound, MK-801, provides an example of the latter. MK-801 blocks sodium currents only slightly under voltage clamp conditions at 10^{-4} mol/liter.[49] Also, it has little effect on intracellularly recorded action potential parameters at room temperature.[50] At 37°C, however, it limits SRF at 5×10^{-7} mol/liter.[51, 52] This marked shift in the concentration dependence of the actions occurs simply because of the temperature. Thus, absence of an effect in vitro with a given technique may reflect inability of a technique to detect an effect under the operant conditions. To be therapeutically meaningful, in vitro effects should occur at concentrations that overlap the clinically useful therapeutic range. Drug effects derived with different techniques should be mutually explicable in order to make predictions about the clinical situation.

Second, the effect is voltage-dependent. At very negative transmembrane potentials, drugs bind to a small percentage of sodium channels, with some reduction of sodium current or action potential rate of rise (tonic block). With depolarization, as occurs at the ictal transition, drug binding becomes more likely, and block accrues more quickly.

Third, the effect on sodium channels is use-dependent, requiring multiple activations of sodium currents or firings of action potentials. It is also frequency-dependent and enhanced at fast rates and less negative membrane potentials, which occur at the depolarizing shift signaling the ictal transition. Channels to which a drug is bound are effectively unavailable to fire the next action potential. At fast rates, action potentials have slower rates of rise and, ultimately, failures occur. Firing at slower rates is possible despite the continuing presence of the drug. That is, AEMs with this action modulate, rather than completely block, sodium channel function.

How does this relate to clinical anticonvulsant effects? Ideally, concentration dependence in vitro should predict the therapeutic range. Limitation of SRF by phenytoin, for example, occurs at concentrations equivalent to therapeutic free (not bound to plasma proteins) plasma levels.[35] Most experiments are performed acutely, however, and may not reflect drug actions that occur after chronic administration in humans. Brain tissue levels increase with time. Slow accumulation in the brain may account for gradual improvement in efficacy on a constant dose of an AEM. Alternatively, an active metabolite may accumulate and add to the efficacy of the parent compound. For example, carbamazepine epoxide[36] and the trans-2-en metabolite of valproic acid[53] both limit high-frequency firing and accumulate in the brain and cerebrospinal fluid. Limitation of high-frequency firing by AEMs has not been shown in vivo, so the repetitive firing assay may be only a pharmacologic model. High-frequency action potential firing is transmitted along projection pathways from a chemically induced cortical focus, however.[54] This firing pattern is thought to underlie the spread of abnormal activity from the seizure focus. These cellular data suggest that limitation of this firing should be a useful antiepileptic mechanism. Brief bursts of fast firing or firing sustained at slower rates will not be blocked. This could explain refractoriness of some seizures to sodium channel-blocking medications. Voltage dependence may explain why ambulatory patients tolerate sodium-channel blocking AEMs chronically with minimal dysfunction. Interictally, the patient may function almost as if the drug were not present. But, when abnormal focal activity commences and prolonged depolarization occurs, drug action becomes more effective and limits high-frequency firing along axons projecting to distant relays in the seizure pathway. In essence, this seems to stop the spread of seizures. Perhaps engagement of these actions underlie brief periods of confusion or the perception of transient impairment patients describe when they "almost had a seizure." Frequency dependence allows drugs to be used clinically as AEMs. Blocking too many sodium channels, for example due to a high concentration of one or an interaction between two sodium channel blockers, could result in sedation, reduced motor speed, and impaired cognition. In the extreme, compounds that bind tightly to sodium channels, such as the marine toxin tetrodotoxin, are lethal. Thus, the same cellular action may be relevant to both therapeutic efficacy and toxicity.

Several of the new AEMs appear to limit SRF. Felbamate[55] and topiramate[56] limit repetitive firing, but sodium channel blockade has not been definitively shown for these AEMs. Oxcarbazepine[57] and gabapentin[58] limit firing frequency and reduce maximal rate of rise. The effect of gabapentin, however, is different because of time dependence (maximal efficacy apparent after 5–12 hours of exposure). Also, gabapentin does not block sodium current in Chinese hamster ovary cells with cloned brain sodium channel alpha subunits.[59] These findings suggest that the effect of gabapentin may be indirect. The strongest evidence for a sodium channel action exists for lamotrigine, which limits SRF and binding of the sodium channel opener batrachotoxinin[60] and blocks voltage-clamped sodium current.[59, 61] Sodium channel blockade is consistent with the demonstrated protection by these new AEMs against MES seizures in animals and clinically against partial seizures with and without secondary generalization.

Voltage-Sensitive Calcium Channels

Four main biophysically and pharmacologically distinct types of voltage-sensitive calcium currents have been identified—T, L, N, and P[15, 16, 62, 63]—and others are being characterized. Calcium influx through the T-type channel is activated at negative potentials near the resting potential (low-threshold calcium current) and is involved in the generation of membrane potential oscillations underlying periodic burst firing behavior. The L-type channel is activated by greater depolarizations (high-threshold calcium current), involved in excitation-contraction coupling in cardiac and smooth muscle and in neurotransmitter release, and blocked by dihydropyridines (e.g., nifedipine). The N and P types are also high-threshold channels involved in neurotransmitter release. Blockade by ω-conotoxin identifies the N type. Neither the N- nor P-type channel is blocked by dihydropyridines.

Effects of AEMs on different types of calcium channels and currents have not been described systematically. Phenytoin blocks L current in neurons and cardiac tissue at therapeutically relevant concentrations.[64] Along with limitation of sustained high-frequency repetitive firing, blockade of L current could contribute to the well known blockade by phenytoin of post-tetanic potentiation, the calcium-dependent enhancement of neurotransmitter release after high-frequency stimulation.[65] Ethosuximide, which is effective only against generalized absence seizures, blocks the T current, which underlies paroxysmal bursting in thalamic and other neurons.[66, 67] The ability to block the T current parallels the ability of drugs to protect against clonic seizures induced by subcutaneous injection of PTZ, which predicts clinical efficacy against generalized absence seizures. Phenytoin blocks T current only at a significantly higher concentration than used clinically.[65] Valproic acid has been reported to have no effect on T current[66] and to block slightly at high concentrations (10–15% at 100–500 μM).[68] Given the broad clinical spectrum of activity of valproate, other mechanisms are likely to contribute to the control of absence seizures. To date, there are no publications about the effects of new AEMs on T current.

GABA-Activated Chloride Conductance

There are two major classes of receptors for GABA: $GABA_A$ and $GABA_B$. Binding of ligands to $GABA_A$ receptors opens a chloride-selective ion channel formed by an array of subunits. The resultant influx of chloride anions quickly hyperpolarizes and decreases excitability of neurons with resting potentials less negative than −70 mV, the reversal potential for chloride[19]; at more negative potentials $GABA_A$ activation results in depolarizing responses. Activation of $GABA_B$ receptors by GABA or baclofen and its analogues inhibits neurons in two ways, principally.[69] Direct inhibition results from G protein–coupled activation of a hyperpolarizing potassium current, a process much slower than $GABA_A$ activation. Indirect inhibition, through other G protein–mediated enzymatic pathways, reduces calcium currents involved in neurotransmitter release (L and N currents) and membrane potential oscillation (T current).[69, 70] A vast literature describing wide distribution of $GABA_A$ receptors lends credence to the view that $GABA_A$-activated chloride current is the most potent inhibitory system in the brain. It may be only a matter of time, however, before the contribution of $GABA_B$-mediated inhibition is realized.

The $GABA_A$ receptor is a channel-forming heteropentameric assembly. Isoforms of 15 candidate subunits of the $GABA_A$ receptor, each with four variable membrane-spanning regions and intra- and extracellular binding domains, have been cloned.[18] Only a few variants have been identified in vertebrate brains, but more than 186,000 receptor/channel complexes could be assembled, calculating on the basis of a 5-subunit array and 15-subunit isoforms.[70a] Variation of receptor subunit composition could result in a diversity of responses to pharmacologic agents at different stages of life and in more dynamic situations, such as disease states. The dependence of benzodiazepine binding on the inclusion of the gamma-subunit[71] illustrates the importance of subunit variation.

The $GABA_A$ receptor–channel complex is modulated by binding of several classes of compounds to separate allosteric modulatory sites. Antagonists of $GABA_A$-mediated inhibition are convulsants; drugs that enhance $GABA_A$-mediated inhibition are anticonvulsants. Benzodiazepines and barbiturates enhance $GABA_A$-activated chloride conductance by binding to different allosteric sites.[17, 18, 72] Benzodiazepines increase the frequency of the opening of chloride channels; barbiturates prolong the openings.[19] Convulsants (e.g., picrotoxin or bicuculline) decrease GABA-stimulated chloride conductance by binding at various sites.[17] Neurosteroids increase (e.g., tetrahydroprogesterone) or decrease (e.g., pregnenolone sulfate) GABA-mediated inhibition by binding to yet another site or sites.[73] The roles of $GABA_A$-mediated inhibition in the suppression of seizures and of reduced GABAergic inhibition in epileptogenesis have been extensively reviewed.[74, 75]

Of AEM effects on GABA$_A$ receptors, barbiturate and benzodiazepine mechanisms have been described in the greatest detail. Phenytoin augments GABA responses at concentrations too high for use in ambulatory patients but that are in the range achieved in the treatment of status epilepticus.[35] Valproate seems to increase brain GABA levels by increasing turnover.[76] It blocks the degradatory enzyme GABA transaminase only at high concentrations.[77] Two of the new AEMs, vigabatrin and tiagabine, were deliberately developed to augment GABA-mediated inhibition, although by different mechanisms. Vigabatrin inhibits the degrading enzyme GABA transaminase. Tiagabine blocks reuptake at GABA synapses. Felbamate[78] and topiramate[79] allosterically augment GABA-activated chloride conductance, presumably by non–benzodiazepine-related mechanisms. Gabapentin may raise interstitial GABA concentrations with synaptic activation by causing efflux from neurons due to reversal of the transporter.[80]

Paradoxically, GABAmimetic agents may be psychotogenic. During extensive trials with vigabatrin, for example, untoward behavioral effects, including frank psychosis, have been reported in a significant number percentage of patients.[81–83] Yet, on the basis of common clinical experience, this probably should come as no surprise. Barbiturates have frequently been blamed anecdotally for adverse behavior in children and benzodiazepines for confusional episodes in the elderly. As a result, the use of GABAmimetic agents, alone or in combination, by the elderly should be undertaken with caution.

Glutamate Receptors

Multiple receptors have been cloned.[84, 85] Ionotropic receptors can be subdivided into subtypes that are activated selectively by NMDA, α-amino-3-hydroxy-5-methylisoxazole-4-propionic acid (AMPA), or kainate.[86] Metabotropic glutamate receptors are linked by stimulatory G proteins to a cascade-generating inositol triphosphate that, in turn, releases intracellular calcium.[23, 87] Prolonged exposure to high concentrations of excitatory amino acids causes neuronal death known as excitotoxicity.[88–90] This process might underlie a number of neurologic disorders[91] and could account for neuronal death in the epileptic focus due to prolonged or repeated seizures.[92, 93]

A rich pharmacology of the family of glutamate receptors is evolving.[20, 21, 94] Selective antagonists of ionotropic and metabotropic receptors are available, but their clinical value remains to be clarified. Much attention has been focused on the NMDA/glutamate receptors/channel complexes and antagonists have been developed for multiple modulatory sites. These include competitive antagonists at the NMDA binding site, such as AP-7 and CPP; 7-chlorokynurenic acid at the permissive strychnine-insensitive glycine modulatory site; and uncompetitive blockers of NMDA-activated ion channels, of which the prototypes include MK-801 and phencyclidine.[95] Similar to benzodiazepines, NMDA antagonists increase the number of stimulations necessary to produce fully kindled seizures in animals.[96] In the future, it may be possible to interfere with the progressive changes that lead to chronic epilepsy after a first seizure or to interfere with epileptogenesis after head trauma or stroke. To date, however, members of two of these classes of antagonists, MK-801[97] and CPP-ene,[98] failed in clinical trials. A series of AMPA antagonists, including 1,2,3,4-tetrahydro-6-nitro-2,3-dioxo-benzo[f]quinoxaline-7-sulfonamide (NBQX) has been shown to protect against seizures and stroke in animals,[99] but there are no published reports of clinical trials in man. Delayed neuronal injury or death due to intracellular processes triggered by NMDA- and AMPA-mediated calcium influx may limit the usefulness of glutamate antagonists as postevent treatment agents.[90] Clinically useful antagonists of facilitatory endogenous polyamines, such as putrescine and spermidine,[100–102] and agents active at the redox modulatory site[103] have not been identified.

Of standard AEMs, phenytoin with intracellular recording techniques[104, 105] and carbamazepine with whole-cell patch clamp techniques[106] have been shown to block NMDA responses and currents, respectively. Of the new AEMs, felbamate may block NMDA channel activation by binding to the glycine permissive site[107, 108] and blocking the channel.[78] Topiramate reduces kainate-activated, but not NMDA-activated, currents in isolated neurons (D Coulter, personal communication, December 1994). This differential effect may have important implications.

The psychotogenic effect of phencyclidine, an uncompetitive antagonist of NMDA-activated channels, in humans[109, 110] suggests that other NMDA/glutamate antagonists may produce adverse behavioral effects in humans or adversely affect learning and memory,[111] processes in which NMDA/glutamate receptors have been implicated. Both MK-801, a channel blocker, and CPP-ene, a competitive NMDA antagonist, were associated with adverse behavioral effects in clinical trials according to anecdotal reports. In addition, mitochondrial vacuolization has been demonstrated in neurons of animals after acute administration of NMDA channel blockers.[112] The significance of these behavioral and structural findings is unclear. Phenytoin and carbamazepine do not cause such effects, although long-term use of phenytoin at high doses has been implicated in cerebellar dysfunction. By the same token, there has been no systematic documentation of adverse behaviors in patients taking felbamate for years during the testing. It may be a matter of degree or potency. Thus, AEMs with multiple actions including glutamate antagonism should be used cautiously and when needed but not necessarily avoided in the elderly, in whom behavior and memory may be altered already by other medications or the aging process itself.

Relevance of Cellular Effects of Antiepileptic Medications

A wide variety of cellular[113] and animal[114–116] models can be exploited as pharmacologic models in the development of novel AEMs. Although the predictive power of these models is not entirely clear, some correlations are fairly strong. There is a reasonably strong correlation among efficacy against MES-induced seizures, ability to limit high-frequency action potential firing, and clinical efficacy against partial and secondarily generalized tonic-clonic seizures. Efficacy against kindling and kindled seizures is generally thought to provide additional support for efficacy against these clinical seizure types,[96] but this test is not yet universally used in screening for novel compounds. There is also fair correlation among preventing clonic seizures induced by PTZ, blocking T-calcium current, and clinical efficacy against generalized absence. Efficacy against seizures in genetic models of absence lends further support. There are, however, no specific animal models or mechanistic predictors of efficacy against atonic seizures. Chemically induced (e.g., with PTZ) jerks and photomyoclonic responses of the ape *Papio papio* are blocked by GABAmimetics in general, although other mechanisms may also suppress these seizures. These animal seizures serve as pharmacologic models of myoclonic epilepsy and suggest a broader spectrum of efficacy against primary generalized seizures. Nonetheless, it should be apparent that cellular and animal models constitute a limited pharmacologic predictor of clinical efficacy of AEMs and probably do not account for the full clinical spectrum of any of the agents in current use. The same actions responsible for therapeutic efficacy may contribute to common central nervous system–related adverse effects, but chronic toxicity and interactions are frequently not anticipated on the basis of preclinical testing. These insights should temper what can reasonably be expected from AEMs, both standard and new.

THE FIRST WAVE OF NEW ANTIEPILEPTIC MEDICATIONS

Felbamate

Felbamate (2-phenyl-1,3-propanediol dicarbamate; Felbatol, Wallace Laboratories) is the first new AEM to be approved by the FDA since valproate in 1978. It is a white crystalline powder that has a molecular weight of 238 (conversion factor: 1 µg/ml = 4.2 µM). In preclinical testing, felbamate was effective against both MES-induced seizures and pentylenetetrazol (PTZ)-induced seizures, more so against MES.[117] The order of potency is opposite that of valproate[118] but suggests a broad spectrum of anticonvulsant activity. It also protected against NMDA- and quisqualate-induced seizures. The protective index of felbamate was greater than that of standard AEMs.[117, 119] Felbamate enhanced GABA-activated chloride conductance and blocked NMDA-activated currents at a channel site (0.1–3.0 µM).[87] Both effects occurred at fairly high concentrations with EC_{50} for GABA of approximately 1 µM, or 238 µg/ml, and the IC_{50} for NMDA of approximately 2 µM, or 475 µg/ml. Felbamate also bound competitively at the strychnine-insensitive glycine site (IC_{50} 374 µM, or approximately 90 µg/ml)[107, 108] and limited sustained high-frequency repetitive firing of cultured neurons (IC_{50} 280 µM, or 67 µg/ml).[55] Felbamate doses of 2,400–3,000 mg/day resulted in effective steady state plasma levels of up to 52 µg/ml.[120, 121] Doses of up to 5,400 mg have been tolerated in studies. Felbamate has also been reported to protect hippocampal slices in vitro from hypoxic injury,[122] as have other AEMs (e.g., phenytoin or carbamazepine).[123–125]

This combination of cellular actions should confer a broad spectrum of clinical use on felbamate. Evidence for this includes already published studies that show efficacy against partial and secondarily generalized seizures[120, 121, 126–128] and atonic seizures of the Lennox-Gastaut syndrome.[129] Also, on the strength of novel study designs,[126, 127, 130] felbamate was approved by the FDA for both monotherapy and adjunctive use. The recognition of aplastic anemia and liver failure in the first year of general use raised saftey issues that limit the use of felbamate to selected cases (see Chap. 20).

The pharmacokinetic properties of felbamate have been reviewed,[117, 131–136] and some of these are summarized below and in Table 19.2. Felbamate is rapidly absorbed after oral administration. Absolute oral bioavailability is approximately 90%; this is not affected by food or antacids.[137, 138] The absorption has been described as linear at doses up to 3,600 mg/day. Doses as high as 4,800–5,400 mg/day have been administered in studies (Wallace Laboratories, data on file). Half maximal absorption (T_{max}) ranges from 2 to 4 hours. Approximately 22–35% of absorbed felbamate is bound to plasma proteins, too little for significant interaction by competition for binding sites. The rest is transported in plasma as unbound drug and in equilibrium with red blood cells (R. Schumaker, personal communication, December 1994). Felbamate is sufficiently lipid-soluble to enter the brain readily. It is metabolized in part in the liver to inactive monocarbamate, parahydroxy, and 2-hydroxy metabolites. The metabolites are inactive in the MES test and very weakly active in the PTZ test (Wallace Laboratories, data on file). There is no evidence of autoinduction of liver enzymes.

Interactions of felbamate with other AEMs were first identified in animals.[139] In humans, felbamate behaves in general as an inhibitor of the metabolism of other antiepileptic drugs. Plasma levels of phenytoin[140] and valproate[141, 142] rise approximately 30% with the addition of felbamate. Carbamazepine levels decrease approximately 21%, but the epoxide may increase as much as 50%.[140, 143–146] Reciprocally, phenytoin, phenobarbital, and carbamazepine, which induce liver enzymes, lower the plasma level of felbamate. Valproate, an inhibitor of metabolism, raises the blood level of felbamate.[141, 147] Approximately 80–85% of an oral dose of felbamate appears in the urine, 40–50% unchanged. An additional 40% consists of unidentified metabolites and conjugates, and approximately 15% appears as parahydroxy felbamate, 2-hydroxy felbamate, and felbamate monocarbamate (Wallace Laboratories, data on file).[148] The relative proportion of felbamate excreted unchanged in the urine is greater than that of the older antiepileptic medications. The complexity of the interactions makes felbamate no more easy to use in polypharmacy than the older medications, however. The interactions limit the rate of introduction of felbamate in the setting of polypharmacy. Abrupt reduction of concomitant antiepileptic medications in the first week, as recommended in the package insert, introduces a risk of increased seizure frequency and status epilepticus. Slower dose escalation and more cautious reduction of concomitant antiepileptic medications could result in more successful introduction of felbamate, particularly in the elderly.

Gabapentin

The second of the new compounds to be approved by the FDA is gabapentin (1-[aminomethyl]cyclohexaneacetic acid; Neurontin, Parke-Davis) in 1993. Its properties have been extensively reviewed[149-152]: Gabapentin is a bitter-tasting, white crystalline material with a molecular weight of 171.34 (conversation factor: 1 µg/ml = 5.84 µM). It has a novel structure that consists of GABA integrated into a cyclohexane ring. It is basically an amino acid and is a zwitterion at physiologic pH. There are no enantiomers. Gabapentin was tested in a wide variety of animal models in preclinical testing.[150, 153] Gabapentin is about as effective as phenytoin against MES-induced seizures. Unlike phenytoin and carbamazepine, gabapentin was effective against PTZ-induced seizures, but not against seizures in a genetic mouse model of generalized absence. Gabapentin was relatively ineffective clinically against absence seizures.[154] Efficacy against compounds that produce seizures in animals by inhibiting GABA synthesis or antagonizing GABA-mediated inhibition suggests that gabapentin is different from standard medications.[150, 153] Gabapentin prolonged the latency to onset of tonic-clonic convulsions and death in the NMDA model, but not in animals injected with kainic acid or quisqualate.[149]

Cellular mechanisms of action of gabapentin are incompletely understood. Gabapentin limits firing frequency and sustained repetitive firing with reduction of action potential rate of rise in time-dependent manner (50% of neurons with limited firing between 1 and 5 hours).[58] Unlike phenytoin or carbamazepine, however, gabapentin did not block sodium currents in Chinese hamster ovary cells with cloned alpha subunits of brain sodium channels under whole-cell patch clamp conditions.[59] This finding and the delay to peak effect (5–12 hours) suggest slow access to or indirect effects on voltage-dependent sodium channels. The delay in the effect on high-frequency action potential firing parallels the delay of peak anticonvulsant effect in animals after intravenous injection of gabapentin.[155] Peak protection occurred at a time when brain interstitial concentrations and plasma concentrations of gabapentin were reduced substantially. Thus, it appears that the anticonvulsant protection depends on accumulation of gabapentin in neurons. As with phenytoin and carbamazepine, limitation of repetitive firing parallels efficacy of gabapentin against MES-induced seizures and partial seizures with or without secondary generalization. Gabapentin may reverse the transport of GABA so that interstitial levels increase, resulting in increased inhibition.[80] Gabapentin may interfere also with the transport of other amino acids, especially excitatory amino acids, and may alter metabolism of amino acids in neurons or glia.[153]

Gabapentin is absorbed from the gastrointestinal tract by the saturable L-amino acid transporter.[156] The same transport system is probably responsible for the transport of gabapentin across the blood-brain barrier and into neurons. A unique binding site for gabapentin appears to be concentrated in regions where glutamatergic terminals abound, principally the hippocampus, cerebral cortex, and cerebellum.[157] The relationship of the binding site to anticonvulsant efficacy is not clear, however. The binding site may be the L-amino acid transporter.[158]

Overall, the indications from preclinical and mechanistic investigations would suggest, as borne out in clinical trials,[159-162] that gabapentin is principally an agent for the treatment of partial seizures with or without secondary generalization. The FDA has approved gabapentin for adjunctive use in individuals older than 12 years of age to treat refractory complex partial seizures with or without secondary tonic-clonic generalization. Preliminary findings suggest that gabapentin is effective in monotherapy.[163, 164] Monotherapy trials and trials in children are in progress.

Pharmacokinetic properties of gabapentin have been reviewed in detail.[136, 150-153, 165-167] Bioavailability is dose-related, probably due to the saturable transport mechanism. The average bioavailability is approximately 60%. At an oral dose of 900 mg, 75% is bioavailable by the oral route, whereas at doses of 1,800 and 4,800 mg, bioavailability falls to 30–35%[167, 168] (also H Bockbrader and A Sedman, personal communication, December 1994). Gabapentin is readily absorbed, with a T_{max} of 2–3 hours.[168, 169] The compound is highly water-soluble and is transported in plasma unbound to plasma proteins.[169] The volume of distribution ranges from approximately 0.65 liter/kg to 1.04 liter/kg, (H Bockbrader and A Sedman, personal communication, December 1994) indicating distribution to tissues that is greater than that to plasma. Gabapentin is not metabolized and has no effect on hepatic enzymes. As a result, there have been no reports of interaction with other antiepileptic drugs[160, 162, 170-174] or oral contraceptives.[175] The only interactions reported so far have been minor reductions of bioavailability by concomitant administration of the antacid, Maalox TC[176] and a 12% decrease in renal clearance due to cimetidine.[167] Gabapentin is excreted quantitatively in the urine, and the package insert contains recommendations for administration to individuals with compromised renal function. The gabapentin dose can be modified in proportion to the creatinine clearance.[177] Oral and renal clearances of gabapentin decrease with age in parallel with declining creatinine clearance.[178] This suggests that lower doses may be effective in treating the elderly.

The pharmacokinetic profile makes gabapentin particularly attractive for use in elderly individuals taking medications for systemic illnesses in addition to epilepsy. Potential disadvantages arise from the dose-dependent bioavailability and short elimination half-life of 5–7 hours.[168, 169] This is an important consideration because elderly patients are more likely to forget their medications. It should be pointed out, however, that patients taking multiple medications are accustomed to multidose regimens. In practice, bioavailability of gabapentin has not been limiting, but safety may be increased. A 16-year-old girl deliberately took 48.9 g (860 mg/kg) of gabapentin at one time.[179] Symptoms, including lethargy, dizziness, and diarrhea, resolved within 18 hours. Thus, the saturable transport system is a protection against accidental or intentional overdose. The maximally tolerated dose and therapeutic range of plasma concentrations have not been determined. In the case of this young woman just mentioned, a plasma level of 62 µg/ml was detected 8.5 hours after ingestion.[179] Plasma levels above 2 µg/ml been have reported to have therapeutic efficacy,[160, 161] and a steady-state peak level of approximately 12 µg/ml was obtained with a daily dose of 1,600 mg tid (H Bockbrader and A Sedman, personal communication, December 1994; Parke-Davis, data on file). As mentioned, gabapentin accumulates in neurons, and the anticonvulsant effect outlasts the peak plasma and interstitial brain concentrations, suggesting that two daily doses may be sufficient for some patients.

Lamotrigine

Lamotrigine (3,5-diamino-6-[2,3-dichlorophenyl]-1,2,4-triazine; Lamictal, Glaxo-Wellcome Co.) is the third new compound to be approved by the FDA (1995). It is a white powder with a molecular weight of 256.09 (conversion factor: 1 µg/ml = 3.90 µM).[180] It is as effective as phenytoin and carbamazepine in the MES test and blocks voltage-dependent sodium current and action potentials. [59, 60, 61] Lamotrigine was shown to block veratradine-induced, but not potassium-induced, release of the excitatory amino acids, glutamate, and aspartate. Release of the inhibitory amino acid GABA was blocked to a lesser extent.[181, 182] This finding is consistent with the blockade of voltage-dependent sodium currents by lamotrigine, since veratradine is a plant alkaloid that activates sodium current.[31] There was dose-dependent reduction of kindled seizures by lamotrigine, although kindling development was not blocked.[180] In the PTZ test, lamotrigine and phenytoin failed to decrease clonus and even shortened the latency to clonus, suggesting proconvulsant activity in this test.[183] Lamotrigine, but not phenytoin or carbamazepine, reduced visually evoked afterdischarges in animals,[184] however, suggesting a wider spectrum of activity. Clinically, lamotrigine has been reported to be effective against complex partial seizures with or without secondary generalization, both as mono- and adjunctive therapy.[185–188] Also, there are anecdotal reports of efficacy against atypical absence with atonic seizures, primary generalized tonic-clonic seizures and status epilepticus.[189–191] Further mechanistic studies will be necessary to account for the broader spectrum of activity anticipated from preclinical studies and clinical experience in the United Kingdom.

Pharmacokinetic features of lamotrigine have been reviewed.[182, 191–196] It is readily absorbed after oral administration. Absolute bioavailability is approximately 95%,[197] and there is no significant food effect.[191] Absorption is linear, with T_{max} of 4–12 hours and a volume of distribution of about 1.1 liter/kg, suggesting wide distribution and concentration in tissues.[198–202] It is approximately 55% bound to plasma proteins, about the same extent as phenobarbital.[203] It is glucuronidated in the liver, but no active metabolites have been identified.[203] It does not appear to induce or inhibit hepatic mixed function oxidase significantly.[204] Moderate autoinduction (37% reduction of lamotrigine levels demonstrated after multiple doses) of unclear clinical significance occurs.[201, 202] Lamotrigine is excreted in the urine principally as the glucuronide (63%), and less than 10% of the compound is excreted unchanged.[203] The elimination half-life is approximately 24 hours.[201] The relatively long half-life allows once or twice daily dosing. Studies of interactions with medications other than antiepileptic drugs have not been reported. Lamotrigine does not consistently reduce or increase levels of other AEMs.[195, 200, 201] Mixed effects on carbamazepine epoxide have been reported.[205-208] Inducers of liver enzymes, such as phenobarbital, phenytoin, or carbamazepine, decrease lamotrigine $t_{1/2}$,[185, 200, 201] however. These interactions can be compensated for by increasing the oral dose of lamotrigine. Valproate more than doubles the $t_{1/2}$ of lamotrigine,[195, 209, 210] perhaps due to competition for glucuronidation.[196] Interactions with another generally inhibitory compound, felbamate, have not been described. The $t_{1/2}$ is also prolonged in patients with Gilbert's syndrome.[211] In a study comparing healthy elderly (65–76 year of age) and younger (27–36 years of age) volunteers, peak plasma levels were 27% higher and clearance was 37% longer ($t_{1/2}$ 31 hours versus 25 hours) in the elderly.[212] Slow-dose escalation has been the rule in clinical studies to avoid serious rashes.

Relative freedom from drug-drug interactions and dosing once or twice daily are the most attractive pharmacokinetic properties of lamotrigine. In some patients, addition of lamotrigine resulted in improvement to the extent that other AEMs could be discontinued. Preliminary reports suggest efficacy and safety in continued monotherapy.[191, 213] This would eliminate some interactions. The only major concern with lamotrigine appears to be rashes. This problem is probably no more difficult to contend with than what is encountered with phenytoin or carbamazepine. It will be useful in treating mixed seizure disorders and in combination therapy of refractory epilepsy in the elderly.

THE SECOND WAVE OF NEW ANTIEPILEPTIC MEDICATIONS

There are several promising compounds in phase three trials in the United States. In this group are vigabatrin, tiagabine, topiramate, and oxcarbazepine. Vigabatrin and oxcarbazepine are currently marketed in Europe. By the time the optimal use of the first wave of drugs is established, the second-wave drugs are likely to be available or nearing final approval by the FDA.

Vigabatrin

Vigabatrin (dl-4-aminohex-5-enoic acid, or gamma-vinyl GABA; Sabril, Hoechst-Marion-Roussel) is freely water-soluble and has a molecular weight of 129.16 (conversion factor: 1 µg/ml = 7.74 µM). Only the (S)-enantiomer of vigabatrin is active against seizures in animal models.[214] It is a substrate for GABA-transaminase that results in irreversible inactivation of the enzyme.[215] No other mechanisms of action have been identified for vigabatrin. Use of other inhibitors of GABA-T, such as amino-oxyacetic acid and L-cycloserine, is limited by reversibility of the block and biochemical actions. As expected, vigabatrin causes dose-related increase in cerebrospinal fluid concentrations of unbound and total GABA in patients.[216-218] Reactivation of GABA transaminase to 50% of the original activity requires approximately 2–3 days,[219] suggesting the potential for intermittent dosing in some patients.

In animal models, vigabatrin protects against a wide variety of seizures, including those induced by MES and bicuculline; PTZ; strychnine (tonic seizures); isoniazid (generalized seizures); reflex seizures, including audiogenic and photic seizures; and amygdala-kindled seizures.[214] This spectrum of activity in animal models would predict a very broad spectrum of clinical anticonvulsant efficacy. Approximately 50% of patients with partial seizures responded to adjunctive treatment with vigabatrin—that is, they experienced a more than 50% reduction of these seizure types.[8, 214, 220-224] Encouraging results have been obtained in uncontrolled trials against childhood seizures, in particular symptomatic infantile spasms.[225-229] There are anecdotal reports that primary generalized seizures are worsened in some patients by vigabatrin.[230-232] Overall, vigabatrin may be used primarily to treat partial seizures with and without secondary generalization, the most common seizure type affecting the elderly.

Recognition of microvacuolization or intramyelinic edema in the corona radiata of the rat and dog brain after long-term treatment[233] resulted in temporary suspension of trials. Lack of significant effects on neurophysiologic parameters and the absence of abnormal histopathologic findings in surgical and autopsy specimens, however, suggested this was a species specific effect.[233-239] As a result, trials recommenced.[240]

Pharmacokinetics of vigabatrin have been reviewed[83, 214, 241-243]: It is absorbed linearly to a maximum within 2 hours, and there is no significant effect of food on absorption.[244, 245] Absolute bioavailability is at least 75%, and the volume of distribution is approximately 0.8 liter/kg.[246] Vigabatrin is highly water-soluble, not bound to serum plasma protein, and has negligible effects on hepatic metabolism.[245, 247] It is not metabolized. It is eliminated in urine unchanged, with an elimination half-life of 5–8 hours.[244-246] The short half-life has less consequence because blockade of the transaminase is irreversible and resynthesis is slow.[219] In the elderly, absorption is delayed, peak levels are increased significantly, and $t_{1/2}$ is prolonged.[248] Elevation of brain GABA is greater when the dosing interval is decreased, and this corresponds with improved seizure control.[215] Therefore, vigabatrin is given in two to four divided doses, depending on the requirements for seizure control. Other antiepileptic drugs have not been shown to alter vigabatrin concentrations, but vigabatrin lowers phenytoin concentrations approximately 20–30% and barbiturate levels to a lesser extent by unexplained mechanisms.[247, 249, 250] Valproate and carbamazepine levels were unaffected in these studies.

Adverse behavioral effects, including psychosis, have been reported during seizure control and on abrupt withdrawal of vigabatrin.[251] Given the altered pharmacokinetics in the elderly, vigabatrin will need to be used with caution, especially with other GABA-enhancing drugs, such as benzodiazepines prescribed for anxiolitic purposes. Such combinations increase the prospect of pharmacodynamic interactions that lead to adverse behavioral effects.

Oxcarbazepine

Oxcarbazepine (10,11-dihydro-10-oxo-carbamazepine; Trileptal, Ciba) is a new medication for treatment of complex partial seizures with or without secondary generalization.[252–254] It differs from carbamazepine in that oxcarbazepine has a ketogroup instead of a double bond at the 10,11 position. It is a lipophilic, white, crystalline substance with molecular weight of 252 (conversion factor: 1 µg/ml = 3.96 µM) and very low aqueous solubility.[255, 256] Oxcarbazepine is rapidly converted in humans to a monohydroxy derivative, which is the principal antiepileptic compound.[257, 258] Oxcarbazepine (ED_{50} 10–20 mg/kg) and the monohydroxy derivative (ED_{50} 50 mg/kg) are about as potent as carbamazepine in inhibiting hind-limb extension in the MES test in rodents; both are ineffective against clonic seizures produced by PTZ.[57, 259] Against chemically induced convulsions, such as picrotoxin and strychnine, both oxcarbazepine and the monohydroxy derivative have ED_{50} values in the range of 150–250 mg/kg PO.[259] Both the parent and the metabolite limit high-frequency action potential firing with use-dependent decrease in rate of rise, suggesting a sodium channel mechanism of action, but suppression of bursting also suggests effects on potassium currents.[57]

Oxcarbazepine is almost entirely absorbed (96%) after oral administration.[255, 256, 260] In the plasma, oxcarbazepine is reduced by ketone reductase to the monohydroxy derivative, which in turn is conjugated by the microsomal enzyme glucoronyl transferase and excreted in the urine.[256] Approximately 50% of the hydroxy compound is bound to plasma proteins and has a volume of distribution of approximately 0.3–0.8 liter/kg.[261] After achievement of steady state, there have been no indications of autoinduction, induction of hepatic mixed function oxidase activity, or accumulation of oxcarbazepine or its monohydroxy derivative.[261] There is no epoxide metabolite. In addition, the elimination half-life of antipyrine increased when patients were crossed over from monotherapy with carbamazepine to oxcarbazepine, suggesting less enzyme induction during treatment with oxcarbazepine. Approximately 96% of oxcarbazepine is excreted in the urine; approximately 70% of the total is free or conjugated monohydroxy derivative. Elimination $t_{1/2}$ of oxcarbazepine is approximately 1.0–2.5 hours; elimination of the monohydroxy derivative is approximately 8 hours.[262] Less than 1% of oxcarbazepine appears unchanged in the urine, and approximately 9% appears as direct conjugates. Other inactive metabolites account for the residual fraction. The elimination half-life ranges from 8 hours to 12 hours. In crossover trials comparing carbamazepine and oxcarbazepine, steady-state plasma levels of valproate (21–27%) and phenytoin (25%) increased due to the lesser enzyme induction by oxcarbazepine.[262] This suggests that oxcarbazepine will have fewer drug-drug interactions than carbamazepine. Oxcarbazepine and its monohydroxide were unaffected by propoxyphene, cimetidine, or erythromycin, which inhibit the biotransformation of carbamazepine.[256] In addition, in the Scandinavian trials of oxcarbazepine, there were fewer serious rashes in those taking oxcarbazepine than in patients taking carbamazepine, perhaps due to the absence of an epoxide intermediate.[253, 254, 257, 258, 263] Hyponatremia has been demonstrated during treatment with oxcarbazepine, as is the case with carbamazepine.[264] This could be a disadvantage in elderly patients, who are already prone to electrolyte abnormalities because of concomitant use of diuretics, for example. Clearance is reduced in the elderly, suggesting that lower doses may be effective in this age group.[265] The principal advantages of oxcarbazepine for the elderly are the reduced potential for drug-drug interactions and lower incidence of rash, with efficacy comparable to that of carbamazepine.

Tiagabine

Tiagabine ([R-]-N-[4,4,-di-(3-methylthien-2-yl)but-3-enyl] nipecotic acid hydrochloride; Abbott Laboratories and Novo Nordisk A/S) is a white crystalline material with a molecular weight of 412 (conversion factor: 1 μg/ml = 2.43 μM). Nipecotic acid is a blocker of GABA reuptake at central synapses. Its anticonvulsant efficacy is compromised by the fact that it does not cross the blood-brain barrier freely. In tiagabine, nipecotic acid is linked to a lipophilic anchor that affords rapid absorption and entry into the brain.[266] Inhibition of GABA uptake into synaptosomes occurs with an IC_{50} of 75 nM. In humans, brain microdialysis studies reveal significant increases in interstitial GABA levels of patients after oral doses of tiagabine.[267] Effects on binding to other neurotransmitter receptors occur at 20- to 400-fold higher concentrations than are required to reduce synaptosomal GABA uptake.[266] Tiagabine is effective against kindled seizures and myoclonic seizures in the photosensitive baboon. It protects weakly against MES- and bicuculline-induced convulsions. Animals given doses of tiagabine of more than 30 mg/kg develop abnormal tone and tremor.[266] Tiagabine is in widespread phase III investigation, and preliminary reports indicate efficacy in the treatment of partial seizures with or without secondary generalization.[268, 269]

Tiagabine is highly lipid-soluble and is absorbed linearly, with a T_{max} of 0.5–3.0 hours.[266, 270] In comparison with volunteers of a fasted control group, nonfasted volunteers had delayed peak levels of tiagabine, but bioavailabilty was not significantly reduced.[271] It is extensively bound to plasma proteins. Tiagabine induces liver enzymes[272] and is oxidized and conjugated in the liver.[273] Active metabolites have not been identified. Approximately 2% of an oral dose of tiagabine is eliminated unchanged in urine along with the oxoderivative with an elimination $t_{1/2}$ of 4.5–13.4 (mean 6.7) hours; more than half of the dose appears in feces as unidentified metabolites and unabsorbed drug.[266, 273] Tiagabine area under the curve increased in patients taking valproate and decreased in patients taking AEMs that induce hepatic enzymes,[272] typical of expected interactions with the other AEMs.

Specific uses for tiagabine in the elderly population must await further characterization of the compound clinically. Little has been described in the way of drug-drug interactions. Again, there is potential for pharmacodynamic interaction with other GABA-enhancing compounds and adverse behavioral effects. Lack of interactions and simple pharmacokinetics are attractive properties of tiagabine for use in the elderly.

Topiramate

Topiramate (2,3:4,5-BIS O-[1-methylethylidene]-β-D-fructopyranose sulfamate; Topamax, McNeill Pharmaceuticals) is a highly water-soluble crystalline derivative of D-fructose, with a molecular weight of 339 (conversion factor: 1 μg/ml = 2.95 μM). The O-sulfamate moiety resembles that of acetazolamide structurally.[274–276] It and several analogs protect against MES seizures in mice[274, 276, 277] and against postischemic injury and seizures.[278] Topiramate blocks kainate-acitivated currents, but not NMDA-activated currents (D Coulter, personal communication, December 1994), limits repetitive firing of sodium-dependent action potentials,[56] and augments GABA-activated chloride conductance.[79] This spectrum of cellular actions suggests a potentially wide range of clinical efficacy. Little clinical information has been published to date, but preliminary reports indicate efficacy against refractory partial seizures.[279–282]

Topiramate has simple linear pharmacokinetics.[283, 284] Bioavailability is virtually complete after oral administration.[285] It is absorbed maximally within 1.5–4.5 hours, and the volume of distribution is 0.6–0.8 liter/kg.[284] Topiramate is less than 20% bound to plasma proteins. It does not affect liver enzymes. Metabolites have not been characterized in detail, but hydroxylation is one mechanism of biotransformation (D Doose, personal communication, December 1994). Topiramate is eliminated predominantly in the urine, with an elimination half-life of approximately 19–23 hours.[283, 286]

Topiramate has not been shown to interact with carbamazepine, phenytoin, or valproate.[284, 287] Slowed cognition has been reported in a few patients taking topiramate with other AEMs, however.[282] This effect may depend on dose, dose escalation rate, seizure frequency, or concomitant AEMs. Much remains to learned about this interesting compound. Early experience suggests that slow rates of initiation and dose escalation may be important ultimately to avoid adverse events in the elderly.[288]

New Formulations

Fosphenytoin,[289] a novel water-soluble prodrug of phenytoin, and a sodium salt of valproate (Abbott Laboratories, data on file) are under development. Availability of these water-soluble compounds will allow parenteral substitution in patients unable to take medicine by mouth, either due to debility or preparation for surgery. Fosphenytoin is anticipated to replace the existing parenteral formulation of phenytoin used to treat status epilepticus. The vehicle in which phenytoin is currently dissolved for intravenous use (40% propylene glycol, 10% ethanol at pH 12) is potentially arrhythmogenic. Availability of fosphenytoin should increase the safety of using phenytoin intravenously, but cardiovascular effects of phenytoin cannot be overlooked and may limit the rate of administration. Examples of settings in which increased safety of phenytoin preparations would be most welcome in treating elderly patients in status epilepticus include polypharmacy with antiarrhythmics or vasodilators and acute myocardial infarction, in which cardiovascular function is altered.

THE THIRD WAVE OF NEW ANTIEPILEPTIC MEDICATIONS

Several compounds are in use outside the United States, such as zonisamide and clobazam, or are in earlier stages of clinical testing (e.g., remacemide) than the AEMs mentioned above. Zonisamide, a benzisoxazole with carbonic anhydrase-blocking activity, was initially tested in the United States, but the appearance of multiple cases of renal calculi led to cessation of testing here. It is currently marketed in Japan, where further evaluation continues. It blocks sodium channels.[290] Variable clinical efficacy against refractory partial[291–295] and myoclonic[295] seizures in children and adults has been reported.

Clobazam is a benzodiazepine with an active N-desmethyl metabolite.[296] Controlled and open studies have shown efficacy against partial and generalized seizures, mixed seizures types of the Lennox-Gastaut syndrome, and catamenial epilepsy.[297] Its use may be limited by the usual benzodiazepine-related problems, including sedation and seizures on abrupt discontinuation. In addition, tolerance has been reported to develop to both sedative and anticonvulsant effects in some patients.[298] Clobazam is marketed in many countries, including Canada. These and other compounds already marketed abroad might be introduced in the United States if further study indicates a favorable side effect profile or greater efficacy than currently available information would suggest.

Remacemide is a diphenyl-ethyl-acetamide derivative with a clinical spectrum very similar to that of phenytoin and carbamazepine.[299] It has an active desglycinated metabolite that is more potent and has a lower therapeutic index than the parent compound. It is currently in phase II trials. Both the parent and the desglycinate block NMDA-activated current under patch clamp conditions.[300] Calcium channel blockers, such as nimodipine and flunarizine, have been studied for antiepileptic properties in humans and animals. Adjunctive use of flunarizine, in particular, has been reported to reduce refractory seizures significantly in approximately one-third of patients, although results of controlled studies and monotherapy studies are not available.[301] Flunarizine has a very long half-life (10–50 days) due to its lipophilicity and resultant concentration in tissues. It also has interactions with other AEMs. The factors complicate any dose adjustments required to avoid side effects for the elderly.[136] Flunarizine is widely used abroad, however, primarily to treat migraine headache, and long-term safety has been good.[301]

These few AEMs represent a host of compounds under development. It is beyond the scope of this chapter to name them all. The interested reader is referred to several recent reviews and texts.[302–307] These promising agents in various stages of development encourage the belief that there will be continuing progress in the pharmacologic treatment of epilepsy. Introduction of the newer agents, however, is likely to depend on the fate of the first and second waves of new AEMs and on the changing disposal of resources under the political and economic pressures of health care reform. Perhaps the future will depend more on studies of mechanisms of epileptogenesis and AEM actions to bring us unique medications for the treatment of patients with still inadequately treatable syndromes and seizure types.

SUMMARY

Development of the new AEMs was motivated primarily by the large number of patients with refractory partial seizures. Although most of the new AEMs were discovered with standard animal screening methods, the development process has yielded several new compounds with unique chemical structures and a mixture of new and old mechanisms of action (Table 19.3). Felbamate, for example, has three cellular actions at therapeutically relevant concentrations that may contribute to a broad spectrum of clinical efficacy to some extent. Felbamate and vigabatrin augment GABA-mediated inhibition by different mechanisms. One can only speculate why vigabatrin has been associated with behavioral adverse effects, whereas felbamate has not. As discussed above with respect to sodium channels, it may be a matter of degree. At therapeutically relevant concentrations, felbamate augments GABA-activated current 20–40%.[78] This degree of enhancement may be beneficial, whereas greater enhancement may result in adverse effects (i.e., "too much of a good thing is bad"). Alternatively, vigabatrin may have additional, as yet unidentified, actions, or preexisting psychopathology may contribute to altered behavior. The single well documented effect on sodium current is not sufficient to explain the broad clinical spectrum of efficacy of lamotrigine. The relevant mechanisms of action of gabapentin have not been conclusively demonstrated, yet it is a useful AEM clinically, especially because of its pharmacokinetics. In all likelihood, additional actions will be discovered for each of the new AEMs. Sheer numbers of actions may not be most important. Current knowledge of these multiple mechanisms does not explain the clinical spectrum of the activity of old or new AEMs completely. Perhaps it is not possible to extrapolate from the available in vitro data, and they represent only pharmacologic models that corroborate or compete with animal models. None of the mechanisms mentioned here has been demonstrated in vivo during a seizure to be involved in the action of an AEM. Ultimately, however, mechanistic investigations should improve understanding of how the new medications differ from the standard ones and how to use these newer agents to maximal effect. Also, in view of the multiplicity of mechanisms of action of most AEMs, polypharmacy cannot truly be rational without a fuller understanding of polypharmacology.

Table 19.3 Candidate mechanisms of action of antiepileptic medications (see text)

	$SRF/V_{max}/I_{Na}$ Blockade	T-Calcium Current Blockade	GABA Enhance-ment	Glutamate Blockade
Old antiepileptic medications				
Carbamazepine	Yes/Yes/Yes	?	No	NMDA current, channel-binding site (?)
Diazepam	Yes/Yes/? At high concentrations only	?	Allosteric increase of chloride current	?
Ethosuximide	No/No/No	Yes	No	?
Phenobarbital	Yes/Yes/? At high concentrations only	?	Allosteric increase of chloride current	Non-NMDA receptors
Phenytoin	Yes/Yes/Yes	Slight	High concentration	NMDA response, channel-binding site (?)
Valproate	Yes/Yes/Yes	Slight at high concentration	Increased GABA turnover (mechanism not proven)	?
New antiepileptic medications				
Felbamate	Yes/?/?	?	Allosteric increase of chloride current	NMDA current channel + glycine site
Gabapentin	Yes/Yes/No	?	Reverse transport	No
Lamotrigine	Yes/?/Yes	?	?	?
Oxcarbazepine	Yes/Yes/?	?	?	?
Tiagabine	?/?/?	?	Increased [GABA]	?
Topiramate	Yes/?/?	?	Allosteric increase of chloride current	Kainate current
Vigabatrin	?/?/?	?	Increased [GABA]	?

GABA = gamma-amino butyric acid; NMDA = N-methyl-D-aspartate; SRF = sustained high-frequency repetitive firing; I_{NA} = sodium current; ? = unknown.
Note: High concentration = above free therapeutic range; such concentrations achieved during treatment of *status epilepticus* with diazepam, phenobarbital and phenytoin.

How well will these new AEMs serve the elderly, who have special needs imposed by altered physiology, diseases of advancing years, and multiple medications? In search of an answer, it may be a useful exercise for the reader to test some of the new and older AEMs against an "ideal" standard. The short list of

Table 19.4 Comparison of properties of the first wave of new antiepileptic medications with an "ideal drug"

"Ideal drug"	Felbamate	Gabapentin	Lamotrigine
Highly effective	Effective	Effective	Effective
Broad spectrum	PS ± GTCS, atonic; primarily generalized; JME (?)	PS ± GTCS	PS ± GTCS; primary generalized; JME (?)
Number of identified cellular actions	2–3	3	1
Simple kinetics	Linear	Saturable uptake, linear elimination	Linear
No dose-related adverse effects	Multiple adverse effects reduce tolerability	Mild, transient	Mild
No organ toxicity	None	None	Rash
Fast titration	Slow	Fast	Slow
Inexpensive	$$$	$$$	$$$

PS = partial seizures; GTCS = generalized tonic-clonic seizures; JME = juvenile myoclonic epilepsy; $$$ = expensive.

Table 19.5 Comparison of properties of the second wave of new antiepileptic medications with an "ideal drug"

"Ideal drug"	Oxcarbazepine	Tiagabine	Topiramate	Vigabatrin
Highly effective	Effective	Effective	Effective	Effective
Broad spectrum	PS ± GTCS	PS ± GTCS	PS ± GTCS	PS ± GTCS, JME (?)
Number of identified cellular actions	1	1	2–3	1
Simple kinetics	Linear	Linear	Linear	Linear
No dose-related adverse effects	Hyponatremia	Mild, transient	Cognitive dysfunction	Cognitive dysfunction
No organ toxicity	None	None	None	Rash
Fast titration	Slow	Slow	Slow	Slow
Inexpensive	$$$	$$$	$$$	$$$

PS = partial seizures; GTCS = generalized tonic-clonic seizures; JME = juvenile myoclonic epilepsy; $$$ = expensive.

properties used in Tables 19.4 and 19.5 is modified from that of Richens.[167] All of the new AEMs must be efficacious to pass the review of the FDA. However, extensive use over a period of years and large comparative studies, for which the two VA cooperative studies set the standard, will ultimately determine which are the most useful ones. The spectrum of efficacy once again will depend on widespread use and further study in the treatment of well characterized patients with specific seizure types or syndromes. Information from available clinical trials gives an initial impression of the spectra, however. Kinetics should be simple if a medication is to gain wide acceptance. Operationally, "simple" means that practitioners do not need to remember a myriad of facts about the medication to optimize therapeutic benefit and avoid adverse events and liability. Absence of interactions is one of the most desirable features in medications for the elderly.[12, 13] Several of the new drugs appear at this stage to lack significant interactions. The new AEMs must inevitably cost more because their development and testing are expensive. The other characteristics determine ease of use and therapeutic benefit and, ultimately, whether cost will be a limiting factor. Reasons to choose one drug over another will become apparent only as each physician gains experience with the new drugs. Many will change their opinions with increasing experience. Before deciding, the reader is referred to Chapter 20, which discusses the clinical efficacy and practical issues for optimal use of the new AEMs.

REFERENCES

1. Hauser WA, Annegers JF, Kurland LT. Incidence of epilepsy and unprovoked seizures in Rochester, Minnesota, 1935–1984. Epilepsia 1993;34:453.
2. Mattson RH, Cramer JA, Collins JF, et al. Comparison of carbamazepine, phenobarbital, phenytoin, and primidone in partial and secondarily generalized tonic-clonic seizures. N Engl J Med 1985;313:145.
3. Mattson RH, Cramer JA, Collins JF, et al. A comparison of valproate with carbamazepine for the treatment of complex partial seizures and secondarily generalized tonic-clonic seizures in adults. N Engl J Med 1992;327:765.
4. Smith DB, Mattson RH, Cramer JA, et al. Results of a nationwide veterans administration cooperative study comparing the efficacy and toxicity of carbamazepine, phenobarbital, phenytoin and primidone. Epilepsia 1987;28(Suppl 3):50.
5. Giagninto S. Aging and the Nervous System. Chichester, United Kingdom: Wiley, 1988.
5a. McLean M. Lecture to the Southern Clinical Neurological Society on Seizures, Neurotransmitters and Aging. Key West, FL, January 1995.
6. Hollister LE. New class of hallucinogens. GABA-enhancing agents. Drug Dev Res 1990;21:253.
7. Cloyd JC, Lackner TE, Leppik IE. Antiepileptics in the elderly: pharmacoepidemiology and pharmacokinetics. Arch Fam Med 1994;3:589.
8. Cacek AJ. Review of alteration in oral phenytoin bioavailability associated with formulation, antacids and food. Ther Drug Monit 1986;8:166.
9. Cramer JA, Mattson RH, Bennett DM, et al. Variable free and total valproic acid concentrations in sole- and multi-drug therapy. Ther Drug Monit 1986;8:411.
10. Mattson GF, Mattson RH, Cramer JA. Interactions between valproic acid and carbamazepine: an in vitro study of protein binding. Ther Drug Monit 1982;4:181.
11. Fernandez MC, Erill S, Lucena MI, et al. Serum protein binding of tolbutamide in patients treated with antiepileptic drugs. Clin Pharmacokinet 1985;10:451.
12. Greenblatt DJ, Sellers EM, Shader RJ. Drug disposition in old age. N Engl J Med 1982;306:1081.
13. Leppik IE. Metabolism of antiepileptic medication: newborn to elderly. Epilepsia 1992;33(Suppl 4):32.
14. Catterall WA. Cellular and molecular biology of voltage-gated sodium channels. Physiol Rev 1992;72(Suppl 4):15.

15. Tsien RW, Tsien RY. Calcium channels, stores, and oscillations. Annu Rev Cell Biol 1990;6:715.
16. Bertolino M, Llinàs R. The central role of voltage-activated and receptor-operated calcium channels in neuronal cells. Annu Rev Pharmacol Toxicol 1992;32:399.
17. Olsen RW, Tobin AJ. Molecular biology of GABA$_A$ receptors. FASEB J 1990;4:1469.
18. DeLorey TM, Olsen RW. γ-Aminobutyric acid$_A$ receptor structure and function. J Biol Chem 1992;267:16747.
19. Macdonald RL, Twyman RE. Kinetic Properties and Regulation of GABA$_A$ Receptor Channels. In T Narahashi T (ed), Ion Channels (Vol. 3). New York: Plenum, 1992;315.
20. Mayer ML, Westbrook GL. The physiology of excitatory amino acids in the vertebrate central nervous system. Prog Neurobiol 1987;28:197.
21. Collingridge GL, Lester RAJ. Excitatory amino acid receptors in the vertebrate central nervous system. Pharmacol Rev 1989;41:143.
22. Wisden W, Seeburg PH. Mammalian iontropic glutamate receptors. Curr Opin Neurobiol 1993;3:291.
23. Schoepp DD, Conn PJ. Metabotropic glutamate receptors in brain function and pathology. Trends Pharmacol Sci 1993;15:13.
24. DeLorenzo RJ. Mechanisms of action of anticonvulsant drugs. Epilepsia 1988;29(Suppl 2):35.
25. Schwarcz R, Whetsell WO, Mangano REM. Quinolinic acid: an endogenous metabolite can produce axon sparing lesions in rat brain. Science 1983;219:316.
26. Snead OC. γ-Hydroxybutyrate model of generalized absence seizures: further characterization and comparison with other absence models. Epilepsia 1988;29:361.
27. Dragunow M, Goddard GV, Laverty R. Is adenosine an endogenous anticonvulsant? Epilepsia 1985;26:480.
28. Bonhaus DW, Laird HE, Mimaki T, et al. Possible Bases for the Anti-Convulsant Action of Taurine. In K Kuriyama, RJ Huxtable, HI Wata (eds), Sulfur Amino Acids: Biochemical and Clinical Aspects. New York: Liss, 1983.
29. Frenk H. Pro- and anticonvulsant actions of morphine and the endogenous opioids: involvement and interactions of multiple opiate and non-opiate systems. Brain Res Rev 1983;287:197.
30. Green AR, Johnson P, Mountford JA, et al. Some anticonvulsant drugs alter monoamine-mediated behaviour in mice in ways similar to electroconvulsive shock; implications for antidepressant therapy. Br J Pharmacol 1985;84:337.
31. Hille B. Ionic Channels of Excitable Membranes (2nd ed). Sunderland, MA: Sinauer Associates, 1992.
32. Hodgkin AL, Huxley AF. A quantitative description of membrane current and its application to conduction and excitation in nerve. J Physiol (Lond) 1952;117:500.
33. Hondeghem LM, Katzung BG. Time- and voltage-dependent interactions of antiarrhythmic drugs with cardiac sodium channels. Biochim Biophys Acta 1977;472:373.
34. Hille B. Local anesthetics: hydrophilic and hydrophobic pathways for the drug receptor reaction. J Gen Physiol 1977;69:497.
35. McLean MJ, Macdonald RL. Multiple actions of phenytoin on mouse spinal cord neurons in cell culture. J Pharmacol Exp Therap 1983;227:779.
36. McLean MJ, Macdonald RL. Carbamazepine and 10,11-epoxycarbamazepine produce use- and voltage-dependent limitation of rapidly firing action potentials of mouse central neurons in cell culture, J Pharmacol Exp Therap 1986;238:727.
37. McLean MJ, Macdonald RL. Sodium valproate, but not ethosuximide, produces use- and voltage-dependent limitation of high frequency repetitive firing of action potentials of mouse central neurons in cell culture. J Pharmacol Exp Therap 1986;237:1001.
38. VanDongen AMJ, VanErp MG, Voskuyl RA. Valproate reduces excitability by blockage of sodium and potassium conductance. Epilepsia 1986;27:177.
39. Courtney KR, Etter EG. Modulated anticonvulsant block of sodium channels in nerve and muscle. Eur J Pharmacol 1983;88:1.

40. Schwarz JR, Grigat G. Phenytoin and carbamazepine: potential- and frequency-dependent block of Na currents in mammalian myelinated nerve fibers. Epilepsia 1989;30:286.
41. Zona C, Avoli M. Effects induced by the antiepileptic drug valproic acid upon the ionic currents recorded in rat neocortical neurons in cell culture. Exp Brain Res 1990;81:313.
42. Ragsdale DS, Scheuer T, Catterall WA. Frequency and voltage-dependent inhibition of type IIA Na+ channels, expressed in a mammalian cell line, by local anesthetic, antiarrhythmic, and anticonvulsant drugs. Mol Pharmacol 1991;40:756.
43. Van den Berg RJ, Kok P, Voskuyl RA. Valproate and sodium currents in cultured hippocampal neurons. Exp Brain Res 1993;93:279.
44. Macdonald RL. Mechanisms of Anticonvulsant Drug Action. In TA Pedley, BS Meldrum (eds), Recent Advances in Epilepsy, 1. London: Churchill Livingstone, 1983;1.
45. Macdonald RL, McLean MJ. Anticonvulsant Drugs: Mechanisms of Action. In AV Delgado-Escueta, AA Ward, DM Woodbury, RJ Porter (eds), Advances in Neurology (Vol. 4). New York: Raven, 1986;713.
46. McLean MJ, Macdonald RL. Benzodiazepines, but not beta carbolines, limit high frequency repetitive firing of action potentials of spinal cord neurons in cell culture. J Pharmacol Exp Therap 1988;244:789.
47. Butterworth JF, Strichartz GR. Molecular mechanisms of local anesthesia: a review. Anesthesiology 1990;72:711.
48. Barber MJ, Starmer CF, Grant AO. Blockade of cardiac sodium channels by amitriptyline and diphenylhydantoin. Evidence for two use-dependent binding sites. Circ Res 1991;69:677.
49. Halliwell RF, Peters JA, Lambert JJ. The mechanism of action and pharmacologic specificity of the anticonvulsant NMDA antagonist MK-801: a voltage clamp study on neuronal cells in cell culture. Br J Pharmacol 1989;96:480.
50. Rothman S. Non-competitive N-methyl-D-aspartate antagonists affect multiple ionic currents. J Pharmacol Exp Therap 1988;248:137.
51. Wamil AW, McLean MJ. Use-, concentration- and voltage-dependent limitation by MK-801 of action potential firing frequency in mouse central neurons in cell culture. J Pharmacol Exp Therap 1992;260:376.
52. Wamil AW, McLean MJ. Effect of temperature on limitation by MK-801 of firing of action potentials by spinal cord neurons in cell culture. Eur J Pharmacol 1993;230:263.
53. Wamil AW, Löscher W, McLean MJ. Limitation by trans-2-en-valproate of firing of sodium-dependent action potentials in mouse central neurons in cell culture. Neurology 1994;44(Suppl 2):235.
54. Sypert GW, Reynolds AF. Single pyramidal tract fiber analysis of neocortical propagated seizures with reference to inactivation responses. Exp Neurol 1974;45:228.
55. White HS, Wolf HH, Swinyard EA, et al. A neuropharmacologic evaluation of felbamate as a novel anticonvulsant. Epilepsia 1992;33:564.
56. Coulter DA, Sombati S, DeLorenzo RJ. Selective effects of topiramate on sustained repetitive firing and spontaneous bursting in cultured hippocampal neurons. Epilepsia 1993;34(Suppl 2):123.
57. McLean MJ, Schmutz M, Wamil AW, et al. Oxcarbazepine: mechanisms of action. Epilepsia 1994;35(Suppl 3):5.
58. Wamil AW, McLean MJ. Limitation by gabapentin of high frequency action potential firing by mouse central neurons in cell culture. Epilepsy Res 1994;17:1.
59. Taylor CP. The anticonvulsant lamotrigine blocks sodium currents from cloned alpha-subunits of rat brain Na$^+$ channels in a voltage-dependent manner but gabapentin does not. Soc Neurosci Abs 1993;19:1631.
60. Cheung H, Kamp D, Harris E. An in vitro investigation of the action of lamotrigine on neuronal voltage-activated sodium channels. Epilepsy Res 1992;13:107.

61. Lang DG, Wang CM, Cooper BR. Lamotrigine, phenytoin and carbamazepine interactions on the sodium current present in N4TG1 mouse neuroblastoma cells. J Pharmacol Exp Ther 1993;266:829.
62. Tsien RW, Ellinor PT, Horne WA. Molecular diversity of voltage-dependent Ca^{2+} channels. Trends Pharmacol Sci 1991;12:349.
63. Spedding M, Paoletti R. Classification of calcium channels and the sites of action of drugs modifying channel function. Pharmacol Rev 1992;44:363.
64. Twombly DA, Yoshi M, Narahashi T. Mechanisms of calcium channel block by phenytoin. J Pharmacol Exp Ther 1988;246:189.
65. Esplin DW. Effects of diphenylhydantoin on synaptic transmission in cat spinal cord and stellate ganglion. J Pharmacol Exp Ther 1957;120:310.
66. Coulter DA, Huguenard JR, Prince DA. Characterization of ethosuximide reduction of low-threshold calcium current in thalamic neurons. Ann Neurol 1989;25:582.
67. Coulter DA, Huguenard JR, Prince DA. Differential effects of petit mal anticonvulsants and convulsants on thalamic neurones: calcium current reduction. Br J Pharmacol 1990;100:800.
68. Kelly KM, Gross RA, Macdonald RL. Valproic acid selectively reduces the low-threshold (T) calcium current in rat nodose neurons. Neurosci Lett 1990;116:233.
69. Bowery NG. $GABA_B$ receptor pharmacology. Annu Rev Pharmacol Toxicol 1993;33:109.
70. Huston E, Scott RH, Dolphin AC. A comparison of the effect of calcium channel ligands and $GABA_B$ agonists and antagonists on transmitter release and somatic calcium channel currents in cultured neurons. Neuroscience 1990;38:721.
70a. MacDonald RL. Lennox Lecture. American Society Annual Meeting. New Orleans, LA, December 1994.
71. Pritchett DB, Sontheimer H, Shivers BD. Importance of a novel $GABA_A$ receptor subunit for benzodiazepine pharmacology. Nature 1989;338:582.
72. Olsen RW. GABA-benzodiazepine-barbiturate receptor interactions. J Neurochem 1981;37:1.
73. Majewska MD. Neurosteroids: endogenous bimodal modulators of the $GABA_A$ receptor. Mechanism of action and physiological significance. Prog Neurobiol 1992;38:379.
74. Gale K. GABA and epilepsy: basic concepts from preclinical research. Epilepsia 1992;33(Suppl 5):3.
75. Meldrum BS. GABAergic mechanisms in the pathogenesis and treatment of epilepsy. Br J Clin Pharmacol 1989;27:3.
76. Löscher W. Effects of the antiepileptic drug valproate on metabolism and function of inhibitory and excitatory amino acids in the brain. Neurochem Res 1993;18:485.
77. Löscher W, Honack D, Taylor CP. Gabapentin increases amino oxyacetic acid-induced GABA accumulation in several regions of rat brain. Neurosci Lett 1991;128:150.
78. Rho JM, Donevan SD, Rogawski MA. Mechanism of action of the anticonvulsant felbamate: opposing effects on N-methyl-D-aspartate and gamma-amino butyric acid A receptors. Ann Neurol 1994;35:229.
79. Brown SD, Wolf HH, Swinyard EA, et al. The novel anticonvulsant topiramate enhances GABA-mediated chloride flux. Epilepsia 1993;34(Suppl 2):120.
80. Kocsis JD, Honmou O. Gabapentin increases GABA-induced depolarization in rat neonatal oprtic nerve. Neurosci Lett 1994;169:181.
81. Sander JWAS, Hart YM. Vigabatrin and behaviour disturbances. Lancet 1990;335:57.
82. Dam M. Vigabatrin and behaviour disturbances. Lancet 1990;335:605.
83. Grant SM, Heel RC. Vigabatrin: a review of its pharmacodynamic and pharmacokinetic properties, and therapeutic potential in epilepsy and disorders of motor control. Drugs 1991;41:889.
84. Barnes JM, Henley JM. Molecular characteristics of excitatory amino acid receptors. Prog Neurobiol 1992;39:113.

85. Monyer H, Sprengel R, Schoepfer R, et al. Heteromeric NMDA receptors: molecular and functional distinction of subtypes. Science 1992;256:1217.
86. Watkins JC, Krogsgaard-Larsen P, Honoré T. Structure-activity relationships in the development of excitatory amino acid receptor agonists and competitive antagonists. Trends Pharmacol Sci 1990;11:25.
87. Schoepp D, Bockaert J, Sladeczek F. Pharmacologic and functional characteristics of metabotropic excitatory amino acid receptors. Trends Pharmacol Sci 1990;11:508.
88. Olney JW. Inciting excitotoxic cytocide among central neurons. Adv Exp Med Biol 1986;203:631.
89. Rothman SM, Olney JW. Glutamate and the pathophysiology of hypoxic-ischemic brain damage. Ann Neurol 1986;19:105.
90. Choi DW. Excitotoxic cell death. J Neurobiol 1992;23:1261.
91. Lipton SA, Rosenberg PA. Excitatory amino acids as a final common pathway for neurologic disorders. N Engl J Med 1994;330:613.
92. Meldrum BS. Metabolic Factors During Prolonged Seizures and Their Relation to Nerve Cell Death. In AV Delgado-Escueta, CG Wasterlain, DM Treiman, RJ Porter (eds), Advances in Neurology (Vol. 34). New York: Raven, 1983;261.
93. Siesjö BK, Wieloch T. Epileptic Brain Damage: Pathophysiology and Neurochemical Pathology. In AV Delgado-Escueta, AA Ward Jr, DM Woodbury, RJ Porter (eds), Advances in Neurology. New York: Raven, 1986;813.
94. Wong EH, Kemp JA. Sites for antagonism on the N-methyl-D-aspartate receptor channel complex. Annu Rev Pharmacol Toxicol 1991;31:401.
95. Rogawski MA. The NMDA receptor, NMDA antagonists and epilepsy therapy. A status report. Drugs 1992;44:279.
96. McNamara JO. Development of new pharmacologic agents for epilepsy: lessons from the kindling model. Epilepsia 1989;(Suppl 1):13.
97. Troupin AS, Mendius JR, Cheng F, et al. MK-801. In BS Meldrum, RJ Porter (eds), New Anticonvulsant Drugs. London: Libbey, 1986;191.
98. Meldrum BS. Glutamatergic Transmission in Epilepsy. Lecture, Karolinska Institute Postgraduate Education Series. Update on Epilepsy: Advances in Pharmacology and Prognosis, Stockholm, Sweden: October 2–3, 1993.
99. Honoré T, Davies SN, Drejer J, et al. Quinoxalinediones: Potent competitive non-NMDA glutamate receptor antagonists. Science 1988;241:701.
100. Rock DM, Macdonald RL. The polyamine spermine has multiple actions on N-methyl-D-aspartate receptor single-channel currents in cultured cortical neurons. Mol Pharmacol 1992;41:83.
101. Williams K, Romano C, Molinoff PB. Effects of polyamines on the binding of [3H]MK801 to the N-methyl-D-aspartate receptor: pharmacologic evidence for the existence of a polyamine recognition site. Mol Pharmacol 1989;36:575.
102. Gilad GM, Gilad VH. Polyamines in neurotrauma: ubiquitous molecules in search of a function. Biochem Pharmacol 1992;4493:401.
103. Aizenman E, Reynolds I. Modulation of NMDA excitotoxicity by redox reagents. Ann N Y Acad Sci 1992;648:125.
104. McLean MJ, Wamil AW. Effects of Anticonvulsant Compounds on Voltage- and Neurotransmitter-Activated Sodium Conductances of Central Neurons in Cell Culture. In MR Klee, HD Lux, E-J Speckmann (eds), Physiology, Pharmacology and Development of Epileptogenic Phenomena. Berlin: Springer Verlag, 1991;211.
105. Wamil AW, McLean MJ. Phenytoin blocks N-methyl-D-aspartate responses of mouse central neurons. J Pharmacol Exp Ther 1993;267:218.
106. Lampe H, Bigalke H. Carbamazepine blocks NMDA-activated currents in cultured spinal cord neurons. NeuroReport 1990;1:26.
107. McCabe RT, Wasterlain CG, Kucharczyk N, et al. Evidence of anticonvulsant and neuroprotectant action of felbamate mediated by strychnine-insensitive glycine receptors. J Pharmacol Exp Ther 1993;264:1248.

108. Harmsworth WL, Wolf HH, Swinyard EA, et al. Felbamate modulates glycine receptor function. Epilepsia 1993;34(Suppl 2):92.
109. Javitt DC, Zukin SR. Recent advances in the phencyclidine model of schizophrenia. Am J Psychiatry 1991;148:1301.
110. Riederer P, Lange KW, Kornhuber J, et al. Glutamate receptor antagonism: neurotoxicity, anti-akinetic effects, and psychosis. J Neural Transm 1991;34:203.
111. Daw NW, Stein PSG, Fox K. The role of NMDA receptors in information processing. Annu Rev Neurosci 1993;16:107.
112. Olney J, Labruyere J, Price MT. Pathological changes induced in cerebrocortical neurons by phencyclidine and related drugs. Science 1989;244:1360.
113. Macdonald RL, Meldrum BS. Principles of Antiepileptic Drug Action. In R Levy, R Mattson, B Meldrum, et al. (eds), Antiepileptic Drugs (2nd ed). New York: Raven, 1989;59.
114. Löscher W, Schmidt D. Which animal models should be used in the search for new antiepileptic drugs? A proposal based on experimental and clinical considerations. Epilepsy Res 1988;2:145.
115. Fisher RS. Animal models of the epilepsies. Brain Res Brain Res Rev 1989;14:245.
116. Kupferberg HJ. Antiepileptic drug development program: a cooperative effort of government and industry. Epilepsia 1989;30(Suppl 1):51.
117. Sofia RD, Kramer L, Perhach JL, et al. Felbamate. In F Pinani, E Perucca, G Avanzini, A Richens (eds), New Antiepileptic Drugs (Epilepsy Res Suppl 3). Amsterdam: Elsevier, 1991.
118. Krall RL, Penry JK, White BG, et al. Antiepileptic drug development: II. Anticonvulsant drug screening. Epilepsia 1978;19:409.
119. Swinyard EA, Sofia RD, Kufperberg HJ. Comparative anticonvulsant activity and neurotoxicity of felbamate and four prototype antiepileptic drugs in mice and rats. Epilepsia 1986;27:27.
120. Leppik IE, Dreifuss FE, Pledger GW, et al. Felbamate for partial seizures. Results of a controlled clinical trial. Neurology 1991;41:1785.
121. Theodore WH, Raubertas RF, Porter RJ, et al. Felbamate: a clinical trial for complex partial seizures. Epilepsia 1991;32:392.
122. Wallis RA, Panizzon KL, Fairchild MD, et al. Protective effects of felbamate against hypoxia in the rat hippocampal slice. Stroke 1992;23:547.
123. Taft WC, Clifton GL, Blair RE, et al. Phenytoin protects against ischemia-produced neuronal cell death. Brain Res 1989;483:143.
124. Boxer PA, Cordon JJ, Mann ME, et al. Comparison of phenytoin with noncompetitive N-methyl-D-aspartate antagonists in a model of focal brain ischemia in rat. Stroke 1990;21(Suppl 3):47.
125. Fern R, Ransom BR, Stys PK, et al. Pharmacologic protection of CNS white matter during anoxia: actions of phenytoin, carbamazepine and diazepam. J Pharmacol Exp Ther 1993;266:1549.
126. Sachdeo R, Kramer LD, Rosenbert A, et al. Felbamate monotherapy: controlled trial in patients with partial onset seizures. Ann Neurol 1992;32:386.
127. Faught E, Sachdeo RC, Remler MP, et al. Felbamate monotherapy for partial-onset seizures: an active-control trial. Neurology 1993;43:688.
128. Bourgeois B, Leppik IE, Sackellares JC, et al. A double-blind controlled trial in patients undergoing presurgical evaluation for partial seizures. Neurology 1993;43:693.
129. Felbamate Study Group in Lennox-Gastaut Syndrome. Efficacy of felbamate in childhood epileptic encephalopathy. N Engl J Med 1993;328:29.
130. Pledger GW, Kramer LD. Clinical trials of investigational antiepileptic drugs: monotherapy designs. Epilepsia 1991;32:716.
131. Perhach JL, Weliky I, Newton JJ, et al. Felbamate. In BS Meldrum, RJ Porter (eds), New Anticonvulsant Drugs. London–Paris: Libbey, 1986.

132. Graves NM, Ludden TM, Holmes GB, et al. Pharmacokinetics of felbamate, a novel antiepileptic drug: application of mixed-effect modeling to clinical trials. Pharmacotherapy 1989;9:372.
133. Leppik IE, Graves NM. Potential Antiepileptic Drugs. Felbamate. In R Levy, R Mattson, B Meldrum, et al. (eds), Antiepileptic Drugs (3rd ed). New York: Raven, 1989.
134. Wilensky AJ, Friel PN, Ojemann LM, et al. Pharmacokinetics of W-554 (ADD 03055) in epileptic patients. Epilepsia 1985;26:602.
135. Brodie MJ. Felbamate: a new antiepileptic drug. Epilepsy 1993;341:1445.
136. Bialer M. Comparative pharmacokinetics of the newer antiepileptic drugs. Clin Pharmacokinet 1993;24:441.
137. Gudipati RM, Raymond RH, Ward DL, et al. Effect of food on the absorption of felbamate (Felbatol) in healthy male volunteers. Neurology 1992;42(Suppl 4):332.
138. Ward DL, Shumaker RC. Comparative bioavailability of felbamate in healthy men. Epilepsia 1990;31:642.
139. Gordon R, Gels M, Wichmann J, et al. Interaction of felbamate with several other antiepileptic drugs against seizures induced by maximal electroshock in mice. Epilepsia 1993;34:367.
140. Graves NM, Holmes GB, Fuerst R, et al. Effect of felbamate on phenytoin and carbamazepine serum concentrations. Epilepsia 1989;30:225.
141. Wagner ML, Leppik IE, Graves NM, et al. Felbamate serum concentrations: effect of valproate, carbamazepine, phenytoin and phenobarbital. Epilepsia 1990;31:642.
142. Wagner ML, Graves NM, Leppik IE, et al. The effect of felbamate on valproate disposition. Epilepsia 1991;32(Suppl 3):15.
143. Fuerst RH, Graves NM, Leppik IE, et al. Felbamate increases phenytoin but decreases carbamazepine concentrations. Epilepsia 1988;29:488.
144. Howard JR, Dix RK, Shumaker RC, et al. The effect of felbamate on carbamazepine pharmacokinetics. Epilepsia 1992;33(Suppl 3):84.
145. Wagner ML, Remmel RP, Graves NM, et al. Effect of felbamate on carbamazepine and its major metabolites. Clin Pharmacol Ther 1993;53:536.
146. Graves NM, Remmel RP, Miller S, et al. The effect of felbamate on the major metabolites of carbamazepine. Epilepsia 1989;30:736.
147. Ward DL, Wagner ML, Perhach JL, et al. Felbamate steady-state pharmacokinetics during coadministration of valproate. Epilepsia 1991;32(Suppl 3):8.
148. Shumaker RC, Fantel C, Kelton E, et al. Evaluation of the elimination of (14C) felbamate in healthy men. Epilepsia 1990;31:642.
149. Bartoszyk GD, Meyerson N, Reimann W, et al. Gabapentin. In BS Meldrum, RJ Porter (eds), New Anticonvulsant Drugs. London–Paris: John Libbey, 1986.
150. Foot M, Wallace J. Gabapentin. In F Pisani, E Perucca, G Avanzini, A Richens (eds), New Antiepileptic Drugs (Epilepsy Res Suppl 3). Amsterdam: Elsevier, 1991.
151. Schmidt B. Gabapentin. In RH Levy, FE Dreifuss, RH Mattson, BS Meldrum, JK Penry (eds), Antiepileptic Drugs (3rd ed). New York: Raven, 1989;925.
152. Goa KL, Sorkin EM. Gabapentin: a review of its pharmacologic properties and clinical potential in epilepsy. Drugs 1993;46:409.
153. Taylor CP. Mechanism of Action of New Anti-Epileptic Drugs. New Trends in Epilepsy Management: The Role of Gabapentin. D Chadwick (ed), Royal Society of Medicine Services International Congress and Symposium Series No. 198, 1993;13.
154. Leiderman D, Garafalo E, LaMoreaux L. Gabapentin patients with absence seizures: two double-blind placebo controlled studies. Epilepsia 1993;34(Suppl 6):45.
155. Welty DF, Schielke GP, Vartanian MG, et al. Gabapentin anticonvulsant action in rats: disequilibrium with peak drug concentrations in plasma and brain microdialysate. Epilepsy Res 1993;16:175.
156. Stewart BH, Kugler AR, Thompson PR, et al. A saturable transport mechanism in the intestinal absorption of gabapentin is the underlying cause of the lack of pro-

portionality between increasing dose and drug levels in plasma. Pharm Res 1993;10:276.

157. Hill DR, Suman-Chauhan N, Woodruf GN. Localization of [^{3}H]gabapentin to a novel site in rat brain: autoradiographic studies. Eur J Pharmacol [Mol Pharmacol Section] 1993;244:303.

158. Suman-Chauhan N, Webdale L, Hill DR, et al. Characterisation of [^{3}H]gabapentin binding to a novel site in rat brain: homogenate binding studies. Eur J Pharmacol [Mol Pharmacol Section] 1993;244:293.

159. Crawford P, Ghadiali E, Lane R, et al. Gabapentin as an antiepileptic drug in man. J Neurol Neurosurg Psychiatry 1987;50:682.

160. UK Gabapentin Study Group. Gabapentin partial epilepsy. Lancet 1990;335:1114.

161. Sivenius J, Kalviainen R, Ylinen A, et al. Double-blind study of gabapentin in the treatment of partial seizures. Epilepsia 1991;32:539.

162. US Gabapentin Study Group No. 5. Gabapentin as add-on therapy in refractory partial epilepsy. A double-blind, placebo-controlled, parallel-group study. Neurology 1993;43:2292.

163. Ojemann LM, Wilensky AJ, Temkin NR, et al. Long-term treatment with gabapentin for partial epilepsy. Epilepsy Res 1992;13:159.

164. Wilensky AJ, Temkin NR, Ojemann LM, et al. Gabapentin and carbamazepine as monotherapy and combined: a pilot study. Epilepsia 1992;33(Suppl 3):77.

165. Chadwick D. Gabapentin. In F Pisani, E Perucca, G Avanzini, A Richens (eds), New Antiepileptic Drugs (Epilepsy Res Suppl 3). Amsterdam: Elsevier, 1991.

166. Vollmer KO, Turck D, Bockbrader HN, et al. Summary of Neurontin (gabapentin) clinical pharmacokinetics. Epilepsia 1992;33(Suppl 3):77.

167. Richens A. Clinical Pharmacokinetics of Gabapentin. New Trends in Epilepsy Managment: The Role of Gabapentin. D Chadwick (ed), Royal Society of Medicine Services International Congress and Symposium Series No. 198. London, 1993;41.

168. Vollmer K-O, von Hodenberg A, Kolle EU. Pharmacokinetics and metabolism of gabapentin in rat, dog and man. Arzneimittel-Forschung 1986;36:830.

169. Vollmer KO, Thomann P, Most M, et al. Pharmacokinetics of the New Anticonvulsant Gabapentin in Man. Presented at the Golden Jubilee Conference and Northern European Epilepsy Meeting. University of York, Great Britain, 1986.

170. Anhut H, Leppik I, Schmidt B. Drug interaction study of the new anticonvulsant gabapentin with phenytoin in epileptic patients. Arch Pharmacol 1988;337(Suppl):127.

171. Graves NM, Holmes GB, Leppik IE, et al. Pharmacokinetics of gabapentin patients treated with phenytoin. Pharmacotherapy 1989;9:196.

172. Graves NM, Leppik IE, Wagner ML, et al. Effect of gabapentin on carbamazepine levels. Epilepsia 1990;31:644.

173. Hooper WD, Kavanagh MC, Herkes GK, et al. Lack of a pharmacokinetic interaction between phenobarbital and gabapentin. Br J Clin Pharmacol 1991;31:171.

174. Radulovic LL, Wilder BJ, Leppik IE, et al. Lack of interaction of gabapentin with carbamazepine or valproate. Epilepsia 1994;35:155.

175. Eldon MA, Underwood BA, Randinitis EJ, et al. Lack of effect of gabapentin on the pharmacokinetics of a norethindrone acetate/ethinyl estradiol-containing oral contraceptive. Neurology 1993;43:307.

176. Busch JA, Radulovic LL, Bockbrader HN, et al. Effect of Maalox TC on single-dose pharmacokinetics of gabapentin capsules in healthy subjects. Pharm Res 1992;9(Suppl 10):315.

177. Comstock TI, Sica DA, Bockbrader HN, et al. Gabapentin pharmacokinetics in subjects with various degrees of renal function. J Clin Pharmacol 1990;30:831.

178. Boyd RA, Bockbrader HN, Turck D, et al. Effect of subject age on the single dose pharmacokinetics of orally administered gabapentin (CI-945). Pharm Res 1990;7(Suppl 9):215.

179. Fischer JH, Barr AN, Rogers SL, et al. Lack of serious toxicity following gabapentin overdose. Neurology 1994;44:982.
180. Yuen AWC. Lamotrigine. In F Pisani, E Perucca, G Avanzini, A Richens (eds), New Antiepileptic Drugs (Epilepsy Res Suppl 3). Amsterdam: Elsevier, 1991.
181. Leach MJ, Marden CM, Miller AA. Pharmacologic studies on lamotrigine, a novel potential antiepileptic drug: II. Neurochemical studies on the mechanism of action. Epilepsia 1986;27:490.
182. Leach MJ, Baxter MG, Critchley MAE. Neurochemical and behavioral aspects of lamotrigine. Epilepsia 1991;32:4.
183. Miller AA, Wheatley P, Sawyer DA, et al. Pharmacologic studies on lamotrigine, a novel potential antiepileptic drug: I. Anticonvulsant profile in mice and rats. Epilepsia 1986;27:483.
184. Lamb RJ, Miller AA. Effect of lamotrigine and some known anticonvulsant drugs on visually-evoked after-discharge in the conscious rat. Br J Pharmacol 1985;86:765.
185. Jawad S, Richens A, Goodwin G, et al. Controlled trial of lamotrigine (Lamictal) for refractory partial seizures. Epilepsia 1989;30:356.
186. Davies G, Kench SV, Clifford JS, et al. Preliminary data from an open multicentre trial of lamotrigine (Lamictal) in patients with treatment-resistant epilepsy on one antiepileptic drug withdrawing monotherapy. Epilepsia 1992;33(Suppl 3):81.
187. Dren AT, Womble GP, Yau MK, et al. Placebo-controlled clinical studies demonstrating the efficacy and safety of lamotrigine (Lamictal) as add-on therapy in patients with refractory partial seizures. Epilepsia 1992;33(Suppl 3):81.
188. Messenheimer JA, Ramsay RE, Leroy RF, et al. Multicenter, long-term study of lamotrigine (Lamictal) in outpatients with partial seizures. Epilepsia 1992;33 (Suppl 3):82.
189. Mims J, Ritter JF, Dren AT, et al. Compassionate plea use of lamotrigine in children with incapacitating and/or life-threatening epilepsy. Epilepsia 1992;33(Suppl 3):83.
190. Brodie MJ. Lamotrigine. Lancet 1992;339:1397.
191. Goa KL, Ross SR, Chrisp P. Lamotrigine: a review of its pharmacologic properties and clinical efficacy in epilepsy. Drugs 1993;46:152.
192. Jawad S, Yuen WC, Peck AW, et al. Lamotrigine: single dose pharmacokinetics, and initial one week experience in refractory seizures. Epilepsy Res 1987;1:194.
193. Miller AA, Sawyer DA, Roth B, et al. Lamotrigine. In BS Meldrum, RJ Porter (eds), New Anticonvulsant Drugs. London: Libbey, 1986.
194. Gram L. Potential Antiepileptic Drugs: Lamotrigine. In R Levy, R Mattson, B Meldrum, et al. (eds), Antiepileptic Drugs (3rd ed). New York: Raven, 1989;947.
195. Binnie CD, van Emde Boas W, Kasteleijn-Nolste-Trenite DGA, et al. Acute effects of lamotrigine (BW430C) in persons with epilepsy. Epilepsia 1986;27:248.
196. Peck AW. Clinical pharmacology of lamotrigine. Epilepsia 1991;32:S9.
197. Yuen AWC, Peck AW. Lamotrigine pharmacokinetics: oral and iv infusion in man. Br J Clin Pharmacol 1988;26:242.
198. Lai A, Wargin WA, Garnett WR, et al. Pharmacokinetics of lamotrigine in epileptic patients following multiple oral dosing. Epilepsia 1986;27:647.
199. Pellock JM, Ramsay RE, Garnett WR, et al. Chronic dose tolerance of lamotrigine in epileptic patients. Epilepsia 1986;27:647.
200. Mikati MA, Schachter SC, Schomer DL, et al. Long-term tolerability, pharmacokinetic and preliminary efficacy study of lamotrigine in patients with resistant partial seizures. Clin Neuropharmacol 1989;12:312.
201. Ramsay RE, Pellock JM, Garnett WR, et al. Pharmacokinetics and safety of lamotrigine (Lamictal) in patients with epilepsy. Epilepsy Res 1991;10:191.
202. Yau MK, Garnett WR, Wargin WA, et al. A single dose, dose proportionality and bioequivalence study of lamotrigine in normal volunteers. Epilepsia 1991;32(Suppl 3):8.
203. Cohen AF, Land GS, Breimer DD, et al. Lamotrigine, a new anticonvulsant: pharmacokinetics in normal humans. Clin Pharmacol Ther 1987;42:535.

204. Posner J, Webster H, Yuen WC. Investigation of the ability of lamotrigine, a novel antiepileptic drug to induce mixed function oxygenase enzymes. Br J Clin Pharmacol 1991;32:658.
205. Graves NM, Ritter FJ, Wagner ML, et al. Effect of lamotrigine on carbamazepine epoxide concentrations. Epilepsia 1991;(Suppl 3):13.
206. Schapel GJ, Dollman W, Beran RG, et al. No effect of lamotrigine on carbamazepine and carbamazepine-epoxide concentrations. Epilepsia 1991; 32(Suppl 1):59.
207. Warner T, Patsalos PN, Prevett M, et al. Lamotrigine-induced carbamazepine toxicity: an interaction with carbamazepine-10,11-epoxide. Epilepsy Res 1992;11:147.
208. Wolf P. Lamotrigine: preliminary clinical observations on pharmacokinetics and interactions with traditional antiepileptic drugs. J Epilepsy 1992;5:73.
209. Yau MK, Wargin WA, Wolf KB, et al. Effect of Valproic Acid on the Pharmacokinetics of Lamotrigine at Steady-State. Presented at the 1992 Annual Meeting of the American Epilepsy Society. Seattle, December 4–10, 1992.
210. Pisani F, De Perri R, Perucca E, et al. Interaction of lamotrigine with sodium valproate [letter]. Lancet 1993;341:122.
211. Posner J, Cohen AF, Land G, et al. The pharmacokinetics of lamotrigine (BW 430C) in healthy subjects with unconjugated hyperbilirubinemia (Gilbert's syndrome). Br J Clin Pharmacol 1989;28:117.
212. Posner J, Holdich T, Crome P. Comparison of lamotrigine pharmacokinetics in young and elderly healthy volunteers. J Pharm Med 1991;1:121.
213. Faught ER, Leroy RF, Messenheimer JA, et al. Clinial experience with lamotrigine (Lamictal) monotherapy for partal seizures in adult outpatients. Epilepsia 1992;33(Suppl 3):82.
214. Mumford JP, Lewis PJ. Vigabatrin. In F Pisani, E Perucca, G Avanzini, A Richens (eds), New Antiepileptic Drugs (Epilepsy Res Suppl 3). Amsterdam: Elsevier, 1991.
215. Jung MJ, Lippert B, Metcalf BW, et al. γ-Vinyl-GABA (4-amino-hex-5-enoic acid), a new selective irreversible inhibitor of GABA-T: effects on brain GABA metabolism in mice. J Neurochem 1977;29:797.
216. Schechter PJ, Hanke NFJ, Grove J, et al. Biochemical and clinical effects of γ-vinyl GABA in patients with epilepsy. Neurology 1984;34:182.
217. Ben-Menachem E. Pharmacokinetic effects of vigabatrin on cerebrospinal fluid amino acids in humans. Epilepsia 1989;30:12.
218. Riekkinen PJ, Pitkanen A, Ylinen A, et al. Specificity of vigabatrin for the GABAergic system in human epilepsy. Epilepsia 1989;30:18.
219. Larsson OM, Gram L, Schousboe I, et al. Differential effect of gamma-vinyl GABA and valproate on GABA-transaminase from cultured neurones and astrocytes. Neuropharmacology 1986;25:617.
220. Rimmer EM, Richens A. Double-blind study of γ-vinyl GABA in patients with refractory epilepsy. Lancet 1984;1:189.
221. Loiseau P, Hardenberg JP, Pestre M, et al. Double-blind, placebo-controlled study of vigabatrin (gamma-vinyl GABA) in drug-resistant epilepsy. Epilepsia 1986;27:115.
222. Tassinari CA, Michelucci R, Ambrosetto G, et al. Double-blind study of vigabatrin in the treatment of drug-resistant epilepsy. Arch Neurol 1987;44:907.
223. Dam M. Long-term evaluation of vigabatrin (gamma vinyl GABA) in epilepsy. Epilepsia 1989;30(Suppl 3):26.
224. Reynolds EH. γ-Vinyl GABA (vigabatrin): clinical experience in adult and adolescent patients with intractable epilepsy. Epilepsia 1992;33(Suppl 5):30.
225. Livingston JH, Beaumont D, Arzimanoglou A, et al. Vigabatrin in the treatment of epilepsy in children. Br J Clin Pharmacol 1989;27:109.
226. Luna D, Dulac O, Pajot N, et al. Vigabatrin in the treatment of childhood epilep-

sies: a single-blind placebo-controlled study. Epilepsia 1989;30:430.

227. Chiron C, Dulac O, Luna D, et al. Vigabatrin in infantile spasms. Lancet 1990;335:363.
228. Chiron C, Dulac O, Beaumont D, et al. Therapeutic trial of vigabatrin in refractory infantile spasms. J Child Neurol 1991;6(Suppl 2):52.
229. Gram L, Sabers A, Dulac O. Treatment of pediatric epilepsies with γ-vinyl GABA (vigabatrin). Epilepsia 1992;33(Suppl 5):26.
230. Besser R, Kramer G, Thumler R. Vigabatrin bei therapieresistenen Epilepsien. Aktuelle Neurologie 1989;16:79.
231. Michelucci R, Tassinari CA, Iudice A, et al. Efficacia a lungo termine del Vigabatrin nell'epilessia farmacoresistente. Bollettino-Lega Italiana contro l'Epilessia 1988;62:393.
232. Mumford JP, Dam M. Meta-analysis of European placebo controlled studies of vigabatrin in drug resistant epilepsy. Br J Clin Pharmacol 1989;27:101.
233. Butler WH. The neuropahtology of vigabatrin. Epilepsia 1989;30(Suppl 3):15.
234. Hammond EJ, Wilder BJ. Effects of gamma-vinyl-GABA on the human electroencephalogram. Neuropharmacology 1985;24:975.
235. Hammond EJ, Wilder BJ. Effect of gamma-vinyl-GABA on human pattern evoked visual potentials. Neurology 1985;35:1801.
236. Pedersen B, Hojgaard K, Dam M. Vigabatrin: no microvacuoles in a human brain. Epilepsy Res 1987;1:74.
237. Hammond EJ, Rangel RJ, Wilder BJ. Evoked potential monitoring of vigabatrin patients. Br J Clin Pract 1988;42(Suppl 61):16.
238. Chiron C, Dulac O, Palacios L, et al. Magnetic resonance imaging in epileptic children treated with γ-vinyl-GABA (vigabatrin). Epilepsia 1989;30:736.
239. Agosti R, Yasargil G, Egli M, et al. Neuropathology of a human hippocampus following long-term treatment with vigabatrin: lack of microvacuoles. Epilepsy Res 1990;6:166.
240. Treiman DA. Gamma vinyl GABA: current role in the management of drug-resistant epilepsy. Epilepsia 1989;30(Suppl 3):31.
241. Schechter PJ. Vigabatrin. In BS Meldrum, RJ Porter (eds), New Anticonvulsant Drugs. London: John Libbey, 1986.
242. Schechter PJ. Vigabatrin. In BS Meldrum BS, RJ Porter (eds), Current Problems in Epilepsy: New Anticonvulsant Drugs (Vol. 4). London: Libbey, 1986;265.
243. Richens A. Potential Antiepileptic Drugs. Vigabatrin. In R Levy, R Mattson, B Meldrum, JK Penry, FE Dreifuss (eds), Antiepileptic Drugs (3rd ed). New York: Raven, 1989.
244. Haegele KD, Schechter PJ. Kinetics of the enantiomers of vigabatrin after an oral dose of the racemate or the active S-enantiomer. Clin Pharmacol Ther 1986;40:581.
245. Frisk-Holmberg M, Kerth P, Meyer PH. Effect of food on the absorption of vigabatrin. Br J Clin Pharmacol 1989;27:23.
246. Schechter PJ. Clinical pharmacology of vigabatrin. Br J Clin Pharmacol 1989;27:195.
247. Rimmer EM, Richens A. Interaction between vigabatrin and phenytoin. Br J Clin Pharmacol 1989;27:27.
248. Haegele KD, Huebert ND, Ebel M, et al. Pharmacokinetics of vigabatrin: implications of creatinine clearance. Clin Pharmacol Ther 1988;44:558.
249. Browne TR, Mattson RH, Penry JK, et al. A multicentre study of vigabatrin for drug-resistant epilepsy. Br J Clin Pharmacol 1989;27:95.
250. Tartara A, Manni R, Galimberti CA, et al. Vigabatrin in the treatment of epilepsy: a long-term follow up study. J Neurol Neurosurg Psychiatry 1989;52:467.
251. Brodie MJ, McKee PJW. Vigabatrin and psychosis. Lancet 1990;335:1279.
252. Houtkooper MA, Lammertsma A, Meyer JWA, et al. Oxcarbazepine (GP 47.680): a possible alternative to carbamazepine. Epilepsia 1987;28:693.

253. Scandanavian Oxcarbazepine Study Group. A double-blind study comparing oxcarbazepine and carbamazepine in patients with newly diagnosed, previously untreated epilepsy. Epilepsy Res 1989;3:70.
254. Friis ML, Kristensen O, Boas J, et al. Therapeutic experiences with 947 epileptic out-patients in oxcarbazepine treatment. Acta Neurol Scand 1993;87:224.
255. Klosterskov Jensen P, Dam M. Oxcarbazepine. In: Dam M, Gram L, eds. Comprehensive Epileptology. New York: Raven Press, 1991; 621-629.
256. Klosterskov Jensen P, Gram L, Schmutz M. Oxcarbazepine. In F Pisani, E Perucca, G Avanzini, A Richens (eds), New Antiepileptic Drugs (Epilepsy Res Suppl 3). Amsterdam: Elsevier, 1991;135–140.
257. Faigle JW, Menge GP. Metabolic characteristics of oxcarbazepine (Trileptal) and their beneficial implications for enzyme induction and drug interactions. Behav Neurol 1990;3:21.
258. Faigle JW, Menge GP. Pharmacokinetic and metabolic features of oxcarbazepine and their clinical significance: comparison with carbamazepine. Int J Clin Psychopharmacol 1990;5(Suppl 1):73.
259. Baltzer V, Schmutz M. Experimental Anticonvulsant Properties of Gp 47 680 and of Monohydroxy Derivative, Its Main Human Metabolite: Compounds Related to Carbamazepine, In H Meinardi, AJ Rowan (eds), Advances in Epileptology. Amsterdam-Lisse: Swets & Zeitlinger, 1978;295.
260. Feldmann KF, Brechbuhler S, Faigle JW, Imhof P. Pharmacokinetics and metabolism of GP 47 680, a compound related to carbamazepine, in animals and man. In H Meinardi, AJ Rowan. Advances in Epileptology. Amsterdam-Lisse: Swets & Zeitlinger, 1978;290.
261. Feldmann KF, Dörhöfer G, Faigle JW, et al. Pharmacokinetics and Metabolism of GP 47 779, the Main Human Metabolite of Oxcarbazepine (GP 47 680) in Animals and Healthy Volunteers. In M Dam, L Gram, JK Penry. Advances in Epileptology: XIIth Epilepsy International Symposium. New York: Raven, 1981;89.
262. Dickinson RG, Hooper WD, Dunstan PR, et al. First dose and steady-state pharmacokinetics of oxcarbazepine and its 10 hydroxy metabolite. Eur J Clin Pharmacol 1989;37:69.
263. Schobben F, Willemse J. Substitution of Carbamazepine by Oxcarbazepine in Epileptic Children. Poster at 16th Epilepsy International Congress, Hamburg, 1985.
264. Johannessen AC, Nielsen OA. Hyponatremia induced by oxcarbazepine. Epilepsy Res 1987;1:155.
265. van Heiningen PNM, Eve MD, Oosterhuis B, et al. The influence of age on the pharmacokinetics of the antiepileptic agent oxcarbazepine. Clin Pharmacol Ther 1991;50:410.
266. Pierce MW, Suzdak PD, Gustavson LE, et al. Tiagabine. In F Pisani, E Perucca, G Avanzini, A Richens (eds), New Antiepileptic Drugs (Epilepsy Res Suppl 3). Amsterdam: Elsevier 1991;157.
267. During M, Mattson R, Scheyer R, et al. The effect of tiagabine HCl on extracellular GABA levels in the human hippocampus. Epilepsia 1992;33(Suppl 3):83.
268. Chadwick D, Richens A, Duncan J, et al. Tiagabine HCl: safety and efficacy as adjunctive treatment for complex partial seizures. Epilepsia 1991;32(Suppl 3):20.
269. Richens A, Chadwick D, Duncan J, et al. Safety and efficacy of tiagabine HCl as adjunctive treatment for complex partial seizures. Epilepsia 1992;33(Suppl 3):119.
270. Leppik I, So E, Rask CA, et al. Pharmacokinetic study of tiagabine HCl in patients at multiple steady-state doses. Epilepsia 1993;34(Suppl 6):35.
271. Mengel H, Gustavson EL, Soerensen HJ, et al. Effect of food on the bioavailability of tiagabine HCl. Epilepsia 1991;32(Suppl 3):6.
272. Richens A, Gustavson LE, McKelvy JF, et al. Pharmacokinetics and safety of single-dose tiagabine HCl in epileptic patients chronically treated with four other antiepileptic drug regimens. Epilepsia 1991;32(Suppl 3):12.

273. Bopp BA, Gustavson LE, Johnson MK, et al. Disposition and metabolism of orally administered 14C-tiagabine in humans. Epilepsia 1992;33(Suppl 3):83.
274. Maryanoff BE, Nortey SO, Gardocki JF, et al. Anticonvulsant O-Alkyl sulfamates. 2,3:4,5-BIS-O-(1methylethylidene)-β-D-fructopyranose sulfamate and related compounds. J Med Chem 1987; 30:880.
275. Shank RP, Vaught JL, Raffa RB, et al. Investigation of the mechanism of topiramate's anticonvulsant activity. Epilepsia 1991;32(Suppl 3):7.
276. Shank RP, Gardocki JF, Vaught JL, et al. Topiramate: preclinical evaluation of a structurally novel anticonvulsant. Epilepsia 1994;35:450.
277. Vaught JL, Maryanoff BE, Shank RP. The pharmacologic profile of topiramate: a structurally novel, clinically effective anticonvulsant. Epilepsia 1991;32(Suppl 3):19.
278. Edmonds HL Jr, Jiang D, Zhang YP, et al. Topiramate as a neuroprotectant and anticonvulsant in postischemic injury. Epilepsia 1992;33(Suppl 3):118.
279. Ben-Menachem E. Double-blind placebo-controlled trial of topiramate as add-on therapy for the treatment of complex partial seizures. Epilepsia 1992;33(Suppl 3):105.
280. Engelskjon T, Johannessen SI, Kloster R, et al. Long-term effect of topiramate in refractory partial epilepsy. Epilepsia 1993;34:123.
281. Mikkelsen M, Ostergaard L, Dam M. Topiramate as long-term treatment in refractory partial epilepsy. Epilepsia 1993;34(Suppl 2):123.
282. Rak IH, Isacoff JM. Topiramate (Topamax) add-on therapy in medically intractable epilepsy: clinical features and cognitive effects. Epilepsia 1993;34(Suppl 6):44.
283. Doose DR, Scott VV, Margul BL, et al. Multiple-dose pharmacokinetics of topiramate in healthy male subjects. Epilepsia 1988;29:662.
286. Wilensky AJ, Ojemann LM, Chamelir T, et al. Topiramate pharmacokinetics in epileptic patients receiving carbamazepine. Epilepsia 1989;31:645.
285. Doose DR, Gisclon LG, Stellar SM, et al. The effect of food on the bioavailability of topiramate from 100-and 400-mg tablets in healthy male subjects. Epilepsia 1992;33(Suppl 3):105.
286. Easterling DE, Zakszewski T, Moyer MD, et al. Plasma pharmacokinetics of topiramate, a new anticonvulsant in humans. Epilepsia 1988;29:662.
287. Floren KL, Graves NM, Leppik IE, et al. Pharmacokinetics of topiramate in patients with partial epilepsy receiving phenytoin and valproate. Epilepsia 1989;30:646.
288. Rosenfeld WE, Holmes GB, Hunt TL, et al. Topiramate-effective dosaging enhances potential for success. Epilepsia 1992;33(Suppl 1):118.
289. Wilder BJ . Antiepileptic drugs used in the emergency management of seizures and introduction of phenytoin prodrug. Epilepsia 1989;30(Suppl 2).
290. Rock DM, Macdonald RL, Taylor CP. Blockade of sustained repetitive action potentials in cultured spinal cord neurons by zonisamide. Epilepsy Res 1989;3:138.
291. Ramsay RE, Wilder BJ, Sackellares JC, et al. Multicenter study on the efficacy of zonisamide in the treatment of medically refractory complex partial seizures. Epilepsia 1984;25:673.
292. Wilensky AJ, Friel PN, Ojemann LM, et al. Zonisamide: a pilot study. Epilepsia 1985;26:212.
293. Takeda A, Inaguma J, Shimizu A. Treatment of intractable epilepsy with a new antiepileptic drug, zonisamide. J Jpn Pharmacol Ther 1987;15:397.
294. Shuto H, Sugimoto T, Yasuhara A, et al. Efficacy of zonisamide in children with refractory partial seizures. Curr Ther Res Clin Exp 1989;45:1031.
295. Sackellares JC, Donofrio PD, Wagner JG, et al. Pilot study of zonisamide (1,2-ben-zisoxazole-3-methanesulfonamide) in patients with refractory partial seizures. Epilepsia 1985;26:206.
296. Meldrum BS, Croucher MJ. Anticonvulsant action of clobazam and desmethyl-clobazam in reflex epilepsy in rodents and baboons. Drug Dev Res 1982; (Suppl 1):33.

297. Shorvon SD. Benzodiazepines. Clobazam. In RH Levy, FE Dreifuss, RH Mattson, et al. (eds), Antiepileptic Drugs (3rd ed). New York: Raven, 1989;821.

298. Oxley J. Tolerance to the Antiepileptic Effect of Clobazam in Patients with Severe Epilepsy. In H-H Freu Froscher, WP Koella, WP Meinardi (eds), Tolerance to the Beneficial and Adverse Effects of Antiepileptic Drugs. New York: Raven, 1986.

299. Muir KT, Palmer GC. Remacemide. In F Pisani, E Perucca, G Avanzini, A Richens (eds), New Antiepileptic Drugs (Epilepsy Research Suppl 3). Amsterdam: Elsevier, 1991;147.

300. Subramaniam S, Donevan SD, Rogawski MA. 1,2-diphenyl-2-propylamine, a major metabolite of the anticonvulsant remacemide, produces a stereoselective block of NMDA receptor currents. Society for Neuroscience Abstracts 1993;19:717.

301. Overweg J, Binnie CD. Flunarizine, In M Dam, L Gram (eds). Comprehensive Epileptology. New York: Raven, 1991;655.

302. Meldrum BS, Porter RJ (eds). Current Problems in Epilepsy 4. New Anticonvulsant Drugs. London: Libbey, 1986.

303. Rogawski M, Porter RJ. Antiepileptic drugs: pharmacological mechanisms and clinical efficacy with consideration of promising developmental stage compounds. Pharmacol Rev 1990;42:223.

304. Levy RH, Dreifuss FE, Mattson RH, et al. (eds). Antiepileptic Drugs (3rd ed). New York: Raven, 1989.

305. Pisani F, Perucca E, Avanzini G, Richens A (eds). New Antiepileptic Drugs (Epilepsy Research Suppl 3). Amsterdam: Elsevier, 1991.

306. Dam M, Gram L (eds). Comprehensive Epileptology. New York: Raven, 1991.

307. Ramsay RE. Advances in the pharmacotherapy of epilepsy. Epilepsia 1993;34(Suppl 5):9.

20

New Antiepileptic Drugs: Age-Related Efficacy

John M. Pellock

Although the seizures of many patients with epilepsy are well controlled with existing medications, perhaps 25% or more patients have either uncontrolled seizures or significant adverse effects.[1] Certain individuals with epilepsy who do not respond to medication should be considered for surgical treatment. This group, however, is limited in number, and a quest for more efficacious medications with fewer side effects continues. Particularly in the elderly, refractory epilepsy significantly limits day-to-day function.

The seizure types most frequently seen in the elderly are characterized by partial (focal) onset with or without secondary generalization. Multiple causes can be responsible, and there is often coexisting medical illness. Consideration of the general state of health of the patient, in fact, makes surgical treatment less likely; thus, chronic antiepilepsy drug (AED) therapy must be the primary treatment modality. Also, because of numerous medications that elderly patients may be taking for concomitant disease, the choice of AED therapy must be considered carefully.

Three new medications have recently been approved by the U.S. Food and Drug Administration (FDA) for the treatment of epilepsy. These are felbamate (Felbatol) (FBM), gabapentin (Neurontin) (GBP), and lamotrigine (Lamictal) (LTG). In addition to these new AEDs, oxcarbazepine, tiagabine, topiramate, vigabatrin (VGB), and zonisamide are in development. Fosphenytoin (Cerebyx), a water-soluble phenytoin pro-drug for parental use, and the extended-release form of carbamazepine (Tegretol XR) using a patented OROS osmotic release delivery system have also been released. In addition, modifications of product formulation are in progress, including intravenous valproate (Depakote) (VPA), and a diazepam preparation for rectal administration (Diastat). Thus, the future management of epilepsy is likely to change for patients with poorly controlled seizures or for those who experience side effects on their current therapies. This chapter concentrates primarily on the three drugs recently approved by the FDA and vigabatrin, which has been marketed outside the United States for a number of years. The discussion focuses on issues of clinical use of the new AEDs and is intended to complement Chapter 19, in which mechanisms of action,

Table 20.1 Probable spectrum of new antiepileptic medications

Antiepileptic Medication	Seizure/Epilepsy Type					
	Partial	Primary Generalized	Infantile Spasms	Lennox-Gastaut Syndrome	Myoclonic	Absence
Felbamate	+	+	+	+	+	+
Gabapentin	+	±	–	–	–	–
Lamotrigine	+	+	?	+	+	+
Oxcarbazepine	+	±	–	–	–	–
Vigabatrin	+	±	+	±	–	–

+ = efficacious, reported or highly suspected; – = no efficacy proven; ± = mixed results in population; ? = needs further evaluation, unknown.

pharmacology, and pharmacokinetics are discussed. Table 20.1 shows the probable clinical spectrum of each compound.

FELBAMATE

FBM was the first AED to be approved by the FDA in more than a decade. Its approval in 1993 is for use as monotherapy and adjunctive therapy in the treatment of partial seizures with and without generalization in adults with epilepsy, and as adjunctive therapy in the treatment of partial and generalized seizures associated with the Lennox-Gastaut syndrome in children.[2] This dicarbamate has a mechanism of action not fully elucidated, but recent studies suggest effects both on excitatory N-methyl-D-aspartate and inhibitory gamma-aminobutyric acid (GABA) mechanisms.[3] Thus, the pharmacologic profile of FBM differs from that of established AEDs and suggests a broad range of clinical activity against both partial and generalized seizures. The efficacy of FBM was therefore assessed in major clinical trials involving several innovative study designs.[2] Four of these trials used FBM as add-on therapy. Before the initiation of controlled studies, an open-label study was performed in 15 patients undergoing presurgical evaluation because of refractory partial onset seizures with and without secondary generalization. FBM reduced the high seizure frequency triggered by rapid reduction of AEDs, improved seizure control despite its substitution for prior AEDs, was relatively well tolerated when rapidly titrated over a 3-day period to 3,600 mg/day, and demonstrated a favorable adverse experience profile. Mean seizure frequency increased from 17 per month during the lead-in phase to 62 per month during the phase of reduction or discontinuation of baseline AEDs. Seizure counts decreased to 36 per month during the 3-day titration period, with a further decrease to nine per month during the 6-week treatment phase. An approximate 50% decrease in overall seizure frequency was observed during the FBM treatment phase compared with the lead-in phase. Seven of the 15 patients had at least a 50% decrease in their seizure frequency, and two patients became seizure-free during the 6-week FBM therapy phase.

A double-blind, placebo-controlled presurgical evaluation in 64 patients with refractory partial seizures followed a similar design.[4] In this trial, patients were randomized to groups who took either placebo or FBM, which was titrated over 3 days. After an 8-day hospitalization, the patients were discharged and followed for 21 days. Using time to occurrence of a fourth seizure as a primary efficacy variable, 46% of the patients in the FBM group had a fourth seizure before completing the 28-day treatment period, compared with 88% in the placebo group. Of the 15 patients taking FBM who successfully completed 4 weeks of double-blind treatment without a fourth seizure, all had at least a 50% reduction in seizure frequency, and four became seizure-free.

The efficacy of FBM as monotherapy in patients with partial onset seizures with or without secondary generalization was assessed in two trials that used low-dose VPA (15 mg/kg/day) as an active control.[5, 6] These trials were not intended to compare FBM with VPA. Rather, the intent of low-dose VPA treatment for the control group was to provide protection against severe seizure exacerbations. A total of 155 patients were treated with these protocols. Standard AEDs were gradually reduced and discontinued after the initial 28 days of treatment. Those taking FBM, 3,600 mg/day in four divided doses, were compared with those taking VPA with respect to those who met escape criteria and those who completed 112 days of treatment. The primary efficacy variable was the number of patients in each treatment group who had any of the following escape criteria: (1) doubling of baseline monthly seizure frequency, (2) doubling of the highest baseline 2-day seizure frequency, (3) a single generalized tonic-clonic seizure if none had occurred during baseline, or (4) significant prolongation of a generalized tonic-clonic seizure (including several seizures or status epilepticus). The difference in percentage of patients meeting escape criteria was statistically significant ($P < .001$) in favor of those taking FBM: 27 (60%) versus 11 (22%) were able to complete the 112 study days. Conversely, 18 (40%) receiving FBM met escape criteria, compared with 39 (78%) of those receiving VPA.

Among the 27 FBM patients who completed 112 study days in the multicentered trial, the average number of seizures per month decreased from 13.2 at baseline to 8.2 at the end of monotherapy, with 70% reporting some reduction in seizure frequency and 48% having at least a 50% reduction.

In 1991, Leppik et al.[7] reported the results of a double-blind, placebo-controlled trial with FBM as add-on therapy in patients with refractory partial onset seizures. The average FBM dose during this study was approximately 2,300 mg/day in three divided doses—a total daily dose below that recommended at present. Nevertheless, the mean seizure frequency decreased by 4.95 seizures with FBM but increased by 0.36 seizures with placebo.

The Lennox-Gastaut syndrome is an extremely difficult to manage encephalopathic epilepsy with typical onset in childhood. Some institutionalized patients, however, continue to suffer from multiple seizure types, both generalized and partial, throughout their lives. Taking FBM versus placebo was evaluated as treatment in this very difficult group. FBM was initiated at 15 mg/kg/day in four divided doses and gradually increased to either 45 mg/kg/day or to 3,600 mg/day, whichever was less.[8] Patients were evaluated according to caretaker seizure counts and comparison of video-electroencephalogram (EEG) telemetry sessions. A total of 73 patients were randomized to either treatment. Three patients treated with FBM had no seizures during the treatment phase, and six had no seizures during the period in which maintenance of optimal dosage occurred. Compared with the baseline phase, FBM patients were reported to experience a mean reduction in atonic seizures of 34%, whereas placebo patients experienced a 9% reduction. Similar decreases were seen for generalized tonic-clonic seizures, myoclonic seizures and atypical absence seizures. Fifty percent of the 36 FBM-treated patients had at least a 50% improvement in the frequency of all types of seizures. In addition, global evaluations during the maintenance period were significantly higher in the FBM-treated group compared with the placebo-treated group, suggesting an overall improvement in the quality of life by increasing alertness and verbal responsiveness in these retarded individuals. The improvement occurring in the double-blind study of Lennox-Gastaut patients has been sustained for at least 12 months in subsequent open-label studies. Those previously randomized to placebo subsequently received FBM, and similar improvement was noted both in seizure reduction and alertness.[9]

In premarketing studies, the adverse experience profile for FBM revealed that this AED was relatively well tolerated. The most common adverse reactions in adults during FBM monotherapy were anorexia, vomiting, insomnia, nausea, and headache. When FBM is administered as adjunctive therapy, dizziness and somnolence were more frequently reported. In all studies and in clinical practice, the incidence of the most commonly occurring adverse experiences was higher when FBM was given as adjunctive treatment rather than monotherapy. This suggests that at least some adverse effects are likely due to drug interactions between FBM and other AEDs. In two of the controlled clinical trials, only anorexia tended to persist when patients were converted from adjunctive to monotherapy. The multiple interactions involving FBM and other AEDs reviewed in Chapter 19 produce a variety of pharmacokinetic and pharmacodynamic effects and thus amplify the reported adverse reactions when FBM is prescribed as adjunctive therapy.

The long-term safety of FBM was initially demonstrated in multiple open-label clinical trials and continues to be monitored as the drug is marketed. During long-term studies in adults, specific events with an incidence of 1% or more associated with patient withdrawal were anorexia, nausea, rash, and weight loss. Although no significant laboratory abnormalities were identified during the initial studies of FBM, postmarketing surveillance has identified more than 30 cases of aplastic anemia associated with FBM administration. Bone marrow aplasia, an apparent idiosyncratic reaction, has typically developed between a few weeks and nearly 1 year after initiation of FBM treatment. The sponsor and the FDA recommended on August 1, 1994, that the use of FBM be suspended unless, in the physician's judgment, an abrupt withdrawal would pose a more serious risk to the patient.[10] In addition, hepatic failure has been reported in patients receiving FBM, perhaps further limiting its use.[10a] For this reason, use is presently limited to patients who accept the risk and seemingly have no other treatment alternatives. Blood counts and clinical symptoms should be monitored on a periodic basis. A small number of patients have developed hyponatremia during FBM therapy, perhaps similar to that associated with carbamazepine, but no mechanism has been identified. Although no exact therapeutic plasma levels for FBM have been established, efficacy has been noted between 18 µg/ml and 150 µg/ml.

In adults, FBM treatment should begin with a dose of 1,200 mg/day orally in two to three divided doses (using the 400- or 600-mg tablets). It is recommended that, within a few days to a week, FBM dosage be increased by 400 mg/day. FBM should then be titrated to clinical response, with the "maximum" dose presently recommended at 3,600 mg/day. This upper limit of dosing is currently being investigated, and some patients show better responses at even higher doses (at least 4,800 mg/day). Limited clinical data in patients older than 65 years old treated with FBM are available, but no restrictions have been placed in this population. FBM is contraindicated in those who have shown hypersensitivity reactions, especially to other carbamates. Most hypersensitivity reactions have been reported during the initial 2–3 weeks of therapy. Symptoms include rash, fever, swelling of mucus membranes, anaphylaxis, leukopenia, thrombocytopenia, elevated liver function testing, arthralgia, myalgia, and pharyngitis. When FBM is used as adjunctive therapy with other AEDs (or other drugs that induce or inhibit hepatic enzymes), special allowance should be made for known drug interactions. Administration of FBM in patients treated with phenytoin, VPA, or both may require dosage decrease of these AEDs. Interactions are dose-dependent and subject to individual patient variability, but both phenytoin and VPA are likely to increase if not adjusted downward. Because FBM decreases CBZ steady-state plasma concentrations by approximately 25% and increases CBZ 10,11-epoxide levels by approximately 50%, CBZ dosage may be kept constant or be adjusted based on clinical observation. The manufacturer suggests that conversion to monotherapy be done whenever possible.[11] Thus, for adults, 1,200 mg/day initial dosing is given during the first week, and doses of original AEDs are decreased by 20–33%. During the second week, therapy is further titrated by increasing FBM to 2,400 mg/day while reducing original dose of AEDs by up to an additional one-third. At the third week, the reduction of initial AEDs is further recommended as indicated, and FBM is increased to 3,600 mg/day. Clinical investigators and other prescribers of FBM have noted that slower initiation schedules of FBM have resulted in fewer adverse effects, especially nausea, rather than the schedules used in studies in which patients were titrated to 3,600 mg over a period of 3 days. For some patients, each dosage change is better done at intervals of 2–3 weeks rather than at weekly epochs. FBM is an efficacious drug for the treatment of both partial and generalized seizures, but the occurrence of idiosyncratic aplastic anemia needs to be further analyzed before widespread use can continue. Drug interactions and the particularly annoying side effects of headache, insomnia, and anorexia and weight loss must be monitored. For some, these symptoms are dose-related, and most adverse effects are decreased by using FBM as monotherapy. Additional information concerning the true incidence and risks for aplastic anemia and other possible idiosyncratic reactions will determine the eventual place of this new AED.

GABAPENTIN

GBP is an antiepilepsy agent structurally related to GABA. Despite its structural similarity to GABA, it does not mechanistically resemble this compound, but instead it binds to a novel high-affinity binding site in the central nervous system (CNS).[12] This agent has shown particular activity against partial seizures with or without secondary generalization. GBP is not bound to plasma proteins and is not metabolized, properties of particular interest with regard to elderly patients, who are likely to be on multiple medications. Thus, it does not interact with AEDs or most medications that undergo hepatic metabolism. GBP is eliminated through the kidneys, and, if renal insufficiently is present, its dosing should be adjusted in accordance with renal function as determined by creatinine clearance.[12]

The efficacy of GBP as adjunctive therapy was established in three multicenter, placebo-controlled, double-blind, parallel group clinical trials involving adults with refractory partial seizures. Effectiveness was assessed primarily on the basis of the percent of patients with a 50% or more reduction in seizure frequency from baseline to treatment. A derived measure termed *response ratio* (RR) was used to express the effectiveness of the drug. RR equals $T - B$ divided by $T + B$, where T is the seizure frequency during treatment and B is the seizure frequency during baseline. Thus, negative values indicate a reduction in the number of seizures during treatment, positive values indicate an increase in seizures, and an RR ratio of -0.33 represents a 50% reduction in seizure frequency from baseline to treatment period. In a study comparing patients receiving GBP, 1,200 mg/day given in three divided doses, with patients taking placebo, the responder rate was 23% in the GBP group versus 9% in the placebo group.[13] A second study compared patients receiving GBP, 600, 1,200, or 1,800 mg/day, with patients receiving placebo.[14] The percentage of patients experiencing at least a 50% reduction in seizure frequency was 8% among placebo-treated patients and ranged from 18–26% for patients who received GBP. As would be expected, there was an incremental improvement from placebo to those receiving 1,800 mg in terms of seizure reduction. The GBP group also experienced improvement in secondarily generalized and simple partial seizures.

In both premarketing studies and reports since the release of GBP, adverse events have been mild and transient, occurring at slightly higher frequency in patients receiving GBP than in those receiving placebo in combination with background AEDs. GBP does not affect serum concentrations of concurrent AEDs and does not produce significant changes in clinical laboratory values. The most frequently occurring adverse events included somnolence, dizziness, ataxia, fatigue, nystagmus, headache, tremor, nausea or vomiting, and diplopia[14] (Parke-Davis, data on file). In the U.S. GBP study comparing patients taking placebo with those taking 600, 1,200, and 1,800 mg/day of GBP, seven (3%) of the 208 patients who received GBP and one (1%) of the 98 patients who received placebo withdrew due to adverse events.[14] The median time for most neurotoxic events to resolve was 2 weeks. Interestingly, reports of adverse experiences did not specifically correlate to GBP dose.

GBP is a novel AED presently recommended for use as adjunctive therapy for the treatment of refractory partial seizures with or without secondary generalization. Because it is not actively metabolized and is instead excreted unchanged in the urine, it has no drug interactions. Thus, GBP is an optimal agent when patients are receiving multiple medications, as is frequently the case with the aged. At present, although doses of 1,800 mg/day are typically recommended, dosage is being extended to 2,400 mg/day routinely and to 4,800 mg/day or more in refractory patients. In the elderly, dosage adjustment may be necessary because of impaired renal function. Monotherapy studies are underway.

LAMOTRIGINE

LTG is chemically unrelated to marketed AEDs. It is a member of the phenylhydrazine class[15] and is one of the major new antiepileptic medications now becoming available throughout the world. Although LTG was derived from a line of drugs that inhibit dihydrofolate reductase and is a relatively weak antifolate compound, it demonstrates anticonvulsant effects in maximal electroshock and pentylenetetrazol models of epilepsy. Similarly, in clinical studies, it has shown a broad range of activity against both partial and generalized seizures of both convulsive and nonconvulsive types.[15, 16]

Efficacy in adults with partial seizures was demonstrated in eight double-blind, placebo-controlled, add-on, crossover, parallel-design studies that produced significant evidence that LTG is effective and safe as add-on therapy in patients with treatment resistant partial seizures.[16] The median reduction in frequency of partial seizures in LTG-treated patients, compared with that in patients who took placebo, ranged from 17% to 59%. These patients received doses that were between 75 mg/day and 400 mg/day. LTG produced a reduction of at least 25% in seizure frequency in 48% and a reduction of at least 50% in 23% of patients studied. A 6-month, parallel-design study[17] revealed a median reduction in frequency of all partial seizures in 8% of placebo controls, in 20% of patients receiving 300 mg/day of LTG, and in 36% receiving 500 mg/day of LTG. During these studies, the investigators' global evaluations further indicated that approximately 50% reported an improved outcome while receiving LTG as compared with those taking the placebo. Some subjects anecdotally, but spontaneously, reported a sense of well being while taking LTG.[18] The conclusions from these studies are that LTG is efficacious when used as add-on therapy in patients with refractory partial seizures, particularly at doses of 200–500 mg/day, and that higher doses may be more beneficial in some patients. In follow-up, open studies, daily LTG doses have been increased to 700 mg/day, with some patients showing superior efficacy at higher doses.[17] We have found that patients better tolerated higher doses when concomitant AEDs were reduced or discontinued. Controlled studies assessing the efficacy of LTG in children are currently in progress. Open-label, add-on studies of both refractory partial and generalized seizures suggest efficacy not only in partial seizures in adults and children, but also in refractory encephalopathic epilepsies such as the Lennox-Gastaut syndrome that begins in childhood and persists throughout life.[19] Thus, in elderly adults with either partial or symptomatic generalized epilepsy, LTG may produce a significant benefit.

The adverse experiences noted in controlled studies were generally minor, and most frequently were of CNS-related neurotoxicity, including ataxia, dizziness, diplopia, and headache. Most were transient and resolved without patients discontinuing treatment. In the controlled add-on clinical trials, 6.9% of patients who received LTG were discontinued due to an adverse effect, compared with 2.9% of those who received placebo. The frequency of treatment-emergent adverse experiences in the study of 98 patients receiving LTG as adjunctive therapy indicates that 5% of the LTG treated patients withdrew, compared with 1% of those receiving placebo. Ataxia, dizziness, diplopia, and somnolence were the neurotoxic symptoms, showing a statistically significant difference between LTG and placebo-treated groups. Besides neurotoxicity, rash has also been experienced in patients receiving LTG. Dermatologic reactions associated with LTG have most frequently been described as maculopapular in nature but have been in rare circumstances more serious, with erythema multiforme or Stevens-Johnson reactions being noted. Rash may be somewhat more common when VPA is administered along with LTG therapy, and with rapid dose escalation after initiating therapy.

Thus, LTG is a promising new AED indicated for the treatment of partial seizures that may secondarily generalize. Ongoing studies also suggest a significant role for LTG in the treatment of generalized epilepsy, including encephalopathic types.[20,20a] The dose administered is dependent on concomitant AED therapy such that recommended daily doses of LTG in adults range from 200 mg to 500 mg in divided doses twice daily. Lower initial and daily maintenance doses should be given to patients receiving VPA, as VPA inhibits the metabolism of LTG. Patients receiving enzyme-inducing AEDs may require slightly higher LTG doses. In most patients, LTG should be adjusted gradually at weekly intervals. If later withdrawal of enzyme-inducing AEDs is attempted, LTG should be reduced. Several studies suggest that a pharmacodynamic interaction that produces slightly more dose-related CNS-associated side effects such as diplopia may be related in part to an elevation in carbamazepine epoxide. Although not consistently shown, the resulting symptoms can be managed by lowering the dose of coadministered CBZ or other AEDs. Continuation studies in the United States have led to the administration of LTG as monotherapy in doses up to 700 mg/day. Increases in doses are sometimes not possible during concomitant therapy, but tolerance is quite good when LTG monotherapy is administered. Monotherapy studies comparing LTG with CBZ and with PHT have demonstrated equal efficacy in partial seizures. In addition, some patients have experienced more efficacious seizure control with these higher doses of LTG. Additional studies showing efficacy in other types of epilepsy and when using LTG as monotherapy are underway.

VIGABATRIN

VGB (gamma-vinyl-GABA) was the first of the new wave of antiepilepsy medications available in many parts of the world. Its development has, however, been slowed in the United States because of findings of toxicity in animals that have not been duplicated in primates or human studies. VGB is a synthetic GABA derivative that acts as an irreversible inhibitor of GABA-transaminase. In animal studies, it demonstrates efficacy in a wide variety of seizure models.[20] VGB was synthesized in 1974, and clinical trials began in 1982. These trials quickly demonstrated the efficacy of this agent in the treatment of partial seizures. Further studies were suspended in the United States for 5 years because of myelin vacuolization seen in rodents and dogs. As no such findings were present in primates or human autopsy or biopsy studies, the FDA has permitted resumption of VGB clinical testing in the United States.

VGB has been mainly studied and used to treat patients with refractory partial epilepsy as adjunctive therapy. In both adults and children, the results have been favorable, particularly in patients with partial seizures. Mumford and Dam[21] reviewed nine European placebo-controlled studies of VGB as adjunctive therapy. The incidence of patients showing at least a 50% improvement in seizure frequency ranged from 33% to 64%, with seven studies revealing at least a 50% improvement in more than one-half of subjects. Most adults do well at doses of 1,500–3,000 mg/day.[20] Adverse experiences associated with VGB administration are usually mild and include sleepiness, fatigue, confusion, and gastrointestinal upset.[22] Sander et al. have reported, however, that a small number of patients have developed depression or psychosis while receiving VGB for epilepsy. Continued monitoring for the exact incidence of behavioral toxicity continues. In some patients with refractory encephalopathic epilepsy (infantile spasms and Lennox-Gastaut syndrome), additional efficacy has been noted. Tolerance does not seem to develop after long-term use and adverse cognitive effects are minimal.[23]

Thus, VGB is an efficacious drug for the treatment of epilepsy, particularly as adjunctive therapy for those with resistant partial seizures. Approval for use in the United States is pending.

CONCLUSION

Numerous medications continue to be investigated for the treatment of epilepsy that is refractory to standard available AEDs. Three new compounds already have been released in the United States: FBM, GBP, and LTG. Aplastic anemia and hepatic failure have been associated with FBM treatment in postmarketing surveillance studies. Long-term use patterns assessing efficacy and tolerance will determine the use of these AEDs in the future. In the meantime, other compounds continue in clinical developmental trials. Special considerations for using these agents in elderly patients with epilepsy require an understanding of pharmacokinetic parameters and possible drug interactions that may affect drug use in this population.

REFERENCES

1. Mattson RH, Cramer JA, Collins JF, et al. Comparison of carbamazepine, pheno-barbital, phenytoin and primidone in partial and secondary generalized tonic-clonic seizures. N Engl J Med 1985;313:145.
2. Pellock JM, Boggs JG. Felbamate: a unique anticonvulsant. Drugs of Today 1995;31:9.
3. Rho JM, Donevan SD, Rogawski MA. Mechanisms of action of the anticonvulsant felbamate: opposing effects on N-methyl-D-aspartate and r-aminobastzrine acid$_A$ receptors. Ann Neurol 1994;35:229.
4. Bourgeois B, Lippik IE, Sackallares JV, et al. Felbamate: a double-blind controlled trial in patients undergoing presurgical evaluation of partial seizures. Neurology 1993;43:693.
5. Faught E, Sachdeo RC, Remler MP, et al. Felbamate monotherapy for partial seizures: an active-control study. Neurology 1993;43:688.
6. Sachdeo RS, Kramer LD, Rosenberg A, Sachdeo S. Felbamate monotherapy: controlled trial in patients with partial onset seizures. Ann Neurol 1992;32:386.
7. Leppik IE, Dreifuss FE, Pledger GW, et al. Felbamate for partial seizures: results of a controlled clinical trial. Neurology 1991;41:1785.
8. Risner ME and the Lamictal Study Group. Multicenter, double-blind, add-on, crossover study of lamotrigine (Lamictal) in epileptic outpatients with partial seizures. Epilepsia 1990;31:619.
9. Ramsay RE, Pellock JM, Garnett WR, et al. Pharmacokinetics and safety of lamotrigine (Lamictal) in patients with epilepsy. Epilepsy Res 1991;10:191.
10. Food and Drug Administration Letter, Felbamate August, 1994.
10a. Brodie MJ, Pellock JM. Taming the brain storms: felbamate update. Lancet 1995;346:918.
11. Felbamate package insert, Wallace Laboratories, Cranbury, NJ, 1993.
12. Taylor CP, Vartanian MG, Yuen P-W, et al. Potent and stereospecific anticonvulsant activity of 3-isobutyl GABA relates to in-vitro binding at a novel site labeled by titrated gabapentin. Epilepsy Res 1993;14:11.
13. U.K. Gabapentin Study Group. Gabapentin in partial epilepsy. Lancet 1990;335:1114.
14. The U.S. Gabapentin Study Group No. 5. Gabapentin as add-on therapy in refractory partial epilepsy: a double-blind, placebo-controlled, parallel-group study. Neurology 1993;43:2292.
15. Goa KL, Ross SR, Chrisp P. Lamotrigine: a review of its pharmacological properties and clinical efficacy in epilepsy. Drugs 1993;46:152.
16. Pellock JM. The clinical efficacy of lamotrigine as an antiepileptic drug. Neurology 1994;44(Suppl 8):S29.

17. Messenheimer J, Ramsay RE, Willmore LJ, et al. Lamotrigine therapy for partial seizures: a multicenter, placebo-controlled, double-blind, cross-over trial. Epilepsia 1994;35:113.
18. Pellock JM, Rao C, Earl N. Lamotrigine efficacy and safety update—U.S. experience. Epilepsia 1993;34:42.
19. Hosking G, Spencer S, Yuen AWC. Lamotrigine in children with severe developmental abnormalities in a paediatric population with refractory seizures. Epilepsia 1993;6:42.
20. Fisher R. Emerging antiepileptic drugs. Neurology 1993;43(Suppl 5):12.
20a. Fitton A, Goa KL. Lamotrigine. An update of its pharmacology and therapeutic use in epilepsy. Drugs 1995;50:691.
21. Mumford JP, Dam M. Meta-anaylsis of European placebo-controlled studies of vigabatrin in drug resistant epilepsy. Br J Clin Pharmacol 1989;27:101.
22. Sander JW, Hart YM, Trimble MR, et al. Vigabatrin and psychosis. J Neurol Neurosurg Psychiatry 1991;54:435.
23. Dodrill CB, Amett JL, Sommerville KW, Sussman NM. Evaluation of the effects of vigabatrin on cognitive abilities and quality of life in epilepsy. Neurology 1993;43:2501.

21

Drug Interactions in the Elderly with Epilepsy

Ilo E. Leppik and Denise Wolff

INTRODUCTION

Medications administered with therapeutic intent have the potential to interact with other exogenously administered medications as well as with endogenous compounds. These interactions can range from alterations in the pharmacokinetic profile of the parent compound and its metabolites to pharmacodynamic changes. These interactions may result in effects such as increased efficacy, decreased efficacy, toxicity, or unexpected adverse effects.

Antiepileptic medications (AEMs) have been found to be involved in many clinically significant drug interactions. When used in combination for the treatment of the refractory epilepsy patient, interactions among AEMs have been well documented.[1] Drug interactions between AEMs and non-antiepileptic medications (non-AEMs) have also been identified.[2–4]

The extent to which a drug interaction occurs varies significantly among individuals. This variability can be due to genetic, environmental, and demographic factors. As might be surmised, the presence of two medications that have the potential to interact with each other pharmacodynamically, pharmacokinetically, or both in combination with potential genetic variability in physiologic and pharmacokinetic response, plus environmental and demographic contributors, makes the anticipation and management of interaction(s) challenging.

Pharmacogenetics is the study of genetically determined variations in drug response.[5] Genetic influences on drug action may be due to effects on an individual's pharmacodynamic and pharmacokinetic response to a particular medication.[5] When pharmacogenetic alteration is identified or suspected, medications should be used with caution in the patient and family.[5] Ethnic origin also has been identified as a factor contributing to genetically based alterations in pharmacokinetic behavior of some drugs and should be a consideration when choosing and monitoring a chosen pharmacotherapy.

Environmental factors have been linked to abnormal medication response and have been shown to have the potential for involvement at sites of absorption, distribution, protein binding, drug-cell interaction, metabolism, and excretion.[5] As one might expect, more than one independent variable may modulate any particular process, and the task of differentiating between genetic and environmental factors is quite difficult.

Demographic parameters such as gender, race, and age are important variables to consider when evaluating the risk for and magnitude of a medication interaction. Gender can be a factor, as males and females have the potential to metabolize and eliminate some drugs differently. The elderly constitute a special patient group having an increased risk for the development of drug interaction. Physiologic aging, although not necessarily paralleling chronologic aging, does occur, thereby having the potential to effect pharmacodynamic and pharmacokinetic parameters of medications. In addition, the elderly have been found to be at greater risk for noncompliance due to omission of doses, errors in frequency of dosing, intentional or unintentional overdosing, taking of medications for the wrong purpose, and use of medications prescribed for others.[6] One study found that approximately 40% of the elderly patients were not using their medication exactly as prescribed and that approximately 90% of those cases were due to underdosing, of which nearly 75% was unintentional.[7, 8] Characteristics that contribute to noncompliance in this population include multiple physicians, multiple pharmacies, multiple chronic diseases, multiple drugs, and multiple doses during the day.[6]

FOCUS ON THE ELDERLY

When correlating patterns of prescription medication use within age groups, it has been observed that the elderly consume a significant amount of medication, due largely to the development of pathologic conditions. In 1981, although 12% of the United States population was older than age 65 years, this group consumed 30% of all prescription drugs.[9] In a group of approximately 3,000 ambulatory people older than age 65 years screened for undetected medical illness, it was reported that 93% of patients took at least one medication within a 5-year period of time, and the mean drug use increased from 3.2 to 3.7 medications per patient during the period of observation.[10] It was noted that women consumed more medications than did men, and medication use increased with age. An increased medication use with age was also noted in the Iowa 65+ Rural Health Study, in which 13% of patients ages 65–69 years did not use any prescription medications, compared with only 7% of the individuals older than age 85 years.[11] The mean number of medications per respondent was 2.9.

It has thus been established that the elderly population, due to the need for medication treatment of various disease states that increase in incidence with age, are at an increased risk for polytherapy. One pathophysiologic disorder that increases in incidence with age is epilepsy.[12, 13] The fact that the primary treatment option for epilepsy is medication therapy creates a special concern for AEM and non-AEM interactions. When assessing the medications at highest risk for potential interaction in the elderly, it is relevant to focus attention on the non-AEM use patterns that have been observed. Table 21.1 lists the top 20 medications prescribed in the elderly in 1989 within the Pennsylvania

Table 21.1 Antiepileptic medication interactions[a] with the top 20 medications used by the elderly[b]

Medication	Antiepileptic Medication	Effect	Mechanism
Diltiazem	CBZ	Increased CBZ serum concentration	Inhibited CBZ metabolism
Furosemide	PHT	Decreased diuretic effect	Possible decreased bioavailability of furosemide
Ranitidine	BZ	Impaired or enhanced effect of BZ	Possible altered bioavailability
Nifedipine	Barbiturates	Decreased nifedipine concentration in the blood	Increased hepatic metabolism of nifedipine
Digoxin	BZ	Increased digoxin serum concentration	Unknown
	PHT	Decreased digoxin serum concentration	Unknown; possible increased digoxin metabolism
Verapamil	Barbiturates	Decreased pharmacologic effect of verapamil	Decreased bioavailability due to increased first-pass metabolism
	PHT	Decreased verapamil serum concentration	Unknown; possible increased verapamil metabolism
Alprazolam	CBZ	Decreased alprazolam pharmacologic effect	Unknown; probable increased alprazolam metabolism
Diclofenac	PHT, VPA	Increased PHT or VPA unbound medication concentration	Protein binding displacement
Propoxyphene	Barbiturates	Increased barbiturate serum concentration	Unknown; probable decreased barbiturate metabolism
	BZ	Additive central nervous system effects	Decreased BZ metabolism
	CBZ	Increased CBZ concentration	Decreased CBZ metabolism
	PHT	Increased PHT concentration	Possible decreased PHT metabolism
Propranolol/ metoprolol	Barbiturates	Altered pharmacokinetic parameters of propranolol and metoprolol	Increased metabolism of propranolol and metoprolol
	BZ	Increased effects of BZ	Inhibited BZ metabolism
Glyburide	PHT	Increased blood glucose levels of PHT	Unknown

CBZ = carbamazepine; PHT = phenytoin; VPA = valproic acid; BZ = benzodiazepines.
Note: Barbiturates also include primidone.
[a]Drug Interactions as reported and published in January 1994 Facts and Comparisons Drug Interaction Index.
[b]From 1989 claims records of the Pennsylvania Pharmaceutical Assistance Contract for the Elderly (PACE) program.

Pharmaceutical Assistance Contract for the Elderly (PACE) program[14] cross-referenced with known interactions with AEMs.

The critical period for an interaction between two medications to develop and become clinically relevant is generally the first few weeks or months of therapy. Attentive clinical and laboratory monitoring during the period after drug initiation is essential for avoidance or management of the interaction.[4]

PHARMACODYNAMIC MEDICATION INTERACTIONS

It has been noted that the elderly generally have increased sensitivity to medications, a phenomenon that is clinically manifested as elevated responsiveness or increased incidence of unwanted side effects. This sensitivity varies with the drug studied and the response measured. Because of the physiologic changes that occur naturally with aging, it is difficult to generalize as to the cause of this sensitivity. A valid study of drug sensitivity requires measurement of drug concentrations at the site of action in order to differentiate between pharmacokinetic and pharmacodynamic alterations. Although this is often difficult, with the advent of detailed pharmacokinetic probes, it is now possible in many cases. Equal concentrations of medication at receptor sites in vivo in young and old individuals have been shown to produce differing effects.[6] This alteration in sensitivity probably relates to altered receptor function or decreased numbers of receptors.[6] Results from these analyses often show that pharmacokinetic rather than pharmacodynamic factors are implicated.[15] Nevertheless, it is thought that pharmacodynamic factors substantially contribute to altered responsiveness.

The most extensively studied AEMs with regard to interactions at the receptor site are the benzodiazepines and barbiturates. Both medication classes have been shown to modulate the activity of the gamma-aminobutyric (GABA)-type A receptor, which is coupled to the chloride channel.[16] This complex has a molecular weight of 215,000–355,000 daltons and contains additional subunits.[16] The action of barbiturates on this receptor involves an apparent increase in the number of high- and intermediate-affinity binding sites for the benodiazepines.[16] Interestingly, barbiturates can also inhibit the binding of benzodiazepine receptor "inverse agonists" or excitatory ligands. From this information, it might be suspected that phenobarbital and the antiepileptic benzodiazepines (clonazepam, nitrazepam, diazepam, clorazepate) might be useful in combination in the treatment of epilepsy. A synergistic anticonvulsant response among these agents has not been demonstrated, however, and, as mentioned previously, in the usual clinical setting the sedative effects of these agents individually often preclude their use in combination. In the treatment of status epilepticus, use of phenobarbital in patients previously treated with a benzodiazepine may increase the risk for respiratory arrest.

Table 21.2   Antiepileptic medication interactions with fluoxetine (Prozac)

Antiepileptic Medication	Interaction	Mechanism
BZ	Increased pharmacologic effect of BZ	Decreased BZ metabolism
CBZ	Increased CBZ concentration	Unknown; possible decreased CBZ metabolism
Hydantoins	Increased hydantoin concentration	Unknown; possible decreased hydantoin metabolism

BZ = benzodiazepines; CBZ = carbamazepine.

PHARMACOKINETIC MEDICATION INTERACTIONS

Changes in the pharmacokinetic parameters of a medication due to a medication interaction usually results from alterations in absorption, distribution, metabolism, or elimination. Some AEMs are very insoluble in aqueous solutions and thus are sensitive to any effects that alter solubility, dissolution, or gastrointestinal motility. Others are characterized by avid binding to plasma proteins, thereby allowing medications that alter protein binding to have an impact on serum concentrations of the unbound, pharmacologically active medication. The majority of AEMs are metabolized hepatically via similar pathways, including hydroxylation and glucuronidation. In general, they are converted from relatively water-insoluble compounds to water-soluble compounds. AEMs such as phenytoin, carbamazepine, and phenobarbital increase the hepatic clearance capability of certain P-450 isoenzyme systems, thereby increasing the clearance of concomitant similarly metabolized medications. Conversely, the AEMs valproic acid and felbamate appear to inhibit the metabolism of similarly metabolized concomitant medications due to a competitive process. Although fluoxetine (Prozac) is not on the 1989 top 20 list for the PACE program as discussed earlier, it is used frequently in many populations and appears to decrease the clearance of phenytoin, carbamazepine, and certain benzodiazepines, necessitating close monitoring (Table 21.2).

Phenytoin

Absorption

Phenytoin is very water-insoluble; however, 85–90% of an orally administered dose becomes bioavailable under normal circumstances. Differences in absorption significant enough to be associated with clinical toxicity occurred in the past due to changes in formulation excipient.[17] This was traced to replacement of calcium sulfate dihydrate with lactose, as the calcium compound interfered with phenytoin absorption. This problem has since been corrected. Data regarding the effect of antacids on the absorption of phenytoin have been conflicting, but in one study antacids containing aluminum hydroxide, magnesium hydroxide, and calcium carbonate decreased the bioavailability of phenytoin.[18] Enteral feedings significantly decrease the bioavailability of phenytoin. Administration of those compounds should occur 1 hour before or 2–3 hours after phenytoin administration.[19] Phenytoin has not been reported to alter the absorption of other drugs.

Binding

Phenytoin is highly bound to plasma protein, primarily albumin, with approximately 90% of the total plasma concentration represented in the bound form.[20] Because a medication must be unbound to be pharmacologically active, in the case of phenytoin, only 10% of the medication present elicits the pharmacologic effect. If another highly protein bound medication were to be added to a phenytoin regimen, displacement may occur, resulting in, for example, 85% of phenytoin bound to protein. The unbound concentration is now 15%, a 50% increase in active medication. Because the liver now has more unbound phenytoin to metabolize, total phenytoin serum concentrations decrease, yet the resulting percentage of free phenytoin is higher than previously, referred to as the free fraction. Thus, a person may exhibit signs of phenytoin intoxication even though the total concentration of phenytoin is similar to or even less that the concentration before the highly protein bound medication was added. In this situation, measuring free phenytoin concentrations before and after the addition of the concomitant medication will assist with interpretation of resultant clinical efficacy and toxicity.

The above-described protein-binding interaction is perhaps most often observed when the AEM valproic acid—90–95% protein-bound—is used with phenytoin. Non-AEMs that are highly protein-bound with the potential for displacement of phenytoin from its binding site include tolbutamide; salicylates; heparin; and nonsteroidal anti-inflammatory medications such as phenylbutazone, ibuprofen, or diclofenac, and warfarin.

Metabolism

Phenytoin also has the capability of inducing hepatic metabolism of certain P-450 isoenzyme systems, resulting in increased clearance of compounds metabolized in the same pathway (Table 21.3).

Carbamazepine

Absorption

Carbamazepine is a neutral lipophilic substance and is virtually insoluble in water. Its bioavailability is 55–86%. Time to maximal concentration (T_{max}) is variable and ranges from 3 to 12 hours after oral dosing. The addition of propylene glycol, polysorbate, or ethanol can accelerate the absorptive process and reduce the T_{max} to 1–4 hours as well as increase bioavailability. No definite interference with absorption due to the use of other medications has been documented.

Table 21.3 Interactions of phenytoin with other substances

Effect	Mechanism
Phenytoin concentrations decreased	
Ethanol (chronic)	Increased metabolism of phenytoin
Folic acid	Same as above
Nicotine	Same as above
Propoxyphene	Same as above
Phenobarbital	Same as above
Phenothiazines	Same as above
Rifampin	Same as above
Antacids	Decreased absorption
Diazoxide	Displacement from protein binding sites
Nonsteroidal anti-inflammatory drugs	Same as above
Tolbutamide	Same as above
Salicylates	Same as above
Valproic acid	Same as above
Phenytoin concentrations increased	Decreased metabolism of phenytoin
Amiodarone	Same as above
Chloramphenicol	Same as above
Chlordiazepoxide	Same as above
Cimetidine	Same as above
Dicumarol	Same as above
Disulfiram	Same as above
Halothane	Same as above
Isoniazid	Same as above
Miconazole	Same as above
Phenylbutazone	Same as above
Propranolol	Same as above
Sulfonamides	Same as above
Trazodone	Same as above
Viloxazine	Same as above
Concentrations reduced by phenytoin	
Carbamazepine	Induction of metabolism of named compound
Dicumarol	Same as above
Doxycycline	Same as above
Folic acid	Same as above
Haloperidol	Same as above
Hormonal contraceptives	Same as above
Theophylline	Same as above
Vitamin D	Same as above

Source: Adapted from IE Leppik, DL Wolff. Antiepileptic Medication Interactions. In O Devinsky (ed), Neurologic Clinics: Epilepsy I: Diagnosis and Treatment. Philadelphia: Saunders, 1993;905; H Kutt. Interactions Between Antiepileptic and Other Drugs. In WH Pitlick (ed), Antiepileptic Drug Interactions. New York: Demos, 1989;39; and P von Book, MA Siegel, NR Jacobs (eds). Growing Old in America. The Information Series on Current Topics. Wylie, TX: Information Plus, 1990;2.

Protein Binding

Carbamazepine is only 68–80% bound to plasma proteins.[21] There is therefore little risk for clinically significant results due to alterations in protein binding with carbamazepine.

Metabolism and Elimination

Carbamazepine undergoes extensive biotransformation in humans.[22] The major metabolic pathway is epoxidation of the 10,11 double bond of the azepine ring catalyzed by the hepatic monooxygenases, leading to the formation of carbamazepine 10,11-epoxide (CBZ-epoxide). As much as 40% of the parent compound is converted to the CBZ-epoxide.[22] The CBZ-epoxide is metabolized to 10,11-dihydro-10,11-dihydroxycarbamazepine by the microsomal epoxide hydrolase enzyme.[23] Use of carbamazepine with other medications may significantly alter metabolite formation as is observed by an increased CBZ-epoxide concentration when valproic acid is used concomitantly. Elimination of carbamazepine is complicated by the fact that it induces its own metabolism. In the original human volunteer studies, half-life values ranging from 18 hours to 55 hours were reported after a single dose.[23, 24] After multiple-dose treatment, the apparent plasma half-life decreases markedly to the 6- to 12-hour range.[24, 25] This effect leads to "time-dependent kinetics" (autoinduction), with higher doses needed to maintain stable plasma concentrations after a few weeks of treatment. Although the autoinduction is dose-dependent, maximal autoinduction occurs within the first 4–6 weeks of therapy.

Carbamazepine undergoes several pharmacokinetic interactions with a wide range of medications. There are four possible types if interactions: Carbamazepine metabolism is increased or decreased by comedication, or carbamazepine increases or decreases metabolism of other medication. Several substances are involved in the first three types of interactions, but no significant occurrences of carbamazepine inhibiting metabolism of other compounds have been reported (Table 21.4).

A clinically significant interaction occurs with some commonly used medications. For example, erythromycin[26] and propoxyphene[27] can markedly increase carbamazepine levels in a day or two after the first dose due to the marked inhibition of metabolism. Fluoxetine can also inhibit carbamazepine metabolism, resulting in increased carbamazepine serum concentrations (see Table 21.4).[28, 29] Careful monitoring of clinical parameters as well as serum concentrations is often imperative after an addition of other drugs to carbamazepine therapy.

NEWLY APPROVED ANTIEPILEPTIC MEDICATIONS

With the recent Federal Drug Administration approval for felbamate (Felbatol) and gabapentin (Neurontin) in 1993 and lamotrigine (Lamictal) in 1994, patients with epilepsy now have a broader slate of AEM options.

Table 21.4 Interactions of carbamazepine with other medications

Effect	Medication	Mechanism
Carbamazepine concentrations increased	Propoxyphene*	Decreased metabolism of carbamazepine
	Erythromycin*	Same as above
	Triacetyloleandomycin*	Same as above
	Phenytoin	Same as above
	Verapamil*	Same as above
	Josamycin	Same as above
	Diltiazem*	Same as above
	Isoniazid	Same as above
	Cimetidine	Same as above
	Nicotinamide	Same as above
	Viloxazine	Same as above
	Imipramine	Same as above
	Fluoxetine*	Same as above
Carbamazepine concentrations decreased	Phenytoin	Increased metabolism
	Phenobarbital	Same as above
	Primidone	Same as above
	Valproate	Same as above
Concentrations of these may be decreased when used with carbamazepine	Phenytoin	Increased metabolism
	Phenobarbital	Same as above
	Valproate*	Same as above
	Coumadin	Same as above
	Doxycycline	Same as above
	Folic acid	Same as above
	Hormonal contraceptives	Same as above

*Often very clinically significant interactions.

With the use of these new medications, we must consider drug interactions (Table 21.5).

Felbamate has a number of interactions with standard AEMs. It increases phenytoin, valproate, and CBZ epoxide concentrations but decreases carbamazepine parent levels.[30] Its interactions with other drugs have not been extensively studied, but one could expect these to occur with any substance metabolized by the pathways used by the AEMs. Gabapentin is unique among AEMs because it is eliminated renally and thus has no interaction with drugs metabolized by the liver. Lamotrigine does not affect the concentrations of standard AEMs, but its elimination is inhibited by valproate.[30] Thus, although little is yet known about interactions between the new AEMs and other classes of drugs, caution will need to be exercised. See Table 21.5 for a comprehensive list of known or strongly suspected drug interactions.

Table 21.5 What is known about interactions between the new antiepileptic medications and non-antiepileptic medications

Antiepileptic Medication	Non-Antiepileptic Medication	Interaction
Felbamate	Antacids or food	No interaction detected
Gabapentin	Aluminum/magnesium hydroxide antacid (Maalox TC)	Slight (<20% decrease in gabapentin absorption[a])
	Cimetidine	Slight (12% decrease in gabapentin clearance[b])
	Probenecid	No interaction detected
	Norethynodrel	No change in norethynodrel concentrations
	Ethinyl oestradiol[c]	No change in ethinyl oestradiol concentrations
	Food	No interaction detected
Lamotrigine	Food	No interaction detected
	Acetaminophen	Increased clearance of lamotrigine
	Oral contraceptives	No interaction detected

[a]Not considered to be clinically significant; however, advisable to separate dosages by 2 hours.
[b]Not considered to be clinically significant; no dosage adjustments necessary.
[c]Ethinyl estradiol with levonorgestrel.

CONCLUSIONS

Due to a combination of decreasing birth rate in combination with economic, social, and medical improvements promoting longevity, the number of elderly populations in developed countries has been increasing during the past several decades[8] and, in fact, has been identified as the most rapidly increasing segment of the population.[31] As of 1990, 12.4% of the population is 65 years or older, with the projection of 21.8% in this age group by the year 2050.[32] The elderly population consumes a significant amount of medication, largely due to the development of pathologic conditions developing with age.

The elderly are at great risk for developing side effects from drug interactions. Some general conclusions regarding drug interactions can be made. One should be aware of the pharmacokinetic properties of the drugs used: their absorption and distribution, hepatic elimination profile, and protein binding. In general, drugs that are hepatically metabolized are more likely to have alterations in their pharmacokinetic profile if administered with other hepatically eliminated medications. Drugs that are completely renally eliminated have a much lower probability of being involved in metabolism-related drug interactions. Caution needs to be exerted in patients with renal dysfunction, however.

Drugs that are at least 90% protein-bound will have interactions with other highly protein bound drugs.

On the other hand, pharmacodynamic interactions may occur between drugs whether or not there are pharmacokinetic interactions. Most drug interactions occur shortly after introducing a drug; therefore, a high degree of suspicion should be exercised at this time. It is important to keep in mind that changes in pharmacokinetic drug effects may also occur when drugs are withdrawn—for example, removing a hepatic inducer such as phenobarbital may increase concentrations of other drugs. Pharmacodynamic changes may also occur when drugs are withdrawn. Appropriate references should be consulted before starting a new drug.[1] Monitoring parameters such as serum drug concentrations and appropriate laboratory tests at baseline and throughout drug therapy are often indicated to maintain optimal patient safety.

Acknowledgments

Preparation of this chapter was supported in part by an NIH grant #P50 NS16308. Liliane R. Dargis provided the word processing.

REFERENCES

1. Leppik IE, Wolff DL. Antiepileptic Medication Interactions. In O Devinsky (ed), Neurologic Clinics: Epilepsy I: Diagnosis and Treatment. Philadelphia: Saunders, 1993;905.
2. Perucca E. Pharmacokinetic interactions with antiepileptic drugs. Clin Pharmacokinet 1982;7:57.
3. Kutt H. Interactions between anticonvulsants and other commonly prescribed drugs. Epilepsia 1984;25(Suppl 2):118.
4. Kutt H. Interactions Between Antiepileptic and Other Drugs. In WH Pitlick (ed), Antiepileptic Drug Interactions. New York: Demos, 1989;39.
5. Meyer UA. Drugs in Special Patient Groups: Clinical Importance of Genetics in Drug Effects. In KL Melmon, HF Morrelli, BB Hoffman, et al. (eds), Clinical Pharmacology: Basic Principles in Therapeutics (3rd ed). New York: McGraw-Hill, 1992;875.
6. DiPiro JT, Talbert RL, Hayes PE (eds). Pharmacotherapy: A Pathophysiologic Approach, East Norwalk, CT: Appelton & Lange, 1993.
7. Cooper PS, Love DW, Raffoul PR. Intentional prescription nonadherence (noncompliance) by the elderly. J Am Geriatr Soc 1982;30:329.
8. Vestal RE, Montamat SC, Nielson CP. Drugs in Special Patient Groups: The Elderly. In KL Melmon, HF Morrelli, BB Hoffman, et al. (eds), Clinical Pharmacology: Basic Principles in Therapeutics (3rd ed). New York: McGraw-Hill, 1992;851.
9. Baum C, Kennedy DL, Forbes MB, Jones JK. Drug use in the United States in 1981. JAMA 1983;251:1293.
10. Hale WE, May FE, Marks RG, Stewart RB. Drug use in an ambulatory elderly population: a five-year update. DICP 1987;21:530.
11. Helling DK, Lemke JH, Semla TP, et al. Medication use characteristics in the elderly: the Iowa 65+ rural health study. J Am Geriatr Soc 1987;35:4.
12. Scheuer MN, Cohen J. Seizures and Epilepsy in the Elderly. In O Devinsky (ed), Neurologic Clinics: Epilepsy I: Diagnosis and Treatment. Philadelphia: Saunders, 1993;787.
13. Hauser WA. Seizure disorders: the changes with age. Epilepsia 1992;33(Suppl 4):6.
14. Snedden TM, Cadieux R. State preserves PACE program for elderly. Pa Med 1988;91:44.

15. Feely J, Coakley D. Altered pharmacodynamics in the elderly. Clin Geriatr Med 1990;6:269.
16. Olsen RW. GABA-benzodiazepine-barbiturate receptor interactions. J Neurochem 1981;37:1.
17. Bochner F, Hooper WD, Tyrer JH, et al. Factors involved in an outbreak of phenytoin intoxication. J Neurol Sci 1972;16:481.
18. Carter BL, Garnett WR, Pellock JM, et al. Effect of antacid on phenytoin bioavailability. Ther Drug Monit 1981;3:333.
19. Fleisher D, Sheth N, Kou JM. Phenytoin interaction with enteral feedings administered through nasogastric tubes. JPEN 1990;14:513.
20. Porter RJ, Layzer RB. Plasma albumin concentration and diphenylhydantoin binding in man. Arch Neurol 1975;32:298.
21. Hooper WD, Dubetz DK, Bochner F, et al. Plasma protein binding of carbamazepine. Clin Pharmacol Ther 1975;17:433.
22. Faigle JW, Feldmann KF. Carbamazepine Biotransformation. In DM Woodbury, JK Penry, CE Pipppenger (eds), Antiepileptic Drugs. New York: Raven, 1982:483.
23. Bellucci G, Berti G, Chiappe C, et al. The metabolism of carbamazepine in humans: steric course of the enzymatic hydrolysis of the 10,11-epoxide. J Med Chem 1987;30:768.
24. Eichelbaum M, Ekbom K, Bertilsson L, et al. Plasma kinetics of carbamazepine and its epoxide metabolite in man after single and multiple doses. Eur J Clin Pharmacol 1975;8:337.
25. Pitlick WH, Levy RH, Troupin AS, et al. Pharmacokinetic model to describe self-induced decreases in steady-state concentrations of carbamazepine. J Pharm Sci 1976;65:462.
26. Wong YY, Ludden TM, Bell RD. Effect of erythromycin on carbamazepine kinetics. Clin Pharmacol Ther 1983;33:460.
27. Dam M, Christiansen J. Interaction of propoxyphene with carbamazepine. Lancet 1977;2:509.
28. Grimsley SR, Jann MW, Carter JG, et al. Increased carbamazepine plasma concentrations after fluoxetine coadministration. Clin Pharmacol Ther 1991;50:10.
29. Pearson HJ. Interaction of fluoxetine with carbamazepine. J Clin Psychiatry 1990;51:126.
30. Graves NM, Leppik IE. Antiepileptic medications in development. DICP 1991;25:978.
31. U.S. Senate Special Committee on Aging. Aging America. Trends and Projections. Washington, DC: US Department of Health and Human Services, 1985–1986.
32. von Book P, Siegel MA, Jacobs NR (eds). Growing Old in America. The Information Series on Current Topics. Wylie, TX: Information Plus, 1990;2.

22

Generic Antiepileptic Drugs in the Elderly: A Special Consideration

Charles E. Pippenger

Administering antiepileptic drugs (AEDs) to the elderly requires special consideration. It is well established that there are marked changes in both the pharmacokinetic and pharmacodynamic parameters of drugs associated with aging. The pharmacokinetic properties associated with drug absorption, distribution, metabolism, and elimination are altered by age-related changes in body composition and organ function.[1–3] In general, the extent of drug absorption is not affected by age, although some orally administered drugs may delay absorption because of altered gastric emptying times and gastrointestinal transit times. Changes in body composition, protein binding, and organ blood flow alter the concentrations of free (unbound) drug, the pharmacologically active component of any drug. The volume of distribution, clearance rates, and elimination half-lives of a variety of drugs also change. It is essential always to remember that drug use patterns also can be markedly altered in a variety of disease processes (e.g., congestive heart failure, hepatic disease, and renal disease) commonly associated with aging.

Alterations in body structure and functions have important consequences on drug distribution in the elderly. There is a significant reduction in total body mass with age. The ratio of lean body tissue mass to lipid tissue mass decreases due to a relative increase in the amount of adipose tissue. Protein binding of drugs is also affected by age. Acidic drugs may be bound less in elderly patients, primarily because of a general decrease in plasma albumin concentrations associated with aging. Elevated free acidic drug concentrations enhance pharmacodynamic effects of these agents, which can result in increased drug toxicity. Conversely, the level of α_1-acid glycoprotein, the major binding protein for basic drugs, is elevated in the elderly. This can lead to a significant decrease in the free concentrations of basic drugs and a loss of therapeutic efficacy. Many antidepressant, psychoactive, and cardiac drugs are bound to $\alpha 1$-acid glycoprotein.

Hepatic microsomal drug metabolism reactions consist of two types: conjugative reactions, which are not significantly altered with aging, and the oxidative (or microsomal drug metabolism) reactions, which may be decreased significantly with aging. For drugs whose major elimination pathway is renal excretion, it should remembered that there are progressive decreases in drug elimination associated with the progressive decline in glomerular and tubular function associated with aging.

The pharmacodynamic effects of drugs also change in association with aging. Elderly epileptic patients often take a wide variety of drugs to regulate age-related disease processes in addition to their seizure-control medications. These agents, particularly at toxic concentrations, can exert central nervous system effects. Often, the clear-cut clinical signs of drug toxicity observed in the normal adult and pediatric populations are obliterated in the elderly. It is wise to remember that the most common clinical sign of AED intoxication secondary to elevated plasma and tissue drug concentrations in the elderly is confusion.

Environmental factors can also significantly alter drug use patterns in the elderly. Of particular importance are the self-induced adverse drug reactions associated with patient noncompliance, inappropriate drug dosage, missed drug doses, improper drug timing, drug-drug interactions, and the ingestion of over-the-counter medications (e.g., laxatives, antacids, pain relievers, etc.). Iatrogenic drug interactions are more common in the elderly because they often are treated by several specialists who may adjust dosages of the drugs they prescribe without appropriate consideration of the patient's total therapeutic regimen.

Altered nutritional status also alters drug use patterns in the elderly. Poor nutrition leads to decreased drug clearance rates. Lack of appropriate nutrients—vitamins and trace elements—can also lead to altered physiologic function, which can alter a drug's toxicity or pharmacodynamic effects. Enteral formula feedings interfere with drug absorption, as drugs can irreversibly bind to the formula components. For example, phenytoin plasma concentrations decrease when phenytoin is administered with enteral feedings.

The narrow therapeutic index of the AEDs has been clearly documented. The necessity for individualization of drug therapy to maintain optimal concentrations and seizure-free status is well recognized by clinicians.[4] Because of their narrow therapeutic index, small changes in AED concentrations can lead to serious clinical consequences, including breakthrough seizures or drug toxicity in the elderly. Routine monitoring of AED concentrations is essential to optimal clinical management of the elderly epileptic.

Generic substitution for brand-name AEDs is currently mandatory in most of the United States. The substitution of one generic manufacturer's product for another generic manufacturer's product without notifying the prescribing physician is commonplace. One rationale for generic substitution is that the active ingredient is exactly the same in both the brand name and generic formulations. Remember, however, that other components of any given drug formulation—binders, fillers, excipients, and lubricants—can significantly alter the bioavailability of a drug.

The published reports of clinical nonequivalence of generic AEDs with breakthrough seizures, increased seizure frequency, or AED toxicity after the dispensing of different AED formulations are well known within the neurologic community.[5–15] These consequences hold for both brand-name-to-generic substitutions and generic-to-generic substitutions. The issues of generic substitution have resulted in controversy within the medical community.[16–25]

The issue of AED generic substitution has been addressed by the Therapeutics and Technology Assessment Subcommittee of the American Academy of Neurology[26, 27] with the following recommendations:

1. "Generic substitution can be approved only if safety and efficacy are not compromised. Patient safety and drug efficacy may be unduly compromised by indiscriminate switching to, from, or between generic drugs for patients taking phenytoin or carbamazepine.

2. "Physicians should avoid switching between formulations of antiepileptic medications except when medically necessary, particularly with carbamazepine or phenytoin. They should also monitor blood levels closely at the time of any known or suspected switch to a different formulation. Medication doses should be readjusted accordingly.

3. "Specific information about each antiepileptic generic drug should be made available to physicians, including area-under-the-curve bioavailability, time to maximum serum concentration, dissolution rate, and reported complications.

4. "Pharmacists should be required to inform patients and physicians when switching a patient between different formulations of antiepileptic medications, and each prescription bottle should be labeled to sufficiently identify the specific manufacturer of the product dispensed.

5. "Any organization that encourages or requires generic substitution of antiepileptic medication, including federal and state agencies, hospitals, health plans, third-party carriers, Medicaid, and Medicare, should evaluate its position regarding this problem.

6. "More research is needed to assess the impact of generic drugs on patients with epilepsy as well as in other clinical situations in which fluctuating drug levels can produce disastrous effects."[26]

Generic drugs present a special problem in the elderly. There are no studies demonstrating the bioequivalency of generic AEDs to brand-name products or between the various different generic manufacturer's formulations in the elderly. This deficit needs our attention. As a general guideline, it is to be emphasized that the same principles associated with the administration of generic drugs that are followed in the pediatric and adult populations must be followed in the administration of generic preparations to the elderly. Particular emphasis needs to be made on the formulation's bioavailability, peak absorption times, and peak plasma concentrations, factors that may predispose to transient toxicity or interfere with maintenance of consistent steady-state AED levels in the elderly. It is essential that plasma AED concentrations be carefully monitored in epileptic patients receiving generic AEDs to ensure maximum therapeutic efficacy with no toxicity.

A good guideline for AED therapy in the elderly is that whenever a patient's therapeutic regimen is changed from a brand name to a generic, from one generic formulation to another generic formulation, or from a generic to

brand name, always carefully monitor the patient's drug levels and clinical status to ensure that appropriate therapeutic adjustments are made in a timely
fashion. Remember that changes in the dosages of an elderly patient's non-AED
regimen can result in drug-drug interactions that can significantly alter that
patient's steady-state AED concentrations and vice versa.

The challenge of optimizing AED drug therapy in the elderly epileptic
patient to ensure efficacy without toxicity is one that must be addressed by
every clinician.

REFERENCES

1. Scharf S, Christophidis N. Relevance of pharmacokinetics and pharmacodynamics.
   Med J Aust 1993;158:395.
2. Williams L, Lowenthal DT. Drug therapy in the elderly. South Med J 1992;85:127.
3. Lowenthal DT. Drug therapy in the elderly: special considerations. Geriatrics
   1987;42:77.
4. Levy RH, Dreifuss FE, Mattson RH, et al. (eds). Antiepileptic Drugs (3rd ed). New
   York: Raven, 1989.
5. Wyllie E, Pippenger CE, Rothner D. Increased seizure frequency with generic primidone. JAMA 1987;258:1216.
6. Sachdeo R, Belendiuk G. Generic versus branded carbamazepine. Lancet
   1987;1:1432.
7. MacDonald JT. Breakthrough seizure following substitution of Depakene capsules
   (Abbott) with a generic product. Neurology 1987;37:1885.
8. Koch G, Allen JP. Untoward effects of generic carbamazepine therapy. Arch Neurol
   1987;44:578.
9. Bell WL, Crawford IL, Shiu GK. Reduced bioavailability of moisture-exposed carbamazepine resulting in status epilepticus. Epilepsia 1993;34:1102.
10. Gilman JT, Alvarez LA, Duchowny M. Carbamazepine toxicity resulting from generic
    substitution. Neurology 1993;43:2696.
11. Jumao-as A, Bella I, Craig B, et al. Comparison of steady-state blood levels of two
    carbamazepine formulations. Epilepsia 1989;30:67.
12. Anonymous. The drugs for epilepsy. Med Lett Drugs Ther 1989;31:1.
13. Nuwer MR, Browne TR, Dodson WE, et al. Generic substitutions for antiepileptic
    drugs. Neurology 1990;40:1647.
14. Welty TE, Pickering PR, Hale BC, Arazi R. Loss of seizure control associated with
    generic substitution of carbamazepine. Ann Pharmacother 1992;26:775.
15. Hartley R, Androwicz J, Ng PC, et al. Breakthrough seizures with generic carba-
    mazepine: a consequence of poorer bioavailability? Br J Clin Pract 1990;44:270.
16. Shulman R. The efficacy of generic primidone [letter]. JAMA 1989;261:2499.
17. Wyllie E, Rotherner D, Pippenger CE. The efficiacy of generic primidone [letter].
    JAMA 1989;261:2499.
18. Nightingale SL, Rheinstein PH, Morrison JL. The efficiacy of generic primidone [let-
    ter]. JAMA 1989;261:2499.
19. Faich GA, Morrison J, Dutra EV Jr, et al. Reassurance about generic drugs. N Engl J
    Med 1987;316:1473.
20. Strom BL. Generic drug substitution revisited. N Engl J Med 1987;316:1456.
21. Levy RA. Therapeutic risks associated with substitution of pharmaceutical alterna-
    tives. N Engl J Med 1985;313:755.
22. Day RL. Therapeutic risks associated with pharmaceutical alternatives [letter]. N
    Engl J Med 1986;314:834.
23. Schwartz LL, Stanton MW. Generic drugs [letter]. N Engl J Med 1987;317:1411.

24. Oles KS, Gal P. Bioequivalency revisited: Epitol versus Tegretol. Neurology 1993;43:2435.
25. Nightingale SL, Morrison, JC. Generic drugs and the prescribing physician. JAMA 1987;258:1200.
26. Therapeutics and Technology Assessment Subcommittee, American Academy of Neurology Assessment. Generic substitution for antiepileptic medication. Neurology 1990;40:1641.
27. Nuwer MR, Browne TR, Dodson WE, et al. Generic substitutions for antiepileptic drugs. Neurology 1990;40:1647.

Part V

Research Findings and Future Directions

23

Antiepileptic Drug Trials in the Elderly: Rationale, Problems, and Solutions

Raymond Tallis

EPILEPTIC SEIZURES IN THE ELDERLY: A GREAT AND GROWING PROBLEM

Elderly-onset seizures are very common. For example, in Rochester, Minnesota, the age-adjusted incidence of epilepsy from 1935 to 1984 was 44 per 100,000, whereas the incidence in those older than age 75 years was 139.[1] This steep rise in incidence in the elderly has been observed in all other recent epidemiologic studies.[2] In the United Kingdom National General Practice Survey of Epilepsy and Epileptic Seizures,[3] a prospective community-based study, 24% of new cases of definite epilepsy were in elderly subjects. Tallis et al. reported an epidemiologic study based on a large computerized primary care database and noted that 35% of all incident cases placed on treatment were individuals older than age 60 years.[4] On the basis of present prevalence, epilepsy is exceeded in frequency only by dementia and stroke among the major neurologic problems of the elderly.

Moreover, epilepsy in the elderly appears to be becoming more common. During the Rochester study (1935–1984), even though the incidence in children younger than age 10 years decreased significantly (by approximately 40%) during these 50 years, this was more than compensated for by a near doubling of the incidence of epilepsy in the elderly population during the same period.[1] The upward time trends for single unprovoked seizures are even more dramatic. As most seizures in the elderly are attributable to occult or overt cerebrovascular disease and as cerebrovascular disease is most common in that part of the population that is rising most sharply,[5] it is to be expected that these upward trends will continue.

EPILEPTIC SEIZURES IN THE ELDERLY: A NEGLECTED PROBLEM

There are many reasons why epileptic seizures in the elderly figure less in the epileptologic literature than they do in "real life." The first is the belief that elderly-onset seizures are comparatively uncommon. The second is the assumption that seizures in the elderly somehow matter less than those in younger people. Nothing could be further from the truth. Aside from the unpleasant and possibly dangerous experience of the seizure, postictal states may be prolonged in the elderly: 14% of subjects in one series suffered a confusional state lasting more than 24 hours, and in some cases it persisted as long as a week.[6] Todd's phenomena are also more common, especially postictal hemiparesis. This may lead to misdiagnosis of stroke. Indeed, in one series, this was the most common nonstroke cause of referral to a stroke unit.[7] Misdiagnosis is particularly likely to happen when seizures occur against a background of known cerebrovascular disease.[8] Although no adequate prospective studies have been undertaken, one might anticipate that seizures more often lead to injury, and these are more likely to be serious in elderly people with osteoporosis.

Seizures may have wider and more chronic consequences. Studies of falls (recently reviewed in Downton[9]) have repeatedly confirmed how a fall may mark a watershed in an elderly patient's life, after which there is a sharp decline in functional independence. In some instances, this decline will be due to the disease underlying the fall, but in many more it will be due to or exacerbated by loss of confidence.

The well-known 3 Fs that may cause an elderly person to become semielectively housebound (fear of further falls) must surely have its analogue in fear of further fits. Moreover, the terrifying experience of a fit may seem like a harbinger of death. This fear may be greater in elderly people not only because they may have known a contemporary who has dies after "a funny turn," but also because they may have distant memories of a childhood when epilepsy was stigmatized; poorly controlled; very much an affair of the street or the institution; and associated with severe chronic impairment of mental function, often partly due to the adverse effects of toxic drugs. The impact of seizures also includes their effect on the attitudes of others, which may lead to decreased activity, exclusion from decision-making processes, less grandparental involvement in child rearing, and more susceptibility to interference in the elderly person's affairs by others; in summary, marginalization, disempowerment, and a shrinkage of life space. So, although the diagnosis of seizures does not usually affect employment and education as is the case in a younger person, the impact on interpersonal relations is no less important. Elderly people may be more dependent on motorized transport for mobility. Thus, if the individual who has the seizure is the only license holder in the family, the consequent ban on driving may mean that two or more people become housebound.

A related misconception is that quality of life is inevitably poor in the elderly, in particular the extreme elderly, and that, against this background, the "minor" adverse effects of seizures or medication are comparatively less important than in a younger person. This also is false. For a start, whatever changes may be attributed to physiologic aging, they do not of themselves lead to clinical symptoms.

Being elderly is not, therefore, inevitably associated with unpleasant symptoms—even though it is characterized by an increased propensity to incur symptomatic disease. Those symptoms occurring in response to disease or its treatment are likely to be more, not less, important, as they more readily translate into dysfunction and loss of independence.

RECENT ENCOURAGING TRENDS

The paucity of separate studies of seizures and their treatment in the elderly reflects in part the belief that what we have learned about seizures in younger patients can be extrapolated to elderly individuals. There are signs that this assumption no longer holds sway and that the era of the neglect of elderly-onset seizures is coming to an end. This is particularly true of epidemiologic and drug studies.

The history of drug trials in elderly people may be summarized as follows:

Phase I: Exclusion of elderly people
Phase II: Accidental "contamination" of study populations with elderly subjects
Phase III: Studies directed specifically at the elderly.

Less than a decade ago, it was usual for elderly people to be excluded from trials of antiepileptic drugs (AEDs). In fact, it is difficult to recall a single AED trial that did not set an age ceiling of 60 or 65 years, and in most adult trials the median age of subjects was in the 20s or 30s. More recently, elderly people have been incidentally included in trials directed at the general adult population. In some cases—for example, the two Veterans Administration (VA) Cooperative Studies—numbers of elderly subjects have been insufficient to permit meaningful separate analysis. Trials targeted specifically at elderly subjects have been mounted only very recently.

There have been promising developments in the United Kingdom, suggesting that the period of neglect of elderly patients in drug trial is now over. For example, a multicenter comparative study of the efficacy of sodium valproate and phenytoin[10] and a single-center comparison of the impact of the two drugs on cognitive function[11] have recently been completed. There are plans to include sufficient numbers of elderly patients in European trials of gabapentin and lamotrigine as first-line monotherapy. Finally, the United Kingdom Medical Research Council Study addressing the question of whether a single unprovoked seizure should be treated is planned to include elderly patients and will involve geriatricians nationwide.

WHY CARRY OUT ANTIEPILEPTIC DRUG TRIALS SPECIFICALLY IN ELDERLY SUBJECTS?

Since drug trials specifically in elderly people are still few and associated with additional problems, it is worth spelling out the case for mounting such trials. The case in brief rests on the fact that elderly adults with epilepsy differ in various ways from the general adult population:

1. The underlying causes will be different, more often being symptomatic and frequently related to focal cerebral lesions, in particular cerebrovascular disease.[3, 12, 13]
2. Seizures may present differently (often without an adequate history), and the problem of diagnosis (in particular that of separating cardiac from cerebral causes of episodic loss of conscious) may be especially difficult.
3. There frequently will be concurrent pathologies unrelated to the seizures, and the patient will be frequently on medication other than antiepileptic drugs. Multiple pathology is one of the characteristic features of illness in the elderly.[14]
4. As elderly patients may be close to the threshold of functional failure, seizures and the adverse effects of their treatment may be more likely to cause loss of confidence and even of independence.
5. There will be differences in drug kinetics and dynamics due in part to age but also (and more importantly) to concurrent illness.

It is appropriate, therefore, that the special problems of monitoring AED efficacy and adverse events in elderly people be addressed. It is necessary to dispose of certain preconceptions, however. The most important of these is that the elderly form a homogeneous group. This is patently untrue. Notwithstanding the special problems of elderly people with epilepsy alluded to above, not all elderly people with seizures can be characterized by all of these features. Being elderly is less a period of predictable change in populations than of increased variance between individuals. Some of this will be due to biological aging and some due to disease. The latter is a much more important source of variance than the former. What proportion of the changes seen with age are due to age per se and what proportion to the increasing burden of disease is a matter of considerable debate.[15]

The complexity of the situation may be illustrated by a specific example. The changes in the pharmacokinetics of AEDs associated with aging are often presented as the differences between the mean values for young and elderly groups. Detailed examination typically reveals wide variation within an age group and substantial overlap between groups; age alone explains only a small proportion of the total variance.[16]

For example, only approximately 25% of the variation among individuals in the maximum rate of phenytoin clearance is attributable to age. Moreover, when one is considering the impact of seizures and the treatment of seizures on cognitive function and quality of life, other sources of variance—current and past life experience, education, social class, and so forth—increase the heterogeneity of the elderly.

In view of the above considerations, AED trials in a general, unselected population of individuals with elderly-onset seizures should be regarded as only a first step. The next stage would be to look at subgroups of elderly people: young-elderly versus elderly, well elderly versus ill and frail elderly, and so forth. We need to take one step at a time, however.

THE SPECIAL PROBLEMS OF ANTIEPILEPTIC
DRUG TRIALS IN ELDERLY PATIENTS

What, then, are the special problems of monitoring the efficacy and adverse effects of AEDs in elderly patients? They may be encapsulated in the assertion that the signal-to-noise ratio is likely to be greatly reduced. The "signal" is the effect of our treatment—either beneficial (control of seizures) or unwanted (adverse drug reactions). The "noise" is composed of all the other sources of variation unrelated to treatment with AEDs.

The obvious measure of the efficacy of treatment is seizure control. Seizure counting may be very difficult in the case of an individual living alone. More sophisticated measures of this crucial endpoint, such as the Seizure Severity Scale,[17] do not circumvent this problem. There are similar problems with the assessment of adverse drug reactions that depend on the patient's making a comparison between symptoms experienced before and those experienced while on the AED.

The reporting of changes in subjective symptoms, such as well-being, depends on accurate recall. It is important not to exaggerate this source of difficulty. Only 5% of individuals older than age 65 years have significant mental impairment (although this will be higher in individuals with seizures due to cerebrovascular disease), and individuals of all age groups have difficulty accurately recalling the occurrence of seizures and adverse drug effects, keeping an accurate diary, or using repeated questionnaires. In the elderly, such difficulties can be overcome by invoking the help of a caregiver or friend.

A more challenging problem arises in relating changes in the patient's condition to medication. There are three major sources of "noise" that need to be taken into account. First, multiple pathology is common in the elderly, and concurrent diseases may fluctuate independently of AED therapy. Such fluctuations may also influence seizure frequency, as in the case of respiratory and cardiac diseases. Cerebrovascular disease may progress and increase the likelihood of recurrence of seizures. In short, it may be difficult to apportion blame when AED therapy fails to improve the patient's functioning and quality of life or even to control seizures. On the other hand, adverse effects of AEDs may be ascribed to being elderly or to the worsening of other medical problems. For example, the adverse neuropsychiatric effects of AEDs may be incorrectly attributed to the effects of cerebrovascular disease. There are more subtle and complex sources of confusion as when, for example, worsening of cardiac failure due to carbamazepine is attributed to progression of ischemic heart disease.

Concurrent medication is the second major source of "noise." Many of the diseases that occur in the elderly are treated with medications that either have a direct convulsive effect (e.g., theophylline, antidepressants, and phenothiazines) or may interact with AEDs, with resulting inhibition of anticonvulsant effect or potentiation of side effects. Polypharmacy (often with unnecessary medication[18]) is a common hazard in the elderly. The difficulty of disentangling the adverse effects of AEDs from that of other medications is exacerbated in the biologically aged patient in whom adverse drug effects may present nonspecifically. For example, both digoxin toxicity and AED toxicity may cause increasing mental confusion and present with increased dependency, falls, immobility, and incontinence.

When we use quality of life measures, which have been advocated strongly in assessment of the quality of care in epilepsy,[19] further sources of "noise" unrelated to medical conditions may be as important as the seizures themselves (e.g., adverse or positive life events such as bereavements, changes of domicile, accidents, etc.). There is a greater incidence of such events late in life. For this reason, quality of life scales may be less useful as a measure of the quality of care of elderly people with seizures.[20] These reservations will have particular force when our concern is to assess only one part of the management package—the use of AEDs. Outcome will be influenced by many other elements of management, including reassurance and explanation, restoration of confidence, rehabilitation, and intervention by the multidisciplinary team.

SOME RECENT TRIALS OF ANTIEPILEPTIC DRUGS IN ELDERLY PATIENTS: LESSONS LEARNED

Lest the catalogue of problems set out above suggests that AED trials in the elderly are impossible, I shall briefly refer to two studies that were undertaken to demonstrate the feasibility and usefulness of such trials.

In a multicenter comparative trial of elderly patients with newly diagnosed epilepsy, 166 patients older than age 60 years (median age of 78 years, age range of 61–95 years) were recruited from 37 collaborating centers and followed for 12 months.[10] One hundred forty-nine patients were available for an efficacy analysis on the basis of intention to treat. Of these, 24 had inadequate seizure records. The remaining patients either completed the trial (86) or had fully documented withdrawal from the trial due to continuing seizures, adverse events (17), or death (18). It was concluded that both sodium valproate and phenytoin were useful broad-spectrum first-line antiepileptic drugs in elderly-onset seizures. Those taking sodium valproate had marginally better seizure control and fewer side effects, although the difference was not statistically significant. Interestingly, actuarial analysis suggested a 6-month remission after a 12-month follow-up would be enjoyed by 78% of the patients taking valproate and 76% of patient taking phenytoin—very comparable to the findings from monotherapy studies in the general adult population.

In a separate, more detailed study of fewer patients, Craig and Tallis investigated the impact of sodium valproate and phenytoin on cognitive function in elderly patients in a single-blind, randomized comparative design.[11] Thirty-eight patients (median age 77 years, age range of 62–88 years) with elderly-onset seizures were entered.

The two groups were matched for age, sex, and seizure type. Attention, concentration, psychomotor speed, and memory were assessed in an extensive battery of tests: twice before treatment (to minimize practice effects) and at 6 weeks, 3 months, 6 months, and 1 year after the start of treatment. We concluded, contrary to previously published data, that there was little difference in impact on cognitive function between phenytoin and sodium valproate. This is consistent with more recent observations in the general adult population.[21, 22] Frequent noncognitive adverse effects were reported, and we concluded that the choice of anticonvulsants in elderly patients may be influenced more by consideration of noncognitive than cognitive side effects.

The results of these trials are less important than the lessons learned in the course of conducting them. The key to any successful clinical trial is recruitment and retention of patients. One way of increasing recruitment is to tap into a larger population of patients through multicenter trials. Such trials may pose problems in that elderly patients with seizures, or presumed seizures, tend to be looked after by physicians who do not have a special interest or diagnostic expertise in epilepsy. It is possible that the study population may be contaminated with individuals who do not have epilepsy but instead other causes of paroxysmal events, in particular syncope due to cardiac arrhythmias. Such patients may be difficult to sort out from those with epilepsy.[23] Such contamination will decrease the power of the study to discriminate between the efficacy and adverse effects of different drugs.

The study will be further weakened if there is a poor retention rate, which will be the case if patients do not believe that they are receiving expert care and if their loyalty to the study is not awakened by the enthusiasm of the physician. These two considerations—the need to avoid contamination and the importance of minimizing drop-out rates—support the argument that favors confining the study to a single center of expertise. We have now come to the conclusion that the best way forward is a "hub-and-spokes" model, whereby recruitment takes place in several centers, with coordination of quality control and detailed testing from a single center. It is important that participating physicians feel ownership of the project and are rewarded for their involvement by increased availability of expert advice and continuous updating on the progress of the study.

If the studies are to contribute to new knowledge, they should not be confined to a small, atypical subgroup of fit elderly people who may not, after all, differ greatly from their middle-age counterparts. Inclusion criteria should not be so stringent as to exclude those kinds of elderly patients who confront us in everyday practice; this will not only affect recruitment, but also will limit the generalizability of the findings. If, however, the study is going to be valid, it should be led by physicians who are familiar with the medical problems of the elderly. This implies either a close collaboration between geriatricians and epileptologists or leadership by a physician with an interest both in epilepsy and the medical problems of elderly people.

CONCLUSION

It is evident that the difficulties attending AED studies in elderly adults should not be regarded as an excuse for not doing such studies. In particular, the new generation of AEDs that have favorable efficacy and side effect profiles should be assessed in elderly people with epilepsy, who may benefit from even minor advances. It must be recognized that any such study will be need to be conducted more painstakingly and with closer monitoring than a study involving younger subjects. Power calculations will have to take into account the many sources of noise. The reward to taking such pains will be progressive improvement in the treatment of this important and growing sector of the population of people with epilepsy.

REFERENCES

1. Hauser WA, Annegers JF, Kurland LT. Incidence of epilepsy and unprovoked seizures in Rochester, Minnesota, 1935–1984. Epilepsia 1993;34:453.
2. Tallis RC. Epilepsy. In JC Brocklehurst, RC Tallis, H Fillet (eds), Textbook of Geriatric Medicine and Gerontology. Edinburgh: Churchill Livingstone, 1992;537.
3. Sander JWAS, Hart YM, Johnson AL, Shorvon SD. National General Practice Study of Epilepsy: newly diagnosed epileptic seizures in general population. Lancet 1990;336:1267.
4. Tallis RC, Craig I, Hall G, Dean A. How common are epileptic seizures in old age? Age Ageing 1991;20:442.
5. Bamford J, Sandercock P, Dennis M, Warlow C. A prospective study of acute cerebrovascular disease in the community: the Oxford Community Stroke Project. 1. Methodology, demography and incident cases of first-ever stroke. J Neurol Neurosurg Psychiatry 1988;51:1373.
6. Godfrey JW, Roberts MA, Caird FI. Epileptic seizures in the elderly: 2 Diagnostic problems. Age Ageing 1982;11:29.
7. Norris JW, Hachinski VC. Mis-diagnosis of stroke. Lancet 1982;1:328.
8. Fine W. Post hemiplegic epilepsy in the elderly. BMJ 1967;1:199.
9. Downton JH. Falls in the Elderly. London: Edward Arnold, 1993.
10. Tallis RC, Easter D, Craig I. Multicenter trial of phenytoin versus sodium valproate [abstract]. Age Ageing [in press].
11. Craig I, Tallis R. Impact of valproate and phenytoin on cognitive function in elderly patients: results of a single-blind randomized comparative study. Epilepsia 1994;35:381.
12. Loisea J, Loisea P, Duche B, et al. A survey of epileptic disorders in southwest France: seizures in elderly patients. Ann Neurol 1990;27:232.
13. Luehdorf K, Jensen LK, Plesner A. Etiology of seizures in the elderly. Epilepsia 1986;27:458.
14. Wilson LA, Lawson IR, Brass W. Multiple disorders in the elderly: a clinical and statistical study. Lancet 1962;2:841.
15. Evan JG. Ageing and Disease. In Research and the Ageing Population Ciba Foundation Symposium 134. Chichester, England: Wiley, 1988;38.
16. Mawer G. Specific Pharmacokinetic and Pharmacodynamic Problems of Anticonvulsant Drugs in the Elderly. In RC Tallis (ed), Epilepsy and the Elderly. London: Royal Society of Medicine Publications 1988:21.
17. Jacoby A, Baker G, Smith D, et al. Measuring the impact of epilepsy: the development of a novel scale. Epilepsy Res 1993;16:83.
18. Lindley CM, Tully MP, Paramsothy VP, Tallis RC. Adverse drug reactions in the elderly; the contribution of inappropriate prescribing. Age Ageing 1992;21:294.
19. Chadwick D, Baker GA, Jacoby A (eds). Quality of Life and Quality of Care in Epilepsy. London: Royal Society of Medicine Publications, 1993.
20. Tallis RC. Through a Glass Darkly: Assessing Quality of Care of Elderly People with Epilepsy Using Quality of Life Measures. In DW Chadwick, GA Baker, A Jacoby

(eds), Quality of Life and Quality of Care in Epilepsy: Update 1993. London: Royal Society of Medicine Publications, 1993.
21. Gilham RA. Cognitive function in adult epileptic patients established on anticonvulsant monotherapy. Epilepsy Res 1990;7:2.
22. Meador KM, Loring DW, Huh K, et al. Comparative cognitive effects of anticonvulsants. Neurology 1990;40:391.
23. Tallis RC. Epilepsy. In RA Kenny (ed), Syncope in the Older Patient. London: Chapman and Hall [in press].

24

Directions of Future Research

Roger J. Porter and Antonio V. Delgado-Escueta

INTRODUCTION

Contrary to previous opinions that epilepsy is uncommon in the elderly, new evidence from the last two decades documents an increased incidence of new-onset epilepsy in those older than age 60 years. In 1975, Hauser and Kurland[1] studied residents in Rochester, Minnesota, and found that both the incidence and prevalence of epilepsy increased after 60 years of age. In Frederiksburg, Denmark, Lühdorf et al.[2] found increased incidence rates (77 per 100,000) for epilepsy after 60 years of age, and Forsgren[3] in Sweden reported even greater prevalence rates (321 per 100,000) after 70 years of age.

Analysis of the etiology of these seizures shows that cerebrovascular disease accounts for approximately one-third of the cases; another third (in most series reported) have an unknown origin (Figure 24.1).[4–8] Half of the patients with cerebrovascular disease have normal examinations; clinically silent cerebral infarctions are frequent. Shorvon et al.[9] reported ischemic lesions and infarctions and low attenuation of periventricular white matter on computed tomography (CT) scans in such patients. Twenty percent of multi-infarct dementia patients develop epilepsy,[10] and Hauser et al.[11] calculates that 20% of patients with Alzheimer's dementia have recurrent seizures and myoclonus during the course of the illness. A large percentage of etiologies of epilepsy in the elderly remain cryptogenic. One important issue is determining which subgroups are genetic and relate to the genetics of aging.

The immediate dilemma of the investigator who is interested in the age-related aspects of epilepsy is the difficulty in separating the fundamentals of genetic epilepsy research from those aspects of epilepsy research that might logically be called age-specific. The task of conducting research—basic or clinical—is daunting enough without the added burden of relating the issues to childhood or to the aged. Assuming, however, that there is merit to such an approach, one need only peruse the literature to note that enormous data have recently accumulated on the "young" side of the equation; developmental neurobiology—and its implications for epilepsy in childhood—is a field that is exploding with new ideas and fruitful investigations.

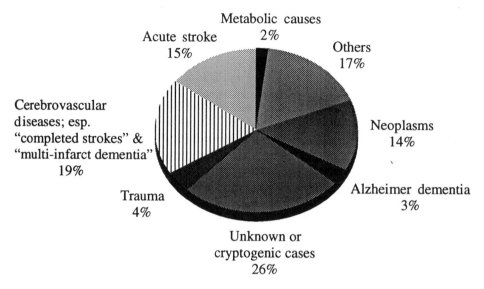

Figure 24.1 Etiology of epilepsy with onset after 60 years of age. Approximate percentages were derived from Hildick-Smith,[4] Schold et al.,[5] Sundaram,[6] Lühdorf et al.,[7] and Roberts et al.[8] The category "other" includes subdural hematoma, contusion, drug withdrawal, Alzheimer's disease, and toxic-metabolic events. (Adapted from MBM Sundaram. Etiology and patterns of seizures in the elderly. Neuroepidemiology 1989;8:234).

Only recently and much more slowly have strides been made to advance our knowledge of the other side of the equation, that of the aging brain and the elderly person with epilepsy. We can take some comfort in knowing, of course, that all investigations, whether age-specific or not, may have implications for the elderly with epilepsy. Nevertheless, acceleration of our understanding of the aging brain and its relation to epilepsy is mandatory if we are to adequately cope with the population of the twenty-first century.

To construct a projection of future research in as giant a field as epilepsy is a task that is inevitably filled with provincialism leading to omission. We can only select a few of the most promising areas of investigation now underway, and estimate the impact on our knowledge and our clinical practice a few years hence. To do this, we have divided the discussion into a continuum of the two classic divisions: preclinical and clinical. Beginning with the preclinical area and moving through preclinical-to-clinical to more purely clinical, we have chosen a few areas of investigations we think are among the most exciting, citing one or two key studies in each that seem to us to indicate the directions of future research. Although most epilepsy research is not targeted toward the elderly population, where implications for the aging brain are present, we will point them out.

PRECLINICAL RESEARCH

Molecular Mechanisms of Normal Aging

Of the different types of neurons in the nervous system, most are subject to age-related changes. With age, both brain weight and total protein decrease; the human brain actually loses neurons in the cerebral cortex and in several subcortical nuclei. Neurons that synthesize and degradate neurotransmitters decrease in number. Neurotransmitter receptors and ion channels also decrease. Examples include neurons in the substantia nigra and locus coeruleus, centers important in the spread and suppression of propagating seizure discharges. Microscopic changes of cell death from aging are accompanied by the accumulation of senile plaques and neurofibrillary tangles, although in numbers considerably fewer than in Alzheimer's dementia.

The molecular mechanisms and consequences of this decrement in neurons are unknown. Three hypotheses have been proposed. First, Medvedev[12] suggests that mutations and chromosomal anomalies accumulate with age; with the exhaustion of reserve deoxyribonucleic acid (DNA), senescence occurs. A second hypotheses suggests that random damage and insults from the wear and tear of time produce errors in DNA duplication. Abnormal messenger ribonucleic acid (mRNA) and proteins are found and senescence soon follows. The third hypotheses suggests that genes program the aging process—a continuum of the genetic control of larger developmental process.

Most intriguing is the question, as yet unanswered, whether the reasons for the cell death that occur in aging are similar to those observed in early development—for example, the elimination of neurons whose axons fail to reach a target, the scaling down of the number of neurons to match target size or presynaptic neuron pool, or the elimination of neurons with connection errors. Other mechanisms of nerve cell death, such as loss of target derived trophic factors or electrical activity or loss of exogenous factors such as sex hormones, may be the same in aging as in early development. Early investigations should focus on whether modifications induced by aging can result in regeneration, collateral sprouting, or unmasking of suppressed synapses. Such plasticity may play a role in the adaptations necessary in aging but could also lead to aberrant learning and epileptogenesis.

Ion Channels: Molecular Structure and Modulation

The concept of ion channels and their importance in cellular function is not at all new. What is new is our rapidly increasing knowledge of how these channels are constructed, what activates and deactivates them, and what modulates their activity. The importance of this subject to epilepsy research is rooted in the well documented thesis that neuronal hyperexcitability is the fundamental element of the epileptic discharge. Given that this hyperexcitability is critical, we may then ask what we know about the fundamentals of neuronal ion channels, how they change with aging, and what role they have in epileptogenesis, and spread and arrest of seizures.

Ion channels are surprisingly conserved in evolution, and much can be learned from species other than the human that bears directly on the human condition. We know that the ion channel is a "pore" surrounded by complex proteins that are divided into subunits that weave in and out of the cell membrane. The number of subunits determines the character of the channel. The sodium, potassium, and calcium channels, for example, have four subunits, whereas other channels may have five or six. The gamma-aminobutyric acid (GABA)-A chloride channel complex has four such proteins, each of which has four subunits. As noted by Olsen, anticonvulsant drugs act on specific receptors on this complex to effect different actions.[13] Olsen divides the various sites of action into five groups, shown in Figure 24.2: GABA site, barbiturate site, benzodiazepine site, steroid site, and picrotoxin site. He characterizes the excitement of the future into four categories: (1) gaining more information about the cellular and molecular mechanisms and specificity of action of anticonvulsant drugs at this target; (2) seeking new partial agonist anticonvulsants such as new benzodiazepines, which have more desirable clinical properties; (3) gaining new insights into the cellular and molecular mechanisms of tolerance, with the aim of avoiding or reversing this effect; and (4) learning more about receptor heterogeneity and receptor subtypes.[13]

There is strong evidence that neuronal ion channels are involved in epileptogenesis and epileptic seizures, but the exact nature of the abnormalities in these channels remains elusive. We do know that glutamate and GABA are the major excitatory and inhibitory neurotransmitters in the brain and that drugs that alter the action of either of these two transmitters can alter the epileptic discharge, both in vitro and in vivo. The above description of a single ion channel complex and its implications for the future are but a very small part of the exciting work ongoing in this arena.

We also need to learn more about changes that occur in ion channels when aging occurs. Do the channels themselves become altered in their function? Or, more likely, are the numbers of functioning channels diminished? How do these changes in aging relate to epileptogenesis? What effects do seizures have on channels of the aging brain? Or is there no change with aging? These critical questions remain unanswered.

Neuronal Migration and Axonal Targeting

In dissecting the brains of patients with epilepsy, it has been common for the neuropathologist to identify—sometimes by gross inspection—abnormalities of the location of various neuronal groups. The obvious observation was that the cells somehow missed their target and ended up in the wrong place during neural development; however, the mechanisms by which such maldevelopment might take place have remained obscure. Less obvious, but perhaps even more important, is the dynamic directing of the nerve fibers themselves. Although we have speculated a great deal about the nature of neuronal misconnections, until

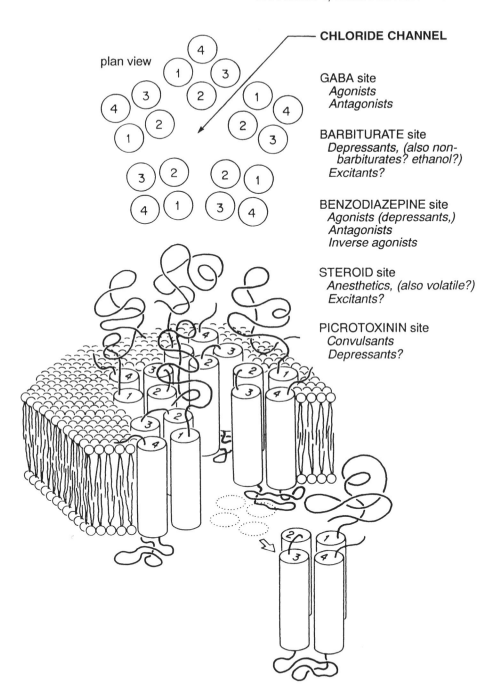

plan view

CHLORIDE CHANNEL

GABA site
  Agonists
  Antagonists

BARBITURATE site
  Depressants, (also non-
    barbiturates? ethanol?)
  Excitants?

BENZODIAZEPINE site
  Agonists (depressants,)
  Antagonists
  Inverse agonists

STEROID site
  Anesthetics, (also volatile?)
  Excitants?

PICROTOXININ site
  Convulsants
  Depressants?

Figure 24.2 Anatomy of the chloride channel. (Adapted from Olsen RW. Advances in GABA pharmacology. Abstract in An Advanced Research Workshop on Basic Mechanims of the Epilepsies. October 24–27, 1993; Yosemite, CA: I-101-4.)

recently, little has been accomplished to elucidate the fundamental mechanisms that may have gone awry.

Goodman and Shatz,[14] in a recent review article, describe the specificity of synaptic connections, beginning with the growing tips of the neurons traversing long distances to seek their eventual home, finally reaching the correct "neighborhood" and ultimately finding the correct target. These investigators have sought answers to some of the most important questions about the nature of this remarkable process and make the following observations:

- Chemoaffinity may be part of the key to understanding the directing of the nerve tips.
- Neural activity is not in itself required for precise patterns of neuronal connectivity.
- The actual mechanisms of guidance of the nerve tips may depend on many factors, including "differential adhesion," diffusible gradients, and repulsion.[14]

Shatz has one special example of his work that documents the excitement of the subject.[15] In studying the characteristics of the developing visual system, the observation was made that each eye has its own territory in the visual cortex. The eye "adopts" this process by stimulation of the neurons. In Figure 24.3, Shatz[15] shows how the process actually works in the cat and how either the administration of tetrodotoxin or the deprivation of stimulation—both of which alter the pattern of normal action potentials of the ganglion cells—alter in a negative way the ability of these ganglion cells to reach their axonal target.

Clearly this system of neuronal wiring is very delicate, and perturbations are undoubtedly at the root of many brain disorders, some of which manifest with epileptic seizures. As we learn more about how the brain becomes "wired," we will also need to study what happens in the aging brain when wiring is "undone" by disease or by the aging process itself. Is the brain capable of rewiring at an elderly age? Might intervention, such as with growth factors, alter connectivity in a positive way? Can we regain the plasticity of the young for the benefit of the elderly? Obviously, a greater understanding of how the brain develops will give important clues about how to cope with altered brain connectivity.

PRECLINICAL-TO-CLINICAL RESEARCH

Certain investigative fields in epilepsy research are difficult to describe in either clinical or preclinical terms, as both are intimately intertwined in the research process. Such is true of the two areas chosen for discussion below: the genetics of epilepsy and the development of new antiepileptic drugs. Genetics of epilepsy is particularly relevant because one-third of seizures in the elderly are idiopathic.

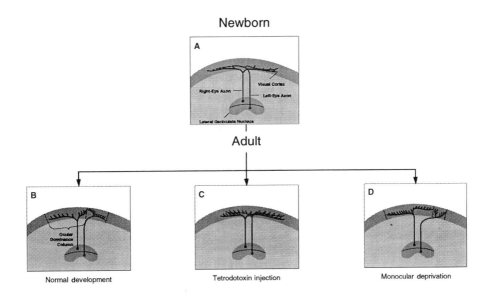

Figure 24.3 One of the characteristics of the developing visual system is segregation of inputs: Each eye adopts its own territory in the visual cortex. The process, however, can be completed if only the neurons are stimulated. In experiments with cat eyes, for example, the axons of the left eye and of the right eye overlap in layer 4 of the visual cortex at birth (A). Visual stimuli will cause the axons to separate and form ocular dominance columns in the cortex (B). Such normal development can be blocked with injections of tetrodotoxin; as a result, the axons never segregate, and the ocular dominance columns fail to emerge (C). Another way to perturb development is to keep one eye closed, depriving it of stimulation. The axons of the open eye then take over more than their fair share of territory in the cortex (D). (Adapted from CJ Shatz. The developing brain. Sci Am September 1992;267:61).

Identification of Genetic Causes of the Epilepsies

Nowhere is the excitement of modern neurobiology greater than in the search for abnormal genes that may cause seizures and epileptic syndromes. Only a few years ago, there were no epilepsy syndromes for which a chromosomal locus had been identified. By the end of 1993, as many as seven epilepsy genes had been localized to various chromosomes using investigative techniques that span both clinical and preclinical efforts (Delgado-Escueta, personal communication, March 1994). Disorders that have been identified are uniformly (thus far) idiopathic generalized epilepsies,[16–37] as one would expect in the early phases of such investigations (Table 24.1). The identification of genetic influences on partial epilepsies will no doubt prove a larger task.

Table 24.1 Epilepsy genes

	Chromosome	Reference Number(s)
Idiopathic generalized epilepsies		
Juvenile myoclonic epilepsy (EJM1)	6p	16–22
Juvenile myoclonic epilepsy (possible EJM2)	Not in 6p	23, 24
Benign familial neonatal convulsions (EBN1)	20q	25, 26
Benign familial neonatal convulsions (possible EBN2)	8q	27–29
Childhood absence epilepsy (possible ECA1)	Not in 6p	30
Progressive myoclonus epilepsies		
Unverricht-Lundborg type (EPM1) (Baltic)	21q	31, 32
Unverricht-Lundborg type (EPM1) (Mediterranean)	21q	33
Juvenile type of neuronal ceroid lipofuscinoses (CLN3)	16p	34
Juvenile Gaucher's disease	1q	35
"Cherry red spot myoclonus" syndrome, or sialidosis type 1	10q	36
Myoclonus epilepsy and ragged-red fibers	Mitochondrial DNA	37

Source: Adapted from AV Delgado-Escueta, J Serratosa, A Liu, et al. Progress in mapping human epilepsy genes. Epilepsia 1994;35(Suppl 1):S29.

Not surprisingly, investigations into the genetics of the epilepsies often result in unexpected outcomes that are complex and reflect the heterogeneity of the disorder under study. In the search for the gene for juvenile myoclonic epilepsy (JME), for example, the first locus was mapped to the short arm of chromosome 6.[17, 18, 20–22, 38] Later studies, however, showed that not all families with JME have their genetic abnormality at this locus. Furthermore, the closely related syndrome, absence epilepsy, also does not localize to 6.[38]

As we become more sophisticated in the search for genetic abnormalities, the limiting factors will probably prove to be clinical—that is, the limiting factors will include the identification of adequate numbers of families with large sibships that can be analyzed by molecular biological techniques. The first step has been to look for discreet genetic abnormalities that cause definitive syndromes, and modest success is at hand. More distant are investigations that involve less discreet clinical data, such as "seizure diathesis." The hope remains that genetic investigations will unlock the door to our understanding of why one person with a head injury acquires epilepsy, whereas another person with an equally severe injury escapes the disorder; the speed with which this new knowledge will arrive is quite uncertain.

One cannot help but observe that genetic investigations have concentrated on the disorders of the young. New and inventive approaches are needed to uncover genetic influences of aging on the epileptic brain as well as genetic influences on epilepsy in the aging brain.

Rational Development of New Antiepileptic Drugs

Historical Notes

Antiepileptic drugs historically have been discovered by one of three different approaches: serendipity, screening, or rational investigation. Each of these three has proved useful in creating the medical armamentarium we have today, and all are in still in use in one form or another.

Serendipity was the manner in which Locock, in 1857, discovered bromides, which he used in the treatment of catamenial seizures. This medication, the first that was useful for the treatment of any epileptic seizure, remained the only therapy until the early twentieth century, in spite of its considerable toxicity. Serendipity was also the manner in which Hauptmann, in 1912, discovered the usefulness of phenobarbital.[39] In treating his patients with depression, he noted the effectiveness of the drug in patients with seizures, thus launching one of the most widely prescribed drugs for epilepsy.

The screening approach came to the fore in 1937, when Merritt and Putnam[40, 41] evaluated a series of compounds sent to them by Parke-Davis for evaluation of their anticonvulsant potential. They used a seizure model based on an electroshock technique for producing convulsions in animals[42] and discovered that the most potent of the new compounds in preventing electroshock seizures in cats was diphenylhydantoin, now called phenytoin. This experimental discovery was a considerable milestone in the development of new drugs, as noted by Swinyard[43]:

- It established that an antiepileptic drug need not be sedative to be effective.
- It demonstrated the value of a systematic experimental laboratory approach to seek new antiepileptic drugs.
- It encouraged the search for drugs with selective antiseizure action.
- It opened a new era of structure-activity relationships.
- It provided a new tool for a wide variety of neurophysiologic and neurochemical investigations of the basic mechanisms of the epilepsies.

In the next two decades, the exploitation of the cyclic ureide moiety resulted in a series of new antiepileptic drugs. These include additional hydantoins and barbiturates and also drugs with selective antiabsence activity such as the tridiones and the succinimides. The era culminated in the United States with the marketing of ethosuximide in 1960; antiepileptic drug development then remained dormant for a decade. The screening approach reemerged as a critical factor in drug development with the discovery of several new compounds such as gabapentin and felbamate.

Facilitation of Inhibition

As noted by Porter and Rogawski,[44] the rational development era of searching for antiepileptic drugs began with attempts to facilitate inhibition. We have long known that neuronal hyperexcitability—in one form or another—is the cellular abnormality responsible for the epileptic event, and it was only natural to search for a dampening process. This was especially true in light of the observed effects of barbiturates and benzodiazepines, which enhance GABAergic inhibition.[45, 46] This approach has been widely investigated.[47]

Many paths may be followed to enhance inhibition of the GABAergic system. The three major approaches have been to (1) create GABA agonists or prodrugs, (2) diminish the activity of the GABA degradative enzyme GABA transaminase, or (3) inhibit the uptake of GABA at the synapse.

The best example of a GABA prodrug is progabide, a lipid-soluble derivative of the amidated form of GABA. Unlike GABA, progabide readily crosses the blood-brain barrier. It is partially converted to GABA itself, but the drug and its metabolites are agonists of brain GABA receptors.[47] Because of hepatotoxicity and marginal efficacy, the drug is no longer being investigated in most countries.

Vigabatrin is the best example of the GABA transaminase inhibitors. It has survived a toxicologic scare—reversible myelinic edema is found in multiple animal species—to be marketed widely in Europe and South America. Approval in the United States is expected within a couple of years. The drug irreversibly inhibits the GABA degradative enzyme, elevating both cerebrospinal fluid and brain levels of GABA. The clinical role of vigabatrin is still uncertain, as some toxic side effects have limited more widespread use.

Tiagabine is the best example of the GABA uptake inhibitors. Tiagabine is a potent, selective inhibitor of neuronal and glial GABA uptake and does not bind to other neurotransmitters.[47] The drug has shown some tendency to cause confusion in volunteers at the higher doses; whether it can overcome this toxicologic deficit remains uncertain.

Diminution of Excitation

Diminution of excitation is a more recent avenue of investigation than is enhancement of inhibition and derives from the longstanding knowledge that both glutamate and aspartate excite neurons cause convulsive activity when placed on the cerebral cortex. Newly discovered receptor subtypes are appearing at a remarkable rate, and compounds that have selective actions on these subtypes are being sought with vigor.

Perhaps the best known compound in this class is MK-801, a drug that was remarkably effective in classic animal screening, especially in the maximal electroshock test. The compound is also potent as an antagonist of N-methyl-D-aspartate (NMDA)-induced seizures in mice. Clues that there were problems with the drug appeared when it was discovered that the drug was much more effective at preventing the development of kindling than preventing already kindled seizures. Although widely studied clinically, it was not highly effective at tolerated doses. In addition, a toxicologic concern (brain vacuolization) became an issue, and the drug is no longer under study. Other drugs with related mechanisms of action such as remacemide are still under development, but their future is also uncertain.

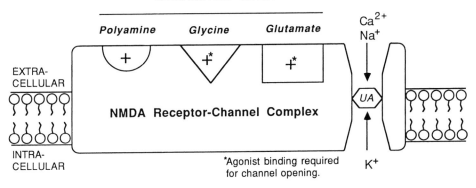

Figure 24.4 Schematic representation of the various anticonvulsant target sites on the N-methyl-D-aspartate (NMDA) receptor–channel complex. Agonist binding to the NMDA-selective glutamate site and the strychnine-insensitive glycine site cause opening of the channel (ionophore) region, allowing passage of Ca^{2+} and Na^+ into the cell and K^+ out of the cell; both the glutamate and glycine sites must be occupied for channel opening to occur. Polyamine binding facilitates activation of the channel but may not be required for opening. Binding of antagonist drugs to any of the three recognition sites diminishes channel activation. Uncompetitive antagonists bind to the ionophore to physically occlude ion transit. In addition, drugs could impair channel opening by binding to an allosteric blocking site (e.g., for Zn^{2+}) unassociated with an agonist binding site. (NMDA = N-methyl-D-aspartate; UA = uncompetitive agonist.) (Adapted from MA Rogawski, RJ Porter. Antiepileptic drugs: pharmacological mechanisms and clinical efficacy with consideration of promising developmental stage compounds. Pharmacol Rev 1990;42:223).

A summary of the complexity of the NMDA-receptor channel complex is shown in Figure 24.4, in which multiple recognition sites can be acted on by agonists or antagonists. See Rogawski and Porter[47] for additional details.

The development of new drugs has tended to be seizure type–specific, with emphasis on seizure types that were easiest to study and that represented the largest market; partial seizures and generalized tonic-clonic seizures are usually chosen for research. Fortunately, these are the most common seizures in the elderly. Although elderly people have rarely appeared in clinical investigations (the climate may be changing), they have benefitted from past investigations of these seizure types. Although the characteristics of a good drug for the elderly are similar to those for the young, worthy of special emphasis are the absence of drug-drug interactions, minimalization of sedative-cognitive issues, and in general, a gentle drug that does not otherwise interfere with the delicate quality of life of the aged.

CLINICAL INVESTIGATIONS: MAGNETIC RESONANCE IMAGING FUNCTIONAL MAPPING AND SPECTROSCOPY

Although CT radiography effected the most radical change in the modern clinical neurology, magnetic resonance imaging (MRI) has provided the continuous advances that have made this latter technique dominant, both in clinical practice and in investigative imaging. These techniques, which have the advantage of being relatively noninvasive, may permit a better understanding of epilepsy in the elderly. Two fundamental advances have import for the patient with epilepsy: functional imaging and spectroscopy. Only functional imaging is considered here.

The original CT and MRI studies were limited to anatomic observations—that is, almost no physiologic observations were possible, as the devices were incapable of measuring function over time. Until the past 2 or 3 years, positron emission tomography (PET) was the functional approach of choice if one wished to image physiologic change in the brain. PET has elucidated much that we currently know about epileptic changes in human brain, including localization of foci[48] and effects of antiepileptic drugs on brain metabolism.[49]

PET, however, is cumbersome and expensive. Its use in clinical localization of epileptic foci, however well documented, has been limited to a few major medical centers. The potential of MRI to begin to measure function has the advantages of better spatial and temporal resolution without the use of ionizing radiation.[50]

A recent study by Connelly et al.[50] has made use of a widely available MRI scanner to visualize functional activation of the human brain. The authors mapped regions of the brain that were activated with visual and motor tasks; in 11 visual and 14 motor studies, activation was seen in all cases, documented by an intensity change, which can be seen in the gray matter. In the accompanying Figure 24.5, one can see the activation of the motor cortex in response to a movement task of the contralateral hand.

If we can see the brain activate with motor or visual tasks, one would think that it might be a relatively easy step to identify the neuronal hyperexcitability of the epileptic discharge. The issue, as usual, is more complex. Neuronal hyperexcitability may become manifest only in a short time window and not in the window chosen by the patient or the radiologist. The location of the lesion may not be easily discovered—certainly not as well correlated as is the motor strip to contralateral motor function. These and other difficulties remain to be solved before functional MRI can be a dramatic breakthrough for the localization of epileptic loci.

The application of this technique to the elderly will require a better understanding of what actually occurs at a functional level when the brain ages. A higher level of resolution may also be required to discern normal brain function from that of early senescence.

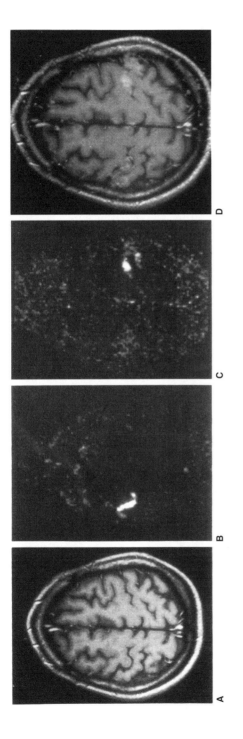

Figure 24.5 Images from a study of motor stimulation involving a hand movement task. A. Anatomy of the selected section. B, C. Effects of left hand (B) and right hand (C) movement. Both B and C were obtained by summing 80 images acquired under control conditions (no movement) and subtracting the resulting image from the corresponding summation of images acquired during hand movement. D. Superimposition of B and C on A. (The original panel D appears in color.) (Reprinted with permission from Connelly A, Jacson GD, Frackowiak RSJ, et al. Functional mapping of activated human primary cortex with a clinical MR imaging system. Radiology 1993;188:127.)

SUMMARY

This chapter highlights a few of the exciting frontiers in epilepsy research, with emphasis and commentary on the applications to the aging process. There seems little doubt that we might improve our current understanding of the senior citizen with epilepsy by more specifically focusing our investigations on issues related to aging.

REFERENCES

1. Hauser WA, Kurland LT. The epidemiology of epilepsy in Rochester, Minnesota, 1937–1967. Epilepsia 1975;16:1.
2. Lühdorf K, Jensen LK, Plesner AM. Epilepsy in the elderly: incidence, social function, and disability. Epilepsia 1986;27:135.
3. Forsgren L. Prevalence of epilepsy in adults in northern Sweden. Epilepsia 1992;33:450.
4. Hildick-Smith M. Epilepsy in the elderly. Age Ageing 1974;3:203.
5. Schold C, Yarnell PR, Earnest MP. Origin of seizures in elderly patients. JAMA 1977;238:1177.
6. Sundaram MBM. Etiology and patterns of seizures in the elderly. Neuroepidemiology 1989;8:234.
7. Lühdorf K, Jensen LK, Plesner AM. Epilepsy in the elderly: incidence, social function, and disability. Epilepsia 1986;27:135.
8. Roberts MA, Godfrey JW, Caird FI. Epileptic seizures in the elderly. Age Ageing 1982;11:24.
9. Shorvon SD, Gilliatt RW, Cox TCS, Yu YL. Evidence of vascular disease from CT scanning in late onset epilepsy. J Neurol Neurosurg Psychiatry 1984;47:225.
10. Lishman WA. Alcoholic dementia: a hypothesis. Lancet 1986;1:1184.
11. Hauser WA, Morris ML, Heston LL, Anderson VE. Seizures and myoclonus in patients with Alzheimer's disease. Neurology 1986;36:1226.
12. Medvedev, ZA. Repetition of molecular genetic information as a possible factor in evolutionary changes of life span. Exp Gerontol 1972;7:227.
13. Olsen RW. Advances in GABA pharmacology. Abstract in an Advanced Research Workshop on Basic Mechanims of the Epilepsies. October 24–27, 1993; Yosemite, CA: I-101-4.
14. Goodman CS, Shatz CJ. Developmental mechanisms that generate precise patterns of neuronal connectivity. Cell 1993;72:77.
15. Shatz CJ. The developing brain. Sci Am September 1992;267:61.
16. Greenberg DA, Delgado-Escueta AV, Widelitz H, et al. A locus involved in the expression of juvenile myoclonic epilepsy and of an associated EEG trait may be linked to HLA and Bf. Cytogenet Cell Genet 1987;46:623.
17. Greenberg DA, Delgado-Escueta AV, Maldonado HM, Widelitz H. Segregation analysis of juvenile myoclonic epilepsy. Genet Epidemiol 1988;5:81.
18. Delgado-Escuta AV, Greenberg DA, Treiman L, et al. Mapping the gene for juvenile myoclonic epilepsy. Epilepsia 1989;30(Suppl 4):8.
19. Delgado-Escueta AV, Greenberg DA, Weissbecker K, et al. Gene mapping in the idiopathic generalized epilepsies: juvenile myoclonic epilepsy, childhood absence epilepsy, epilepsy with grand mal seizures, and early childhood myoclonic epilepsy. Epilepsia 1990; 31(Suppl 3):S19.
20. Durner M, Sander T, Greenberg DA, et al. Localization of idiopathic generalized epilepsy on chromosome 6p in families of juvenile myoclonic epilepsy patients. Neurology 1991;41:1651.

21. Weissbecker K, Durner M, Janz D, et al. Confirmation of linkage between a juvenile myoclonic epilepsy-locus and the JLA-region of chromosome 6. Am J Med Genet 1991;38:32B.
22. Liu A, Delgado-Escueta AV, Weissbecker K, et al. Juvenile myoclonic epilepsy and reference markers of chromosome 6p [abstract]. Epilepsia 1992;33 (Suppl 3):73.
23. Whitehouse W, Rees M, Curtis D, et al. Linkage analysis of idiopathic generalized epilepsy (IGE) and marker loci on chromosome 6p in families of patients with juvenile myoclonic epilepsy: no evidence for an epilepsy locus in the HLA region. Am J Hum Genet 1993;55:652.
24. Leppert M, Anderson VE, Quattlebaum T, et al. Benign familial neonatal convulsions linked to genetic markers on chromosome 20. Nature 1989;337:647.
25. Malafosse A, Leboyer M, Dulac O, et al. Confirmation of linkage of benign familial neonatal convulsions to D20S19 and D20S20. Hum Genet 1992;89:54.
26. Lewis TB, Leach RJ, Ward K, et al. Genetic heterogenicity in benign neonatal convulsions: identification of a new locus in chromosome 8q. Am J Hum Genet 1993;53:670.
27. Ryan S, Wiznitzer M, Hollman C, et al. Benign familial neonatal convulsions; evidence for clinical and genetic heterogeneity. Ann Neurol 1991;29:469.
28. Ryan S. Benign Familial Neonatal Convulsion: Evidence for Chromosome 8q Locus. Presented at the Alsace International Workshop on Idiopathic Generalized Epilepsies, April 1993.
29. Serratosa JM, Delgado-Escueta AV, Pascual-Castroviego I, et al. Childhood absence epilepsy: exclusion of genetic linkage to chromosome 6p markers. Epilepsia 1993;34(Suppl 2):149.
30. Lehesjoki A-E, Koskiniemi M, Sistonen P, et al. Localization of a gene for progressive myoclonus epilepsy to chromosome 21q22. Proc Natl Acad Sci U S A 1991;88:3696.
31. Lehesjoki A-E, Koskiniemi M, Pandolfo M, et al. Linkage studies in progressive myoclonus epilepsy: Unverricht-Lundborg and Lafora's diseases. Neurology 1992;42:1545.
32. Malafosse A, Lehesjoki A, Genton P, et al. Identical genetic locus for Baltic and Mediterranean myoclonus. Lancet 1992;339:1080.
33. Gardiner M, Sandford A, Deadman M, et al. Batten disease (Spielmeyer-Vogt disease, juvenile onset neuronal ceroid lipofuscinosis) gene (CLN3) maps to human chromosome l6. Genomics l990;8:387.
34. Barnveld RA, Keijzer W, Tegelders FPW, et al. Assignment of the gene for human b-glucocerebrosidase to the region of q21–q31 of chromosome 1 using monoclonal antibodies. Hum Genet 1983;64:227.
35. Mueller OT, Henry WM, Haley LL, et al. Sialodosis and galactosialidosis: chromosomal assignment of two genes associated with neuroaminidase deficiency disorders. Proc Natl Acad Sci U S A 1986;83:1817.
36. Shoffner JM, Lott MT, Lezza AMS, et al. Myoclonus epilepsy and red-ragged fiber disease (MERRF) is associated with a mitochondrial DNA tRNA(Lys) mutation. Cell 1990;61:931.
37. Delgado-Escueta AV, Serratosa J, Liu A, et al. Progress in mapping human epilepsy genes. Epilepsia 1994;35(Suppl 1):29.
38. Delgado-Escueta AV, Enrile-Bacsal FE. Juvenile myoclonic epilepsy of Janz. Neurology 1984;34:285.
39. Hauptmann A. Luminal bei epilepsie. Muncher Medizinische Wochenschrift 1912;59:1907.
40. Merritt HH, Putnam TJ. A new series of anticonvulsant drugs tested by experiments on animals. Arch Neurol Psychiatry 1938;39:1003.
41. Merritt HH, Putnam TJ. Sodium diphenylhydantoinate in the treatment of convulsive disorders. JAMA 1938;111:1068.

42. Spiegel EA. Quantitative determination of the convulsive activity by electrical stimulation of brain with the skull intact. J Lab Clin Med 1937;22:1274.
43. Swinyard EA. Introduction. In DM Woodbury, JK Penry, CE Pippenger (eds), Antiepileptic Drugs (2nd ed). New York: Raven, 1982;1.
44. Porter RJ, Rogawski MA. New antiepileptic drugs: from serendipity to rational discovery. Epilepsia 1992;33(Suppl 1):1.
45. Olsen RW. Barbiturates. Int Anesthesiol Clin 1988;26:254.
46. Haefely W. Benzodiazepines: Mechanisms of Action. In R Levy, R Mattson, B Meldrum, et al (eds). Antiepileptic Drugs (3rd ed). New York: Raven, 1989:721.
47. Rogawski MA, Porter RJ. Antiepileptic drugs: pharmacological mechanisms and clinical efficacy with consideration of promising developmental stage compounds. Pharmacol Rev 1990;42:223.
48. Theodore WH, Fishbein D, Dubinsky R. Patterns of cerebral glucose metabolism in patients with partial seizures. Neurology 1988;38:1201.
49. Theodore WH, Ito B, Devinsky O, et al. Carbamazepine and cerebral glucose metabolism. Neurology 1987;37:104.
50. Connelly A, Jacson GD, Frackowiak RSJ, et al. Functional mapping of activated human primary cortex with a clinical MR imaging system. Radiology 1993;188:125.

Index